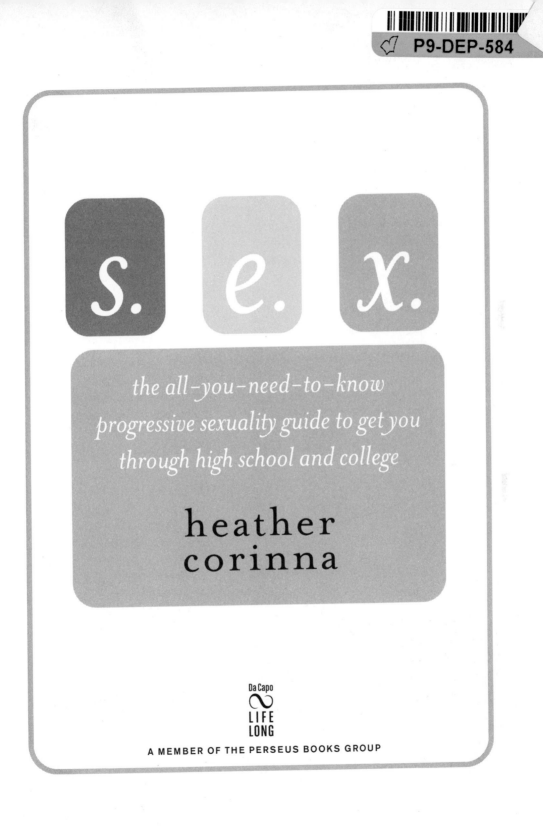

s. e. x.

the all-you-need-to-know
progressive sexuality guide to get you
through high school and college

heather corinna

Da Capo
LIFE
LONG

A MEMBER OF THE PERSEUS BOOKS GROUP

Designed by Pauline Neuwirth, Neuwirth and Associates, Inc.
Set in 11 point Bembo by the Perseus Books Group

Cataloging-in-Publication data for this book is available from the Library of Congress.
ISBN: 978-1-60094-010-1

Published by Da Capo Press
A Member of the Perseus Books Group
www.dacapopress.com

Da Capo Press books are available at special discounts for bulk purchases in the U.S. by corporations, institutions, and other organizations. For more information, please contact the Special Markets Department at the Perseus Books Group, 2300 Chestnut Street, Suite 200, Philadelphia, PA, 19103, or call (800) 810-4145, ext. 5000, or e-mail special.markets@perseusbooks.com.

10 9 8 7 6 5 4 3

PRAISE FOR SCARLETEEN.COM AND

S.e.x.

"Not only would my own adolescence have been vastly less painful and confusing if I'd had access to the accurate, comprehensive, and above all nonjudgmental information that Heather Corinna so carefully provides, but *S.E.X.* is, literally, a lifesaving book: Corinna's vast commonsense wisdom—especially on topics relating to gender roles, queer sexuality, and gender identities—has the potential to improve the physical and emotional health of anyone who reads it, and to help heal our culture's unhealthy, conflicted approaches to sex, sexuality, and gender."

—LISA JERVIS, cofounder, *Bitch: Feminist Response to Pop Culture*

•

"*S.E.X.* is a positive and informative all-embracing guide to sexuality by a dedicated author. Heather Corinna challenges adolescents and young adults alike to be proactive in owning their sexuality by being true to themselves, all the while laying the foundation of knowledge and acceptance—key factors for the development of a healthy sexuality."

—DR. LYNN PONTON, author of *The Sex Lives of Teenagers* and *The Romance of Risk*

•

"Scarleteen editor and founder Heather Corinna is my new hero! Her Web site, 'committed to delivering the best contemporary teen sex ed on the Net,' is easily the most impressive sex education tool I've seen. . . . Scarleteen will appeal to adults and adolescents alike."
—Utne.com

•

"Scarleteen won't send any kids rushing to high-school swingers parties. . . . Corinna does a good job of debunking sex myths and discussing sexual responsibility."
—MSNBC.com

•

"[A] straightforward and no-BS teen-sex advice and info site to counter the 'abstinence only' school programs."
—SFGATE.com

•

"The atmosphere of Scarleteen is a casual, funky, welcoming oasis in a topic that often suffers from a bad case of squeaky, white-tiled Clinical-osis."
—KIM LANE, Oxygen (Moms Online)

about the author

HEATHER CORINNA is a queer writer, artist, educator, activist, peaceful warrior, professional rabblerouser, former musician and early childhood educator, Internet publisher, and community organizer. She has been bringing original, inclusive, informative, feminist, creative, and radical sexuality and women's content—and an awful lot of commas—to the Web since 1997. Natively Chicagoan, she currently lives in Seattle with her partner, too many books, a scrappy old cat, and a terminally precious pug. Scarleteen is her full-time job and cause célèbre.

dedicated to the readers of scarleteen . . .

For bravely asking the questions that have helped millions more to find answers, support, and empowerment; for your trust, your honesty and for giving this educator the biggest, most challenging classroom around and a heightened sense of purpose that she wouldn't trade for all the world.

This book is *because* of all of you—so, this book is *for* all of you.

disclaimer

The information in this book is intended to help
readers make informed decisions about their health
and the health of their loved ones. It is not intended
to be a substitute for treatment by or the advice and
care of a professional healthcare provider. While the
author and publisher have endeavored to ensure that
the information presented is accurate and up-to-date,
they are not responsible for adverse effects or consequences sustained by any persons using this book.

contents

s.e.x.

t-h-a-n-k y-o-u

FROM IDEA TO bookshelf, the process of riffing, writing, proposing, researching, writing some more, editing, surveying, researching again, rewriting, editing again, shopping, shopping again, researching *again,* and editing once more (with feeling) has taken nearly six years.

There're a lot of people in six years of work, and not enough paper to thank all of them properly. Those who cannot fit into these few pages have substantial real estate in my heart. To all of you, my humblest thanks and deepest gratitude. I am incredibly lucky to have a wide, caring, and supportive network with so much faith in me.

Here's to you.

To the Grand Pooh-bah and their staff at Marlowe & Company for making my decade by taking this on, and for making the arduous process of publishing so painless. Boundless thanks to Renée Sedliar, who found this book a great home when I was sure it would remain ever homeless, fought the good fight, wielded her editorial machete like a peaceable ninja, took my serious stuff seriously, and laughed at my jokes. I could not have asked for a better advocate and editor; this is a book made far, far better for your irreplaceable part in it.

To Christopher Schelling, for his tireless attempts over many years to find a home for this book, his incredible patience with me (and everyone else), and his magnanimous support.

To my wonderful, patient, and hard-working volunteers at Scarleteen, for their dedication to sex education, young adults, and sexual health and their faith in my unique approach.

To Clare Sainsbury, who saved—and keeps on saving—the day.

To the generous people who gave me invaluable aid and information, especially editorial assistants Laurel Martinez and Kythryne Aisling, and consultants Rebecca Trotzky-Sirr; Janel Hanmer, MD, PhD; Richard Fraser, APNP; Laura Jones; Kerrick Adrian; Erin Seiberlich, MD; Terri Rearick, RN, BS, CIC; Ben Wizner of the ACLU; and Hollie West, RN, BScN.

To my friend and assistant Brandon Sutton, for his fantastic editorial assistance during the maddening first round of edits, his willingness to camp out and work for weeks, and his much-appreciated companionship and good humor throughout.

To the Scarleteen users who trusted me with very personal information in surveys for this book, to ensure everyone got what they really needed, and to the young readers who read faster than they ever had in their lives to participate in the final focus group for the book, especially Celine, Joey, Joanna, Caylin, Matt, Irmelin, Maggie, Vero, Hannah, Kelly, and Emily.

To Peter Mayle, author of *Where Did I Come From?* If it wasn't for the unbearable cuteness of those wiggly, pink sperms with roses in their teeth, and his tale of reproduction for the littlest readers, which was my favorite book at the age of five, I suspect that I and this book might not have wound up where we did.

To Joss Whedon, for providing me (and everyone else) many, many hours of the sort of productive, inspiring downtime a young-adult-sexuality author requires to sustain her sanity.

To the incredible women who have played an integral part in providing mentorship for me in this area of work, supported what I do, and shared at least one afternoon of wine and whine with me over the years, most notably: Anne Semans, Cathy Winks, Carol Queen, and Cheryl Lindsay Seelhoff. To the women of my sexual, political, and intellectual ancestry, without whose work mine would not have been possible: Victoria Woodhull, Simone de Beauvior, Shere Hite, the Boston Women's Health Collective, the Jane project, Sarah Weddington, Natalie Angier, Joani Blank, Anne Fausto-Sterling, Marge Piercy, Adrienne Rich, Anaïs Nin, Betty Dodson, Susie Bright, Dorothy Allison, Alice Walker, Germaine Greer, Robin Morgan, Audre Lorde, Marie Stopes, Margaret Sanger, and every woman who has fought against the tide to express, champion, and protect equality, balance, and inclusion in human sexuality.

To my community and all of the cherished friends who lent me their eyes and ears, shut the computer and dragged me outside, boosted me up when I needed it, supported my endeavors, accepted my utter lack of attention to them for weeks on end, and otherwise participated in the care, watering, and feeding of me, especially Megan Anderson, Elise Matthesen, Kathleen Kennedy, Jeyoani Wildflower, Lauren Bacon, Jane Duvall, Al Potyondi-Smith, Mya Wagener, Heather Spear, Kythryne Aisling, Jenny Lobasz, Emira Mears, Michelle Demole, Beppie Keane, Stephen Luntz, Jennifer Andrade-Ward, Molly Bennett, Caroline Dodge, Kaari Busick, Briana Holtorf, and last-so-as-to-clearly-be-most, Becca Nelson.

To the incredible, ingenious, and always inspiring Hanne Blank, who was there at the beginning of all of this, there at the finish line, and there in all the stages in between, always with insight and support;

whom I am always honored to call friend, sister, and comrade.

To my partner, friend, and big, big love, Mark Price, for everything: for accepting the necessary interruptions of this book's journey during our courtship, holding my hand (or other bits) during the hard parts, keeping me in cookies, providing some needed romantic optimism readers should thank him for, and for making the whole of my life, of which this book is part, better than I ever expected. And to all of the Prices, for Mark (thanks!) and for just being that darn awesome.

My mom and my dad are two of the most wildly different people one can imagine, whose mean average somehow = me. I have my mother to thank for my unstoppable work ethic, for my understanding of enough medical mumbo-jumbo so that I could translate it for everyone else, for my fierce loyalties, and for being one seriously ass-kicking lady to look up to. Thanks to my dad for instilling in me the strong spirit of revolution, for empowering my voice in however I wish to use it, for our amazing friendship, and for never letting me forget for a minute (even when I wanted to) that if I think something's broken, I've always got to keep trying to fix it.

I love all of you immeasurably.

To that girl I once was: I *finally* found you that book that you wanted. Sorry it took me so long.

S.E.X.

about scarleteen.com

SINCE DECEMBER OF 1998, Scarleteen has been used by millions of teens and young adults internationally to find real answers to their sexuality and relationship questions. Scarleteen provides comprehensive, fully inclusive, feminist, and nonjudgmental information on sexual anatomy and health, masturbation, arousal and orgasm, safer sex and contraception, reproductive options, gender and orientation, rape and abuse, body image, relationships, and sexual politics. Via both static content and an active message board, users can discuss their questions and concerns with staff and volunteers and get immediate answers, needed resources, and support. Scarleteen is a grass-roots, independent medium that has been applauded by the *Utne Reader,* the *Chicago Tribune,* the American Civil Liberties Union, *GLAAD,* the *Minneapolis City Pages,* the Oxygen Network, the Sexuality Information and Education Council of the United States, and other publications and organizations.

foreword

ANNE SEMANS

YOU ARE one lucky reader. And a deserving one. You are lucky because you hold in your hands the key to a lifetime of good sex information. And a happy, healthy sex life is something everyone deserves. You are lucky because someone cared enough about you to give you this book, or because you, my friend, were resourceful enough to seek it out on your own.

You might be thinking, "I can get sex information anywhere, what's so special about this book?" The problem, of course, is that "sex information" comes in all shapes and sizes—not all of it accurate or complete. And it won't come as any surprise that sex is not a subject you learn in school along with the rest of your ABCs. You can learn about the mating habits of whales, or how plants pollinate, but ask your school to put Sexual Response 101 on the curriculum and the responses run the gamut.

S.E.X.: The All-You-Need-to-Know Progressive Sexuality Guide to Get You Through High School and College believes that you deserve access to all the facts. Remember "knowledge is power?" This book gives you the knowledge so that you have the power to make good choices about your own body and those of your partners.

Imagine what it would be like if you had taken a sexuality class at school, one where the teacher just focused on the facts, and the students were free of embarrassment and could listen in rapt amazement. Sure you would have learned the usual stuff, like how your body works, what your genitals look like, how babies are made, how contraception works, and how STDs get passed around. But you also would have learned that each person's sexuality is unique, and that gender identity and sexual orientation fall on a continuum. You would have learned that sex is a gift you give as well as receive, that it is based on mutual respect and responsibility, that it is about pleasure, that it is more than intercourse, and that being good at it has nothing to do with penis size or tight vaginas, but practice and presence. Imagine that by the time you graduated from high school you had learned all this and more, so that you were able to enter into your sexual relationships with confidence and care.

While that's not the current model of sex ed, this book, along with the author's Web site, Scarleteen, are the next best things. You will find these subjects, and so many more, discussed a lot like you might imagine the teacher of this mythical sex ed class would discuss things—with a bit of science geekiness, mixed with candor and an honesty that only someone who's been in constant communication with teens for the past ten years can bring.

I know I wish I'd had a resource like this as a teen. As a sexually active teen in a Catholic family, I was given no sex information other than the nun who advised our 8th grade class to "think of a hamburger when you have impure thoughts." Fortunately, luck spared me from dealing with teen pregnancy, and my curiosity eventually let me into a career as a sex educator. Now I find myself with a daughter fast approaching her teen years, and I'm not kidding myself that she'll confide her every sex question or dilemma to me.

Lucky for me, lucky for her, and lucky for you, we have this book.

—Anne Semans,
sex educator, author, parent

s.e.x.

who's this book for, anyway?

THIS BOOK IS for adolescents and young adults.

This book is also for parents, teachers, aunts and uncles, Mom and Dad's cool best friends, mentors, allies, grandparents, friends, for anyone with an interest in the emotional and physical health and well-being of young people today.

Anyone who's got a grip on history and current events, basic physiology, psychology, and sociology—and anyone with simple life experience—knows that sexuality is inevitable, important, and integral. Anyone with that knowledge and experience also knows that sexual choices, sexual identity, and sexual health have a huge impact on our world, interpersonally and globally. Poor sexual choices, sexual dissatisfaction, power inequities, sexual shame, aggression, vio-

lence and victimization, and the like all contribute to the personal and global problems of unprepared and unwanted parenting, negative body image and low self-esteem, the perpetuation of abusive and unhealthy relationships, unending cycles of rape and abuse, chronic physical and mental illness, sexism, homophobia, and sexual objectification and exploitation.

Accurate, accessible sexuality information offers important and needed protections for young adults. When young people know what consensual, enjoyable, and egalitarian sex is, they can understand what is not consensual, what is not enjoyable—physically, emotionally—and what is not mutual or balanced. Learning preventative care that addresses sexuality—reproductive healthcare, safer sex practices, birth control—teaches them to care for their bodies as a whole, as well as protecting them from sexually transmitted infections or unwanted pregnancy. Learning to love and accept their *whole* bodies—including, but not limited to genitals and reproductive systems—promotes their lifelong sexual and general health, well-being, and self-esteem. Learning how to assess and improve the quality of intimate relationships, to figure how they do or don't mesh with individual wants and needs—which may differ from cultural standards—and to advocate for oneself within a relationship is vital for anyone to be healthy, happy, and whole. Knowledge and acceptance of the range of positive, realistic human sexuality offer young adults protection from others who would—and often do—prey upon sexual ignorance or shame. All of these aspects and more open the door not only to a safer sexual life but to one that is enjoyable, beneficial, satisfying, and empowering.

Chances are good that when it comes to matters of my opinion, my cultural and social analysis, or my assessments of teen sexual life and general sexuality, you won't always agree with me. That's okay.

A few years ago, I got an unforgettable letter from a parent. He wrote that while he supported the work that I did, he didn't share a lot of my personal views. He told me he was a "once-player," now an avowed "Jesus freak," and that he'd raised his daughter conservatively. But he also told me that he was glad as heck I was around, and that he, quite gladly, directed her to the information I gave out. He'd explained to her that she'd heard all the things he had to say, and she should go read very different views—with accurate information throughout—and thus,

be best equipped to make up her own mind, to make her own decisions, wherever they fell along that whole spectrum.

what's in this book and what isn't—the short list:

- The term *abstinence* is very rarely used, although discussion about celibacy and waiting until partnered sex can happen in a healthy, responsible way is paramount.
- It is not set forth as a given that saying no to partnered sex is always better than saying yes.
- Sexuality is not discussed in a context that requires or champions one specific sexual orientation, gender or gender identity, relationship model, set of values, religion, or age.
- It is presumed and asserted that all living beings are entitled to their sexuality, sexual identity, and fully consensual sexual partnership choices, to the degree that they have the agency to make them.
- Because the current pervasive cultural approach to human sexuality and young adult sexuality is often considerably flawed, alternative approaches are often presented.
- I do not claim to have all the answers, nor do I assert that there is one set of sexual choices or behaviors that are best for everyone.

Ultimately, this book aims to provide information to help lay a solid foundation for clear, usable, informative, and healthy sex education to benefit individual readers and their support networks.

▪ HOW CAN YOU USE THIS BOOK? ▪

READ IT YOURSELF, FIRST, AND GET UP TO DATE.

Many of us—parents, teachers, and mentors—didn't get accurate, inclusive sex education ourselves, and haven't kept up with current information. If you're going to talk to the young adults in your life about birth control and safer sex, you will want to make sure that you're not unintentionally endangering them when you want to help protect them. Not only is it challenging to obtain accurate and sound sex information in the first place, but the information is constantly changing, both because of new research and new social contexts. I do this work full-time; I am constantly checking new reports, studies, and books, and reading new questions, and even *I* have a tough time keeping up.

Read this book yourself before you set it out for teens or young adults. Check out information available from other reliable, comprehensive sources such as the Sexuality Information and Education Council of the United States (SIECUS), the Guttmacher Institute, or Planned Parenthood and other sound organizations and clearinghouses listed in the Resources section at the end of this book. You can get on mailing lists so that new information and studies are delivered right to your Inbox. Build a small library at home of accurate sexuality information. Ask your family doctor to help you learn what you need to know.

Not only can the information in this book be useful to you in discussions about sexuality with the teen in your life, but you may even find that the information benefits your own sex life, as well.

NORMALIZE SEXUALITY DISCUSSION.

To foster comfort, trust, and calm communication, discussions about aspects of sex and sexuality should be casual, ongoing, and commonplace from the get-go, rather than taking place when the issue is fever-pitch or personal. There's no need to wait for a time, year, or event to have that One Big Talk—have regular discussions about general health, body issues, development, relationships, and sexuality. Discussions about sex that concern cultural or world events, or rules and policies at school, can take place over dinner, for instance, and are excellent ways to take a lot of steam out of the overheated engine that is parent/teen sex talk. By the time your kids are developing sexually, when they are thinking about or having sexual partners, very little of this should be new to them, and talking about it should be pretty old hat, even if there are still some (inevitable) rough spots.

It can be trickier if you're feeling that NOW is the time to start these discussions. A whole lot of teens' sexual information and personal sexual ethics and values are ingrained even before they start puberty. (You might be pleasantly surprised to know how many reported parents as their sexual relationship role models in the surveys for this book.) But just as any birth control is better than no birth control, any time you choose to foster open, honest, and sensitive sexual discussion with a child or teenager is far better than never doing it at all.

s.e.x.

IF YOU'RE PICKING THIS BOOK UP TO START TALKING TO YOUR TEEN OR YOUNG ADULT FOR THE FIRST TIME:

▶ You might want to open by explaining why the subject hasn't been discussed before (for instance, because you were worried about bringing it up at the wrong time, or in the wrong way, and lousing it all up).

▶ You might want to ask more questions at first, rather than doling out answers.

▶ If you've avoided talking about sex until now, or if you tried before and gave up because of embarrassment, know that you're not the first one. Talking about something so intimate is difficult for a lot of people. It may have been tricky for you to figure out how to talk about it without feeling that you're crossing boundaries or grossing your teen out. Let them know that. If you feel embarrassed, say so. If you're worried about boundaries, tell them. That sort of humility can be a real icebreaker because, often, they feel *exactly* the same way.

▶ You can let your teen know you'd be open to and interested in discussing the book or other sexuality information with them, and ask whether they'd like to initiate those discussions or have you do it. You could even organize an informal family or group book club about it, if that's your usual dynamic. As with anything else, the best approach is going to depend a lot on your family and your kid: what's empowering for one teen may be embarrassing for another.

"i" statements are your best friend

 VOICING what your subjective viewpoints and ethics are, and explaining that they are yours—not theirs, not universals—is a very big deal. One of the easiest ways to isolate a young person in the process of forming a personal identity is to give the impression that your choices and experiences must or should be everyone's.

Remarks like "casual sex is disrespecting yourself" and "you'd be better to focus on your homework than boys/girls right now" are not "I" statements and probably won't be welcomed. Statements like "sex before marriage is wrong" or "you just think you're bisexual, you can't know that" are dogmatic and subjective. Teens aren't stupid; they know these sorts of statements are based on your opinion. Strident presentations often leave them with resentment, with a feeling of being controlled, with disrespect for the differences between your generation and theirs. If you've made the same choices you're telling them they shouldn't make, they may feel (validly) that you're being hypocritical.

Try this on for size: "I feel that starting to have sex at fifteen was too early for me because I didn't understand the risks or consequences of sex, and it kept me from achieving my goals." Or this: "I don't understand how you can know you're bisexual now, because I'm forty-one and even *I'm* still not sure about my orientation." Or, "I'm concerned that if you're dating now, other things I know are important to you are going to get the shaft," or "I feel sex before marriage is wrong because I'm Catholic, and in our religion, premarital sex isn't okay." Then follow any statement like that with: "What do YOU think? Why do you feel that way?"

s.e.x.

▪ THE SILENT TREATMENT ▪

One of the toughest things many adults face when it comes to talking to teens about sex is that many of their teens either aren't going to—or just plain don't want to—talk to them. That can happen to even the most open, honest parent, to the parents who have great relationships with their kids and have had good talks about aspects of sex throughout their kids' lives. It can happen to the parent whose kid truly thinks of them as their best friend. And it can be heartbreaking for that adult, understandably.

Most of our sex lives are private; for a teenager, there's no exception. (One teen in the surveys for this book said, "My parents don't talk to me about their sex life, why should I talk to them about mine?") Beyond that, for many teens, talking to parents about their sex lives is just a little too intimidating. They may not be toddlers anymore, and they may say they don't care, but to many teens parents are still the sun, moon, and stars. That can make it difficult even for a teen who is behaving very responsibly, or who isn't even sexually active yet. Even voicing doubts about whether or not they want to be active in the future, and how, can be uncomfortable if they're worried about parental judgments.

Many young adults are far more likely to talk to almost everyone else before their parents: friends, partners, other relatives, teachers, you name it. That's not necessarily a bad thing, even though it might make you feel like you're out of a loop you should be in, or that you've erred in your parenting somehow.

Allowing them the freedom to talk to someone else can help open the doors of communication between you, so they can know you're available and you CAN have productive discussions with them.

And if you're waiting for your teen to be the one to initiate discussion, stop waiting! One of you has got to take the leap, after all, and it's harder for them to do so than you.

▪ GIVING THIS BOOK ▪ TO YOUNG ADULTS

This book is intended for a readership between approximately the ages of sixteen and twenty-two. There are many readers who could utilize and absorb it at younger ages, and plenty of readers will still find a good deal of this information new at older ages. If you've been an involved parent or mentor, you probably have a pretty good idea of when a book like this is appropriate for the young adults in your life. Trust your instincts.

I suggest you make this book and others like it readily but casually available: don't hide it or pass it over as if it were the Dead Sea Scrolls. Dedicate an area of your bookshelf to books that concern shared family issues—or heck, books about sex, period—and when they're curious and interested, your kids will seek the information out. If your teen asks a question about sex you don't know how to answer, pull out this book, or another like it, and find the answer with them. Not only will doing this show them where and how to find accurate information, it has the added benefit of showing them that you are invested in providing them with this information. Further, this approach illustrates the fact that sex is a very big and complex topic to which none of us has all the answers: not them or their peers, not the media, not you.

is it ever too early?

 GIVING a book like this to a ten- or eleven-year-old—maybe with the idea of being as supportive and proactive as possible—is unlikely to be in any way damaging, but it probably won't be very helpful, either. For instance, even very intelligent ten-year-olds are very unlikely to read information about birth control, STIs, or communication with sexual partners and store it in their minds for later, because it just isn't likely to be applicable to them *now*. For some preteens and even plenty of teenagers, making a big presentation of a book like this too early may actually feel like pressure, or a statement that they SHOULD be ready for or interested in these issues. If they're not interested yet, this can make them worry about what stage of development and sexual interest they should be in. For a list of a range of age-appropriate sexuality books, see the Resources section.

You may not need to hear this, but I'm going to say it anyway: I have **never**—not in years of reading tens of thousands of teenagers posting online about these issues, not in hundreds of e-mails—seen even one teen express that a parent who was down-to-earth, honest, compassionate, respectful of boundaries, and primarily concerned with their well-being had seriously screwed things up in addressing sex with them. Never.

I certainly have heard more than few express that they felt embarrassed or insulted when parents brought up sex in any number of ways, or with sexuality books or items parents gave them, of course. But that "Ugh!

My super-uncool mom/dad/aunt!" stuff has never struck me as overriding the positives teens glean from caring parents doing their level best to ensure that their teens are comfortable with their sexuality and have all the information possible to make the best choices about a healthy, happy sex life. And even if you do stumble—maybe you freak out at a teen coming out as gay, becoming sexually active, taking up with a partner you feel is unsuitable, or even starting puberty—most of the time, brushing off your knees and plopping a Band-Aid on the wounds heals them up in no time. Ultimately, if you care about your kids, accept they're becoming adults, and love the adults they're becoming just as much as the children they were, you're going to do just fine, and so are they.

Every teen is different. Some of the "facts" in this book might surprise you, in various ways. You may have thought, for instance, that the average age when teens are becoming sexually active these days was younger *or* older than in the past. Some of the issues addressed in this book may be pertinent to the young adult in your life, some may not. Some parts of this book may make you feel much more comfortable about young adult sexuality; some may make you more *un*comfortable. You may have various levels of comfort with your teen even reading parts of this book at all.

But they do need this information. Right now, every day, the Scarleteen.com Web site is visited by between ten thousand and thirty thousand readers—readers who looked so intensely for the answers to their questions that they made Scarleteen.com the number one search engine result for sex ed. The information at the Web site and in this book is based on all the questions we've been asked over the years, on discussions the teens themselves are initiating and sustaining. We field as many pregnancy scares, rape crises, and anal sex questions in a day as we do questions about breast development, weight, gender inequities, bisexuality, or how to ask someone out; what teens want to know about sexuality at any given time is incredibly varied and individual. Given the number of unplanned pregnancies in young adults in a year, given that high-school and college-age people have been the fastest growing number of STI sufferers for quite some time, given the body-image and self-esteem issues so many teens grapple with, given the rates of sexual assault and abuse, given the dangerous social isolation of many gay youth, given the endless mixed messages from the media and the inaccuracy and politicalization in so much school-based sex ed, as well as the misinformation peers and partners disseminate, *they need this stuff.* At this point in their lives, they are establishing the patterns in their sexual identities and behavior that will be the primary foundation of their adult sex lives. If they feel unable to say no *or* yes now when they want to, if they feel ashamed or confused now, if they don't learn how to practice contraception or safer sex now, if they don't learn what they do or don't want sexually now, they may well never learn it.

They need this information.

And they need you.

This book, and others like it, paired with proactive, informed, and relaxed (as relaxed as it gets, anyway, when it comes to sex) parenting and modeling, in loving environments, will nurture a *much* different world than we have now: a much *better* world.

In other words, this book is very valuable, but it increases in value substantially when you—parents, extended family, mentors, teachers, role models, and other caring adults—are just as big an influence as it is.

So, who's this book for?
Everyone.

s.e.x.

I pledge allegiance . . . to myself and the united state of my sexuality

AN INTRODUCTION FOR READERS

AS YOU START to read this book, I want you to make a bold choice: I want you to choose to create a healthy, happy and fulfilling sexual life that is fantastic for you and for everyone else in it.

You *have* the power to do that, no matter your age or your gender, whether you're currently choosing to be sexually active with partners or not, or even if it feels too soon for you to do *anything* in terms of your sexuality just yet. You have the power to make every choice you make about sexuality support your happiness, health, and wellbeing, based on your own, unique criteria.

Sure, spelling out sexuality isn't simple: it's a big, bubbling stew of biology and chemistry, physical and emotional development and individuality, nature and nurture. Each person's sexual self is not only often shifting and evolving, but is a very individual com-

bination of personal preferences and desires, gender identity and sexual orientation, body image, relationship needs, interpersonal patterns, ideals and previous experiences, and emotional, chemical, physical, and hormonal states. Add to that simmering pot personal and public health issues, reproductive issues and choices, laws, cultural and community values, attitudes, and expectations, personal ethics, and sexual fantasy and reality. That's a whole lot to sort out, process, and start learning to juggle and fit into the rest of your life. Take it all on the road with other people in relationships, add all of THEIR stuff to yours, and it's pretty easy to see why a whole lot of people can feel pretty overwhelmed by sexuality.

But when you make smart, healthy, and informed choices that really feel right for you, it's actually pretty easy not only to stay safe and sound, but to *enjoy* your sexuality and your sexual life, which is what it's there for in the first place.

In fact, you have more freedom to create and claim what is best for you sexually than your grandparents did, and more agency to do that than your parents had. We now have more complete and accurate information than ever before, about sexuality as a whole, about infection and disease, about reproduction and birth control. We have greater access to that information, and to sexual health services and support. Even though the mass media, public health, politics, and the ever-changing values of our world add extra complications and confusion—especially given the mixed messages we so often get about sexuality—you can pick and choose what you expose yourself to and support. You even have the ability to positively impact the media and public health policies when it comes to sex, both with your personal choices and your collective actions as a generation.

You have a unique opportunity to create, explore, nurture, and enjoy an authentic, personal sexuality that is beneficial to you and others, that is healthy and balanced, that is informed and empowering, and that allows you to find and express intimacy, joy, and pleasure in your life.

So, make a choice to do just that. That choice alone nearly guarantees that every other sexual choice you make will be a good one.

Maybe you picked up this book because at some point you felt that you wanted to begin exploring your sexuality, or because you felt that you couldn't get away with ignoring it any longer. Maybe someone else gave you this book because you've asked about sex, because you're at an age when you are likely to, or just because they're a cool person who loves you to bits and wants you to have all the sexuality information you might need when you do want or need it.

No one person, group, or book can—or should—tell everyone what choices are right for them, because there is no *one* right set of sexual choices for everyone. What is absolutely right for one person can be absolutely wrong for someone else. Only you can find out what your sexuality should be like, and define it accordingly.

What this book *can* do is to give you a solid foundation of information so that you can make those choices more soundly for yourself. I may be something of an expert when it comes to general young adult sexuality, but the only person who is an expert when it comes to *your* sexuality is you.

There's no one right way to use this book. You might find that some parts of the book are more useful to you than others, that you're already past some of it, or that some of it isn't information you need just yet. (You might feel ambivalent about some parts of it, or even feel a little scared, weirded out, or overwhelmed by it now, and that's okay, too.) Some parts may be more useful to a sibling, friend, or partner than they are to you. Some of what's addressed may be within your personal experience, some may be outside it. The information in here might be something you want to digest and process alone, or you might want to use it to initiate or further discussions with friends, partners, or family. It should give you a whole lot of answers, and it should also give you some new questions. However you use it to help you make choices that are best for you at any given time is the right way.

My wish is that this book will help you

to enter into or continue your sexual life gladly and comfortably—and with as much empowerment and support as possible for what's best for **you**. It's intended to help *you* spell out what *your* sexuality is and what *you* want it to be.

If I have any agenda, it isn't for me to be the expert. It is for *you* to be the expert, for you to have a healthy, happy, and fulfilling sexual life that is great for you and for everyone else in it, because that's not only the right thing for you, but the right thing for all of us.

s.e.x.

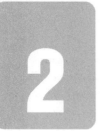

2

your body:
an owner's manual

▪ WHAT IS "SEXUALITY"? ▪

SEXUALITY ISN'T TECHNICALLY "adult," or something that pops out of the blue when anyone reaches a certain age: it's been with all of us from day one. When as infants we comforted ourselves by sucking on our thumbs, by nursing, by touching our own bodies, even our genitals, we were experiencing our sexuality, even though infant sexuality is very different from adult sexuality. When as children we enjoyed the smell, the feel, and the sound of things, when we learned about the world by putting everything we could grab into our mouths, when we peeked in underpants other than our own and asked about our parents' bodies, we were experiencing some of our sensual and sexual nature and curiosity. When we played

doctor, experienced our interest in being physical with others, when we masturbated or examined our own bodies, began getting crushes on peers or adults, when we started to become more and more curious about sexuality, our soon-to-be-adult sexual selves were developing.

Sexuality isn't just about your genitals. It is a mix of many different things—of physical, chemical, emotional, intellectual, social, and cultural aspects—and that mix is different for, and unique to, everyone.

Our physical and emotional development from children into adults substantially changes our sexual wants, needs, and identity. By the time we're well into or finished with puberty, our bodies are fully capable of healthy solo or partnered sexual activity

so, what is "sexuality"?

- **Physical:** The development, health, and function of our sexual organs and reproductive system, the brain and nervous system (the big drivers of sexual arousal and function), and the whole of the body.
- **Chemical:** AKA hormones, which take the blame for a lot of hasty or poor sexual choices—choices there seems to be no other way of accounting for, as in, "Those dirty hormones made me do it!" Sex hormones include testosterone, the big chemical libido driver, and estrogen, but there are also others that take part in sexuality, like adrenaline, serotonin, oxytocin, dopamine, and endorphins.
- **Emotional and intellectual:** Feelings, values, and ideas about sexual anatomy; sexual self-image issues such as body image, gender, sexual orientation, and relationships; masturbation, sexual activity with oneself, and partners. The emotional and intellectual side of sexuality concerns the ways all of those drive us sexually, and the way we feel about ourselves, our sexuality, our sexual choices, and our sexual relationships.
- **Social:** Sexuality in the context of our relationships—with partners, friends, family—and the influences those relationships have had and have now on our feelings about our sexuality, our sexual wants and needs, and our sexual choices with others.
- **Cultural:** How the rest of the world—including peers, as well as local and larger communities, like the government and the media—views sexuality. The messages it gives overtly and covertly, what it allows and disallows, what it idealizes or punishes, the effect and influence it has on us, consciously and unconsciously. Where and how we fit within cultural attitudes toward, approaches to, and presentations of sexuality, in terms of our own sexuality, sexual identity and ethics, body image, gender identity, orientation, and relationships.

and reproduction—whether or not our emotions, minds, and goals agree or are in alignment.

LET'S TALK ABOUT SEX

"Sex" is often used to mean heterosexual intercourse or partnered sex. But what the word "sex" *really* refers to is the categories into which a species is divided, by the appearance of the external sexual anatomy, and more accurately, by chromosomal structure. This usually refers to the binary (or two) categories male and female.

The basic aspects of human sexual development and anatomy differ for different biological sexes: for the male and the female. So, before we get started talking about the stages of puberty, it's helpful to know where we stand when it comes to our gonads.

We are sexed at birth by visual examination of the genitals, but the most accurate way we are sexed is via the chromosomes in the nucleus of every cell. Sex chromosomes determine what kind of genitals and internal reproductive system we have, but they also guide the endocrine system as it generates sex hormones and other chemicals.

s.e.x.

The classic sex chromosome pattern for males is called XY (because that's what they look like under a microscope), and for women, XX. So the difference between men and women, chromosomally, is the Y chromosome.

Most of us can go through the following chapter with a pretty easy understanding of which parts apply or applied to us. If our sex wasn't obvious enough before puberty, it usually becomes all the more so once it begins.

did you know . . . ?

There are also other chromosomal combinations, though they're far more rare than XX and XY. There are sex chromosome structures like XO or XXY, XO/XY, and XYY, and there are individuals with even rarer patterns. Those with such genetics are known as intersexed. Some intersexed conditions are Klinefelter's syndrome, androgen insensitivity syndrome, adrenal hyperplasia, Sawyer's syndrome, and Turner's syndrome. These can occur in as many as one in every thousand to twenty thousand births. But, because reports of intersex are often based on ambiguity in genital appearance, which doesn't always occur to intergendered or intersexed people, and because many of us will never have our chromosomes investigated, it's hard to have accurate figures.

While many intersexed people's bodies at birth look like anyone else's, some intersexed and intergendered people are born with what are commonly called "ambiguous" genitals—those that cannot easily be typed as male or female. Many infants born with ambiguous genitals have been given surgery at birth or nonelective hormone therapy to "correct" the variation, rather than simply accepting it as a normal variation, which is what intersex is. Some intersexed people, at a certain age, may want surgical or hormonal adaptations, but plenty may not. Those who had corrections done at birth or in early childhood, or those who did not have ambiguous genitals, may not even be aware they are intersex, though they may have a feeling that there is something different about them.

As growing and grown people, intersexed individuals may look slightly different than we'd expect someone sexed a certain way to look, but most look like anybody else, with differences that are very subtle or none you can see at all.

If you suspect you may be intersexed—either in terms of your sexual development, fertility, or general appearance, or if you're experiencing what seems like a serious delay in the onset of puberty, or if you just have a profound feeling that your sex doesn't "fit" you, talk to your doctor. Intersexed conditions often don't require any sort of medical treatment, but it can be important for intersexed people to know, both in terms of fertility, if that's a priority, and in terms of forming their own identity.

s.e.x.

MEGA-METAMORPHOSIS: •
Puberty

Puberty doesn't start and end with breast growth and getting a period, or with a voice that has deepened. During puberty, the entire body goes through growth spurts until it completes its maturity in bone mass and overall size and shape, and the sexual organs and secondary sexual characteristics also finish their basic development.

On average right now, puberty begins for girls between the ages of eight and eleven, and for boys, usually between the ages of ten and fourteen. In some girls, puberty might begin as early as age six; puberty is currently considered to be "precocious," or early, if it begins before the age of eight for girls and nine for boys. Puberty is currently considered to begin late if NO sexual development has occurred for girls by the age of thirteen, or for boys by fourteen. No matter when puberty begins, most men and women are finished with puberty by the time they're in their twenties. Overall, the entire process—whenever it starts and ends—tends to occur in a similar order for everyone.

basic stages of puberty in girls and young women:

- **Breast development:** The first part of puberty for girls is most often initial breast growth, called "breast budding," because the growth starts with small lumps just under the nipples (and not always at the same time; sometimes one begins before the other). Breast development includes changes in the size and shape of the *areola,* or nipple area, as well as the rest of the breast.

- **Vaginal discharges:** At or around the same time as breast budding, vaginal discharges will become apparent. As a woman gets further into puberty, or after she becomes sexually active, it's common to become far more aware of what's going on down there, so if you've just noticed discharges, it's likely nothing new.

- **Body hair and pubic hair growth:** After breast budding, pubic hair and other body hair will usually begin growing. For some, pubic hair may appear before breast growth.

- **Menarche:** Usually about two years after breast budding, the menstrual cycle begins, starting with first ovulation and then with the first period, called menarche. Menstruation may be delayed if a young woman is underweight, malnourished, overexercising, excessively dieting, or experiencing an eating disorder.

- **Body size and shape changes:** The body will both grow taller and change shape. By the time a woman has her first period, the peak growth in terms of height and bone mass is usually complete. It's normal during puberty to be gaining weight, to be eating more than before and probably more than after puberty. It's also normal for the shape of the body to feel a bit disproportionate sometimes, which is one reason why teen body ideals should not be based on adult bodies.

s.e.x.

basic stages of puberty in boys and young men:

- **Penis and testicles:** Puberty in boys commonly starts with testicular growth. During the whole of puberty, the penis and testes will grow to their adult size. It's common for the length of the penis to grow faster than the width of the penis, and for testicle growth to start before penis growth. Growth of the penis and testicles often is not complete until the end of puberty.

- **Growth spurts:** Because puberty starts later in boys, it's normal for young men to be shorter than their female friends of the same age, for a while. Through puberty, men become taller, muscle mass increases, and, as with girls, it's normal to be gaining weight, and normal to feel out of proportion at times. While men don't develop breasts, it is also common to experience nipple swelling, and larger young men may see some breast development, which is normal.

- **Erections:** While even infants can get erections, during puberty, they often occur frequently and involuntarily—something that is a source of embarrassment for many young men, but is completely normal. Most men get erections several times a day, and young men often get them even more regularly. Plenty of times, it isn't about sex or arousal; it can happen due to friction, temperature changes, and hormone fluctuations. Every erection does not mean a guy wants or needs sex right at that moment, and sex or masturbation isn't required to make an erection go away. They can just be waited out, and will pass in a relatively short amount of time.

- **Ejaculation:** When ejaculation begins—well after the ability to achieve erection—it's typical to have "wet dreams": ejaculation that occurs while sleeping, due to sexual dreams, high levels of semen accumulation, stimulation from sheets and blankets, and/or having a full bladder. First ejaculation is sometimes called "spermarche," just like a woman's first period is called menarche.

- **Body and pubic hair:** Pubic hair—around the base of the penis, as well as on the thighs and around and between the buttocks—is usually the first adult body hair to crop up, and continues growing around the anus, buttocks, and legs. Growth of underarm hair usually follows, and chest and facial hair often develop last, sometimes even after the end of puberty. For some men, body hair is sparser than others: for instance, many fully-developed men have little to no chest hair at all.

- **Voice changes:** During puberty, the male voice deepens, and may go through stages of being all over the place. At times, men may experience voice cracking or croaking.

It's normal and common for anyone to feel awkward or to have body image issues during puberty. People gain weight as a necessary part of puberty, and that can be hard in a culture where thinness is idealized. Acne, voice changes, body hair, various stages of breast development (or slow development), unwanted erections for young men and the unexpected arrival of monthly periods in young women can all be sources of body image woes. Adults and peers, often without even realizing it, may call unwanted attention to your changing body. A parent may feel a daughter needs a brassiere before she wants

in both men and women:

Skin changes: As everyone goes through puberty, it's normal for the skin to become oilier, and for perspiration and body odor to become stronger, because hormones are shuttling through the body at higher levels than before. Adolescent acne (pimples and zits), suck as it may, is as common as the sun in the sky.

one (if she ever wants to wear one at all), or may inadvertently make public a son's wet dreams—and things like that can seriously up the social discomfort of puberty.

Our bodies feel pretty simple during childhood. We don't have to worry about body odor, acne, wet dreams, or menstruation. Sexual feelings and maturation, and the attention from others that comes with those things, can be big-time uncomfortable. Plenty of folks going through puberty have times when they truly hate their bodies, or feel that certain developing parts—like breasts, pubic hair, or erections—are gross, and feel ashamed of them. Some may even wish they could avoid becoming adults altogether, physically and otherwise. The ideas other people have about young adult bodies as they're developing can be hard to deal with sometimes: like insistence you should be excited about development that doesn't thrill you at all, or that you should hide things you either really can't or don't want to hide.

There are other added stresses for teens who start developing either far earlier or later than most of their peers. Late bloomers may feel like babies—or be treated like them—compared to their friends or siblings. Early developers may find themselves the center of a lot of unwanted or inappropriate sexual attention or teasing. Since boys start puberty later than girls, and many girls aren't aware of

that, boys may encounter expectations of sexual development or desire from their female peers that they don't feel ready for yet, or don't want at all.

Puberty is unavoidable, and there's no healthful way to curb certain parts of it. Excessive dieting, for example, in an attempt to prevent normal weight gain or breast development, or to try to make menses stop, is only going to make you sick. You also can't make it hurry up by using herbal supplements or hormones, by weight training, or by behaving in certain ways.

Puberty has its own timetable for everyone, and no matter what you do, it's going to stick to that individual schedule. But puberty is also temporary: it does end, and you only have to go through it once.

• WHAT'S UP DOWN THERE? •
Male and Female Sexual Anatomy

Quick: what's the name for the external female genitals? The vagina, right?

Bzzzzzt. **Nope.**

Even if you think you know all about sexual anatomy—yours or that of the opposite sex—you might be surprised to find that even some of the most basic things you've learned aren't accurate.

So, what's the name for the external female genitals?

s.e.x.

▪ FEMALE SEXUAL ANATOMY: ▪
From the Outside In

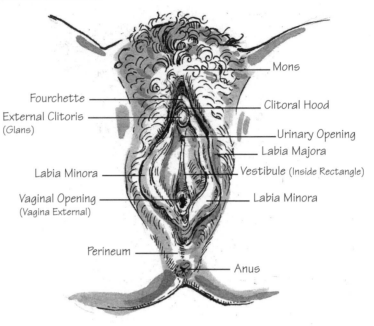

Mons

Fourchette

Clitoral Hood

External Clitoris
(Glans)

Urinary Opening

Labia Majora

Vestibule (Inside Rectangle)

Labia Minora

Labia Minora

Vaginal Opening
(Vagina External)

Perineum

Anus

Vulva is the name for the external female genitalia. Cunt, pussy, fanny, twat, coochie, muff, and snatch are some common slang names for the vulva.

The vulva begins with the *mons,* a fatty area of skin below the lower abdomen, where most of the pubic hair is. The mons continues downward, to form the *labia majora,* or outer labia (Latin for *lips*). The mons and outer labia are skin like that on our arms and legs, rather than the mucous membrane of other parts of the genitals. The size of the labia majora varies a good deal among women, as does the flatness or puffiness of the mons, depending on body size and shape, and on bone structure, as the pubic bone is just beneath the mons. (If you've ever been horseback or bicycle riding for a long time, you know *exactly* where your pubic bone is, because it can feel mighty sore afterward.) And it's normal for

the mons to be a bit puffier for teens than it is in fully grown women.

Between the labia majora, you may see the *labia minora,* or inner labia, peeking out. Because the length of the inner labia varies a lot—not just between women, but between one woman's own pair—some women's inner labia will peek out even when her legs are closed, and others will have shorter inner labia that aren't visible unless the legs or outer labia are spread open. The inner labia are made of mucous membrane, contain sebaceous glands and sensory nerve endings, and tend to look a lot like flower petals or two little tongues. They can vary a lot in color, from pink to red, brown to violet. Many women have asymmetrical labia minora, with one labium longer than the other. The labia minora also aren't very uniform in shape—some may have ragged looking edges, and that's normal.

s.e.x.

The inner labia are important: not only do they help to keep bacteria and other ickies from getting into the *vestibule*—the area between the inner labia, which houses the clitoris, urethra, and vaginal opening—they're also connected to the clitoral hood, so they play a part in genital stimulation and sexual arousal.

Clit Lit

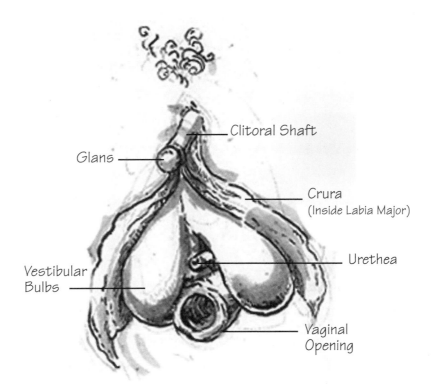

Glans

Clitoral Shaft

Crura
(Inside Labia Major)

Urethea

Vestibular Bulbs

Vaginal Opening

Just inside the vestibule—beneath the *fourchette,* where the inner labia connect—is nestled the visible part of infamous *clitoris* (sometimes called the *clit*). Beneath the clitoral hood (a little skin fold), is the *glans,* or the tip of the clitoris, often mistaken for the whole of the clitoris. If you explore your own clitoris with your fingers, you'll usually feel an intense tingle or a tickle. Pressing down on it, you may be able to feel a firm portion that is the *shaft* of the clitoris. The clitoris also has little "legs" inside the body, called the *crura,* which run down the sides of the vulva, inside the labia majora. There is one more portion of the clitoris, the *vestibular,* or *clitoral, bulbs.* Those are also internal, beneath the inner labia, and surround the vaginal opening (the bulbs—which are erectile tissue, much like the penis—and the crura can provide some clitoral stimulation during vaginal sex). You can see, then, that the clitoris is a *whole* lot bigger than she looks. The whole of the clitoris is similar in size to the penis.

The clitoris is usually the most sensitive spot of the vulva. In fact, the tiny glans of

S.e.x.

the clitoris alone has more sensory nerve endings than the penis or any other part of the human body—and it is the only organ of the human body whose ONLY purpose is to provide sexual pleasure. It's attached to ligaments, muscles, and veins that become filled with blood during sexual arousal and contract during orgasm.

The clitoris is the area that most women give the most airplay during masturbation, and what most women like to have stimulated during oral or manual sex (sometimes called *fingering*) and during intercourse. Because of differences in sensitivity, preference, and tolerance, women differ in how and where they like the clitoris touched.

Right below the clitoris is a little dot or slit, which is the *urethral opening,* the door from the *urethra,* where a woman urinates (pees) from. You may or may not be able to see it easily, especially since it's so tiny. Just inside the urinary opening, and on the upper wall of the vagina inside, are glands called the *Skene's glands,* or *paraurethral glands,* which drain into the urethra. The male equivalent of the Skene's glands is the prostate gland.

Below that is the *vaginal opening,* the opening to the *vagina.*

Around the vaginal opening, there may or may not be a *hymen.*

It's a pretty safe bet that all women are born with hymens, and before puberty, barring injury or sexual assault, the hymen usually covers the vaginal opening completely or partially. It isn't a full seal, as it contains small holes and perforations called *hymenal orifices,* the size and shape of which vary widely. After puberty starts, estrogen, menstruation, and physical and sexual activity

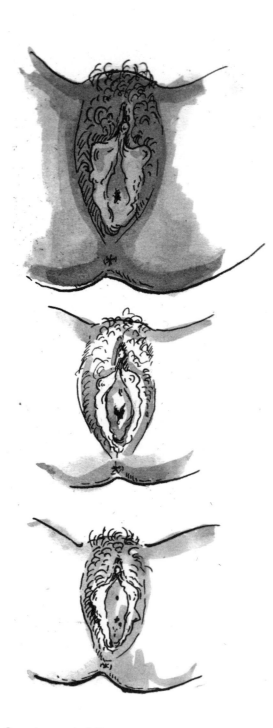

Some hymens look like . . .

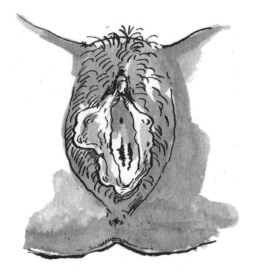

to the *anus,* the external opening to your *rectum,* through which bowel movements pass.

Life on the Inside

If you slide your finger inside the vaginal opening (whether that's into your own vagina or someone else's), you're in the *vagina.* The vagina is the muscular tube between the external genitals and the internal reproductive system: the cervix, uterus, and fallopian tubes. It's where the action happens during vaginal play or intercourse, and it's where an infant passes through during a vaginal childbirth.

Just inside the vaginal opening are glands called the *Bartholin's glands.* During sexual arousal, these glands may provide some lubrication.

The vagina isn't a passive object. In other words, it DOES things, rather than simply being an empty place that just sits around like a slacker. When nothing is inside it, the walls of the vagina lie together, closed. When something is inserted within it—be it a tampon, fingers, a penis, or a dildo—it can hold whatever it is pretty intensely: it's flexible and muscular! When whatever was inside it is removed, it goes right back to its collapsed, "resting" state. You or a sexual partner can feel that yourself, with your fingers, and you can feel some of the muscles that surround the vagina, the PC—*pubococcygeus* (and if you want to sound like a smartypants, it's pronounced pew-bo-cock-se-GEE-us)—muscles, too. If, while urinating, a woman squeezes to stop the flow of urine, those are the PC muscles at work.

The vaginal canal is curved, rather than straight—if you could see it inside in profile, you'd see a soft U-shape from opening to cervix—and there are a lot of different

start to wear the hymen away. When someone talks about "popping a cherry," they are referring to the hymen. Really, hymens are rarely "popped" or "broken." Instead, they simply wear away, often gradually and without much notice, especially since the hymen doesn't have any sensory nerve endings in it. Some young women who experience pain or discomfort during initial vaginal entry or intercourse may be feeling hymenal microtearing or stretching, which can put pressure on the parts of the vaginal opening the hymen is attached to, and these parts DO have plenty of nerve endings. That's normal, and it's just as normal NOT to feel pain or discomfort—or for the hymen to be stretchy enough or worn away enough by that time so that it's not in the way at all. (Pain and discomfort can also happen for different reasons altogether; for more on pain or discomfort during vaginal sex, see page 160).

Even after the hymen has been worn away, little folds of tissue from it often remain just inside the vaginal opening.

Below the vaginal opening, there is an area of skin called the *perineum.* That leads

s.e.x.

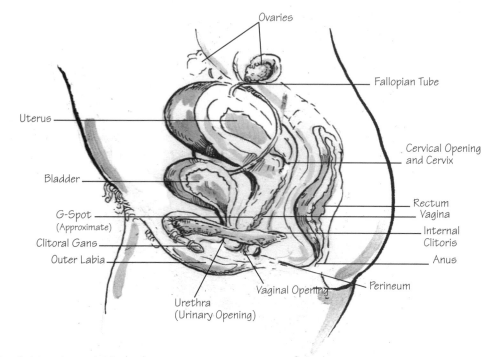

Ovaries

Fallopian Tube

Uterus

Cervical Opening and Cervix

Bladder

Rectum
Vagina

G-Spot
(Approximate)

Internal
Clitoris

Clitoral Gans

Outer Labia

Anus

Vaginal Opening

Perineum

Urethra
(Urinary Opening)

Female internal reproductive anatomy

textures within it. On the front wall of the vagina, you may be able to feel a small, spongy or textured area, kind of like the roof of your mouth. That is the infamous *G-spot,* or *Gräfenberg spot,* another potential contributor to sexual pleasure and orgasm.

Even farther back into the vagina, you might feel something deep inside, sticking out a bit, the edge of which will have a little dimple. This is the *cervix* (Latin for *neck*), and the dimple is the opening of the cervix, the *os* (Latin for *mouth*). The cervix is the passage from the uterus to the vagina. There's no reason to ever worry about losing a tampon, a toy, or anything else in the vagina: the os is very, very small. The very back of the vagina, slightly above and around the base of the cervix, is called the *fornix.* During sexual arousal, the fornix gets larger, or "tents," to

make extra room for whatever might be inside the vagina.

Inside the body, the cervix leads into the *uterus* (also called the *womb*), a pear-shaped and muscular internal organ that's about four centimeters thick and about eight centimeters long. The uterus is the area of the female sexual anatomy where a fetus develops and grows. The lining of the uterus, called the *endometrium,* builds up every menstrual cycle to prepare for a fertilized egg, and this is what a woman sheds each cycle when she does not become pregnant and has her period.

On either side of the uterus is a *fallopian tube.* Eggs travel through the fallopian tubes, also called the *oviducts,* to get to the uterus. Fingerlike structures called *fimbrae* at the end of the fallopian tubes sweep the eggs from the ovary into the tubes. At the end of each

honorably discharged

VAGINAL DISCHARGE and secretions are a normal, healthy part of the female reproductive system and reproductive cycle.

The vagina is a passageway between the outside of the body and the internal reproductive system. The pH balance of the vagina is acidic, with "good" bacteria that help keep infections away. The vagina is a self-cleaning organ. Secretion is its way of cleansing and regulating itself, in the same sort of way that secreting saliva helps keep our mouths clean and healthy. So, while we need to wash the external genitals, there's no need to try to clean inside the vagina with soap or douching. It does it best all by itself!

Normal vaginal discharge:

- Can be clear and thin–that sort of discharge usually occurs around ovulation, and vaginal secretions during sexual arousal also tend to have this appearance and consistency.
- Can be white or slightly yellowish and thick, much like the consistency of school paste. This sort of discharge tends to occur during less fertile times in the monthly cycle.
- Often has a mild but not a strong or unpleasant odor.
- May have a brown or reddish tint just before or just after menses.
- Will appear on underpants, around the vaginal opening, and/or on the inner labia a lot of the time.

Normal discharge is just that: **normal**. It's nothing to be worried or embarrassed about, there's nothing wrong with it, and you need it to stay healthy. During times when vaginal secretions are especially profuse, or more "wet" than at other times, some women feel more comfortable using a washable or disposable panty liner, but there's no need to do that if you don't want to: your underpants are more than absorbent enough to handle most normal vaginal secretions.

Bacterial, yeast/fungal, or sexually transmitted infections (STIs) can create changes in the amount, consistency, color, or scent of vaginal discharges, so when in doubt, ask your healthcare professional. For more information on general vaginal infections, see page 194, and for information on STIs, see chapter 9 and Appendix A.

fallopian tube is an ovary, which both stores and releases eggs, or *ova,* one at a time during each menstrual cycle (though some women may ovulate more than once in a cycle, and women may also sometimes release more than one egg at a time). The ovaries produce the hormones estrogen and progesterone, which are responsible for the development of sex characteristics, but also keep the genitals flexible, elastic, and lubricated and help keep the vaginal lining healthy. Some estrogen is also produced by fat tissue.

The hormone testosterone, which is partially responsible for libido, or sexual desire, is also produced in the ovaries (and by the adrenal glands elsewhere in the body).

s.e.x.

Oocytes—the name of ova, or eggs, before they are released—aren't created every month, but are all lying in wait by the time puberty begins, around a half-million of them. They then mature, one at a time, in one of your two ovaries randomly, and will continue to be released until menopause, when you're around fifty. If you do the math, you'll find that a whole lot of them that never see the light of day; that's because, during each cycle, about a thousand of them naturally degenerate, and the cells are just absorbed by your body. There are ova still remaining at menopause, so no one is likely to "run out" of ova before then.

The Menstrual Cycle. Period.

The menstrual cycle isn't just something that happens when a woman is on the rag. Periods are only one part of a complex hormonal, physiological, and emotional fertility cycle that takes place about every month, and some parts of it have effects on women every single day.

The menstrual cycle is divided into three phases: the menstrual phase, the proliferative phase, and the secretory, or luteal, phase.

Every monthly cycle is considered to begin on the first day of each menstrual period, starting the **menstrual phase**. A menstrual phase, or period, might last anywhere from just a couple of days to around seven days, with both light and heavy flows. During a period, there may be days when there seems to be no flow at all, and then it

reappears the next day. It is also normal to find that vaginal discharge, which may be scanty or thick during menstruation, has a brownish hue a couple of days after the end of a period, because it is carrying slight residue from the previous days. On average, menstrual flow is only about 35 percent blood. The rest of its contents are endometrial tissue and other vaginal and cervical secretions, so it's perfectly normal to sometimes see globs, rather than simply liquid.

The next phase is the **proliferative phase**. In a section of the brain called the *hypothalamus,* substances are produced and released that travel down to the pituitary gland and stimulate it. The pituitary then releases two hormones: the *follicle-stimulating hormone* (FSH) and the *luteinizing hormone* (LH). These create changes that cause an ovum to mature and be released. It is at the end of the proliferative phase that this occurs, and a woman ovulates: the egg is released from the ovary and begins its slide down to the uterus.

The majority of women are most fertile during the end of the proliferative phase and the start of the secretory phase; sometimes the time just before and during ovulation is called the **ovulatory phase**.

Right at ovulation the **luteal**, or **secretory**, **phase** begins. At this time, the hormone *progesterone* is produced by the ovary, and this hormone is what prepares the lining of the uterus, the endometrium, to nourish and house an egg, should it be fertilized. During this phase, vaginal secretions will become thinner and more fluid, with a stretchy, egg-white consistency. This happens because that type of mucus provides the best environment for sperm to reach an egg. If an egg is fertilized by sperm and implants on the uterine wall—creating a

s.e.x.

pregnancy—even more progesterone is released. If there's no fertilized egg, then the level of progesterone drops; it is that hormonal drop, and the shedding of the endometrium—a period—that starts the cycle all over again. It is typical at the end of this phase, before the next cycle begins, for vaginal secretions to be thick, sparse, or pretty nonexistent.

Menses Management

Menstrual flow—only about three or four ounces total over the course of each period—has gotta go somewhere, and there are many options to help women manage menstrual flow. That choice boils down to personal preference when it comes to ease of use, environmental and health concerns, certain situations (for instance, a pad while swimming isn't usually a good option), cost, and availability. When used properly, all of the following methods are safe and healthy. Some women find that combining a few methods works best for them; others feel that one alone does the job.

Pads: Pads are usually the best choice when first starting menstruation, for heavy flow, and/or while sleeping. Disposable pads come in various levels of absorbency, and have an adhesive backing that attaches to underwear. If using disposable pads, avoid any with added perfumes, as these can irritate the vulva. Most pads are a blend of natural and synthetic fibers, but organic, unbleached cotton pads are also available. Some women may experience vulval irritation due to the synthetic fibers, bleaching, plastic backing, or casing of some commercial pads.

Washable, reusable pads are a better choice for the environment and the body than disposable pads. In the long run, they're also much less expensive, even though they cost a bit more at the outset. Most are constructed with a cotton outer liner over an inner absorbent core, and come in different levels of absorbency. Some brands have a heavier "filler" you can remove, as well. Some have snaps on little wings that wrap around underwear, and others attach like a pair of underwear, with a little g-string. They are washed for reuse, and doing so is just as sanitary as any other menstrual product. When you wash your underwear, it's clean enough again for wearing—same with washable pads. Menstrual flow is really no different from daily vaginal discharge when it comes to germs. You can find washable pads at most natural foods markets or health stores, and some standard pharmacies have started to carry them, as well. They're also available via the Internet, or you can even make them yourself. See the Resources section for some sources.

Tampons: Tampons are good for swimming, for very active women, for use during special occasions or during outercourse (sexual activities like manual or oral sex), or if you just don't like pads. As with pads, tampons without fragrance or perfumes are healthiest. While menstrual flow, like other vaginal fluids, does have its own scent, the idea that it is a "bad" or foul scent is nothing but a marketing ploy—and at the expense of vaginal health. A woman smells just fine so long as she's good with basic hygiene and changing menstrual supplies often enough. Perfumes aren't meant to be inside the vaginal canal, and

S.e.x.

flow chart

IT'S A GREAT idea to keep track of menstrual cycles each month, whether you have to worry about pregnancy or not. The first day of a period, just make a little red dot on your calendar. Continue the dots until the period ends. After that, pay attention to vaginal secretions, or discharge, and note those however is most sensible for you. For instance, you can mark a letter "D" when mucus and discharge are dry or thick, and an "O" when discharge seems thinner, a sign of being more fertile. Charting cycles over time will help you to best understand them, and to be more alert when you may have any problems you'll want to talk to your doctor about. If and when in your life you're ready to conceive a child, being familiar with charting will help you to do so most easily.

This month is....

S M T W T F S

ON VACATION FROM MY PERIOD

s.e.x.

TSS

Tampon use can pose a risk of toxic shock syndrome (TSS). TSS has been on the decline over the last decade, and is rare, but it can cause severe medical problems and even death. TSS is caused by a staph organism that can produce toxins that colonize on the fibers of the tampon. Staph in and of itself is a nasty infection, but the added toxin production of TSS is serious bad news.

Symptoms of TSS are nearly immediate and pretty obvious, so during tampon use, should you suddenly feel dizzy, nauseated, weak, or faint, or develop a sudden high fever or body rash, you need to seek medical attention immediately. But if you only use tampons during the day, change them often, and use the lowest absorbency you need, you don't have to worry much about TSS. If you use any type of pads or a menstrual cup, you don't have to worry about TSS.

but 100 percent unbleached organic cotton tampons are available at most natural foods stores and markets. While it's unclear if they're any better for your body than commercial brands, they are certainly better for the environment.

Sometimes tampons—especially those left in for too long—may separate or shred when removed, and extra fibers may be found coming from the vagina even a week later. While that's nothing necessarily major, if you discover you've got other symptoms, like itching, redness, soreness, extra spotting, headaches, dizziness, or a foul scent, you should see your doctor or gynecologist.

Natural sea sponges: They're reusable, natural, and all you do is soften them with a little water, curl them up, and insert them inside the vagina. To change them, just pull the sponge out gently, rinse it with warm water, and put in a fresh one. At the end of each cycle, sponges can be cleaned by soaking them for a few hours in a cup of warm water with a teaspoon of baking soda, a half-cup of hydrogen peroxide, or a few drops of tea tree oil. Sponges are a good alternative for someone who feels "poked" by tampons, or is looking for an alternative that creates less waste. Natural sponges can be found at most natural foods stores, and should be replaced every few months.

may cause infections that truly ARE stinky. Because tampons are absorbent, however, they may increase vaginal or menstrual scent, as well as cramping.

Some tampons come with plastic or paper applicators, and some come without; which to use is a personal preference. Nearly all commercial brands of tampons contain cotton, as well as rayon fibers and bleaches used on the fibers. The jury is still out in terms of hard data, when it comes to the dangers of bleaches and synthetics,

Menstrual cups: Reusable cups have the adaptability and ease of a tampon, but without the waste and the downsides of fibers, or the endless cost. A menstrual cup (like The Keeper or the Divacup, see Resources), may well last your entire reproductive lifetime for one modest

S.e.x.

payment. Made of gum rubber or silicone, they collect and hold menstrual flow within the cup until you remove it, empty the cup, and reinsert. At the end of a period, menstrual cups are boiled before they're used again. Disposable menstrual cups are also available, but tend to work less well and are far less cost-effective.

Because they collect flow rather than absorb it, they don't disrupt the moisture balance of the vagina, and some users report less cramping than when using tampons. Menstrual cups can often also be used safely for longer periods of time than tampons.

To date, cups have not been associated with TSS. Menstrual cups are often harder to obtain, but as with washable pads, natural foods stores often carry them, and they can be ordered internationally from a handful of online vendors.

For very light flow, for the end of your period, or for someone who just doesn't want to use anything at all—no one *has* to. Some women have undergarments they keep just for menses, or wear dark skirts; some have special sheets set aside for flow at night so they can go product-less. Doing so generally doesn't work very well for work or school, but there isn't a thing wrong with just letting flow go, if that works for you.

When the Rag's a Drag

Cramps: It's normal to experience cramping just before and/or during a period, generally due to chemical and hormonal changes during menstruation (namely, increased prostaglandin, which decreases blood flow to the uterus and causes it to contract). It also is common

for young women to have more painful periods than they will once they're older.

There are many ways to relieve cramps. Over-the-counter anti-inflammatories, like ibuprofen or another analgesic, are often very effective. Warm baths, beverages, or compresses can be very helpful with cramps. Deep stretching, yoga, other exercise, activity, or self-massage are helpful, and acupuncture can also save the day. Calcium, magnesium, and vitamins E and K, which are usually in a regular daily multivitamin, can be of help with cramping and other menstrual discomforts. Some foods that tend to make cramping and other menstrual discomforts worse are caffeine, processed foods, sugar, salt, alcohol, and dairy products, so it's best to pay special attention to diet and consume light, healthy meals while menstruating. An herbal tea of red raspberry leaf, strawberry leaf, peppermint, and ginger can help minimize cramps and balance cycles (and it tastes nice, too).

Irregularity: The menstrual cycle can take a few years to become regular. It's typical during the first few years of menstruating to go a few months without a period sometimes, or have shorter cycles, or bleeding every three weeks instead of every four.

If periods go missing for more than a couple of months outright, or if after a few years of menstruation they're still occasionally very late or missing, diet or exercise can also be the cause. Not eating enough, being very inactive, or overexercising (more than four hours a day, or running over ten miles a day) can throw a body out of whack, and you may begin to miss periods. Stress can also make you miss a period, and sometimes stress because a woman *thinks* she may be pregnant can actually fool her body into acting like it is, thus causing a missed period. Obviously, if there has been a pregnancy risk and a missed period, a pregnancy test is in order.

PMS: Symptoms of PMS, or premenstrual syndrome, include acne, bloating, feeling very tired, backaches or general body soreness, tender breasts, headaches, constipation or diarrhea, food cravings, mood swings, serious crabbiness or depression, and troubles with concentrating or managing normal stresses. Some degree of PMS is normal, and can usually be managed. Track your cycles so you know when to expect it, and do your best during that time to get plenty of rest and exercise, reduce the amount of sugar and caffeine you're taking in, and take basic good care of yourself. Some women also find that a blood-thinning medication, like simple aspirin, helps with PMS symptoms and may reduce cramps at the onset of a period.

Severe effects: If your period produces more severe side effects, such as highly painful and constant heavy cramping (dysmenorrhea), deep abdominal pain, very heavy flow (menorrhagia) or irregular vaginal bleeding during other times in your cycle, heavy-duty acne, strong loss of appetite, very intense mood swings or depression, extensive PMS symptoms—or if you have stopped getting your periods altogether (amenorrhea)—talk to your doctor. Many menstrual maladies can be remedied with the proper treatment or medication, and some may be a result of other conditions, like pelvic inflammatory disease (PID) or endometriosis, which require treatment.

BREAST BASICS

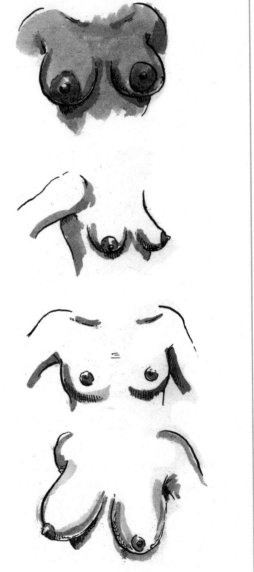

Some breasts look like . . .

s.e.x.

Post-puberty, female breasts are composed of four different things: connective tissue, fat, mammary (milk-producing) glands known as *lobules,* and lactiferous (milk-carrying) ducts. The breasts sit on the rib cage, over the chest or pectoral muscles, and are connected to the body by ligaments.

There's no muscle in the breast itself. The parts of the breasts that create their size and shape are fat and glands. Between the ligaments of the breast are pockets of fat that contain the mammary glands (lobules), and those lead to the lactiferious ducts.

The area of the breast that is darker and surrounds the nipple is called the *areola.* Milk ducts behind the areola—about fifteen to twenty of them in each breast—lead to the nipples from the mammary glands, and during and after pregnancy, those glands will produce milk, which comes through the ducts to nourish a baby. There are also glands called *Montgomery glands* within the areola, which can sometimes be seen, and look like little bumps. Most women's nipples protrude slightly (and noticeably when a woman's aroused or cold), but some women have what are called inverted nipples, which turn inward into the breast—a totally normal variation.

Breasts come in a lot of different shapes: some look round or globelike; other breasts may appear more triangular. For women with very small breasts, only the areola and nipple may protrude or have visible shape. Some women have what are called tubular breasts, which have less glandular tissue than other breasts and look a little long and cylindrical. No one breast shape is necessarily more functional or better than another.

Areola size doesn't necessarily correspond to breast size. Women with large breasts can and do have small areolas; women with smaller breasts can and do have larger areolas. It's normal for breast size and shape to differ slightly in one set of breasts. Areola and nipple size, however, tend to be pretty symmetrical.

bogus boob stuff

- Bras aren't needed for good health, and there has yet to be any viable data that shows that brassieres prevent breasts from sagging over time. Wearing them is an individual preference based on comfort. For those who like wearing a bra to bed, there's little to suggest that it's unsafe, especially if the bra is soft and flexible.

- There are no supplements or creams on the market that can increase breast size. Using some of them may cause the skin to swell, but not only are those results temporary, but many such supplements contain compounds dangerous to long-term health.

- Cosmetic breast surgery and implants in teens are on the rise. Breast implants, while safer than they used to be, still pose risks such as inability to nurse a baby properly, rippling (wrinkling), scarring, sensory loss, and serious and even life-threatening infections. FDA scientists have found a significant link between silicone gel implants and fibromyalgia, a disorder that causes pain and fatigue in the muscles, tendons, and ligaments. According to the FDA, 43 percent of all implant patients have complications within just three years of surgery. The BBC reported in 2003 that scientists at the University Medical Centre in Utrecht found that suicide rates in women who had breast implants were considerably higher than in the general population. They attributed this to profound self-image problems that implants did not correct. Considering that the cost of breast implants—usually thousands of dollars—can be equivalent to the cost of a full four-year college education at a state school, and that breast implants are not one-time surgeries but require upkeep every few years, even removal or replacement, and all the risks they pose, they're pretty iffy stuff.

The size and shape of breasts vary so widely because each person's breasts are made of up different amounts of the various sorts of fatty, mammary, and fibrous tissue, and because the individual fat and muscle composition and structure, as well as the hormones in the body (estrogen, progesterone, and prolactin), vary so widely. That's one reason why even in one person, in a given month, breast size can vary slightly, as can the tenderness of the breast. Most of breast size and shape is determined by genetics, but because genetic combinations are so unique, it's still possible for a given woman's breasts to look nothing like her mother's or sister's.

▪ MALE SEXUAL ANATOMY: ▪
From the Outside In

Let's start from the top, or rather, from the tip. [circumcised penis]

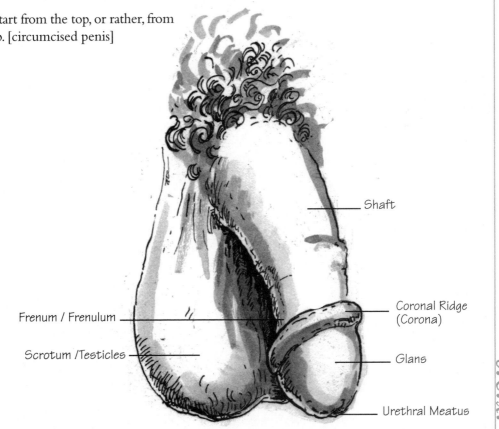

Shaft

Frenum / Frenulum

Coronal Ridge
(Corona)

Scrotum /Testicles

Glans

Urethral Meatus

s.e.x.

At the end of the penis—the name for the external male genitalia, not including the testicles and anus, sometimes called the dick, boner, cock, willie, johnson, or schlong—you'll see the *urethral meatus,* or the opening of the *urethra.* All fluids from the penis, including urine, come through the urethra; unlike a woman's, a man's urethra has both a urinary function *and* a reproductive one: semen and pre-ejaculate come out through the urethra, too.

The urethral meatus is at top and center of the *glans,* or the head of the penis. The glans is mushroom-shaped, and the ridge along the edge at the bottom of the glans is called the *corona,* or coronal ridge. On the underside of that ridge, on the side of the penis facing the stomach when erect, is the *frenum,* or *frenulum.* For many men, this and the glans are the most sensitive areas of the penis.

At birth, the *shaft,* or area of the penis from beneath the coronal ridge to the base, is covered by a loose tube of skin, called the *foreskin.* This is attached to the penis in two ways: at the base, and along the length by the *frenar band,* which extends from the frenulum and runs in a long loop within the foreskin.

The foreskin is chock-full of sensory nerve endings, and looks a lot like a little sleeping bag for the penis. When a penis is flaccid—not erect—the whole of the shaft and glans are covered by the foreskin. When erection occurs, the foreskin retracts: it slides backward down the shaft of the penis, so that the glans and some of the shaft are visible outside the foreskin. When an intact (uncircumcised) penis is erect, the foreskin essentially blends in with the shaft, so it is generally easier to see the difference between circumcised and uncircumcised penises when they're flaccid. The foreskin should slide and retract comfortably, both by

itself, with the hands, or during sexual activity; if you've got a foreskin and yours doesn't do this, check in with your doctor, as most infections and conditions that cause foreskin problems are easily treatable.

Intact penises are self-lubricating to allow the foreskin to move comfortably along the shaft (though men with foreskins may still find they or their partners want or need additional lubrication). It's normal for *smegma,* a white and waxy substance, to be found beneath and around the foreskin. It's made up of shed skin cells and secretions from glands within the foreskin, called the *Tyson's glands,* and the glands of the testes. Basic gentle hygiene takes care of most of smegma, but it's likely to be present in some amounts at all times, and that's both normal and healthy.

All men are born with foreskins. However, about 20 percent worldwide, and about 80 percent in the United States., have been circumcised: their foreskins were removed, usually in early infancy, due to cultural traditions or the belief that a circumcised penis is healthier. However, in 1999, the American Academy of Pediatrics (AAP) made clear that there is *no* medical basis for infant circumcision.

Penises with and without foreskins are healthy and hygienic. It's both normal to have one and not to have one.

In men who have been circumcised, the frenulum isn't attached to the foreskin or frenar band, so it may look like a small V-shaped area. Because circumcisions vary, different degrees of the frenulum, and sometimes the frenar band, may remain. On both circumcised and uncircumcised men, a line, called the *raphe,* can be seen on the side of the penis that faces downward and that follows through the testicles and down to the anus.

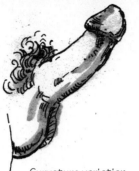

Curvature variation
when erect

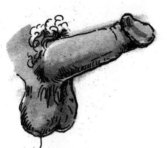

Curvature variation
when erect

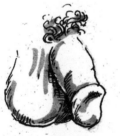

Circumcised flaccid

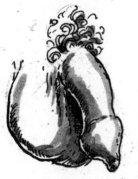

Uncircumsised flaccid

Some penises look like . . .

It's normal for the skin and shaft of the penis to be several shades darker than the skin of the rest of the body, either all the time or just when the penis is hard. It's also normal to have the penis change color somewhat when it gets hard. The coloration should return to normal once the erection goes down. The shaft, when erect, can also look veiny and bulgy in places: that's normal, too.

how big is it supposed to be?

PENISES vary in size pretty widely when they're not erect, but the average is a little over three inches in length. The size of a flaccid penis doesn't dictate the size it may be when erect. According to most studies, the average fully grown penis is about five to six inches long when erect, and four to five inches in circumference. The way averages work, that means there are an awful lot of adult men with penises both smaller and larger than that size.

How big or small someone's penis is, is a lot like how big or small a woman's breasts are. In other words, weight or height doesn't dictate size, genetics do.

Don't get too obsessed about the size of your penis. If you're convinced you've got a serious health concern, deformity, or abnormality, talk to your doctor. Otherwise, you've got bigger fish to fry, and better ways to spend your time—like finding out what's really going on in there.

LIFE ON THE INSIDE

Despite being called a boner, the penis has no bones. In fact, there isn't even any muscle, except the *bulbospongiosus,* a small muscle used to squeeze out urine and ejaculatory fluids, and some muscles and ligaments at the

s.e.x.

33

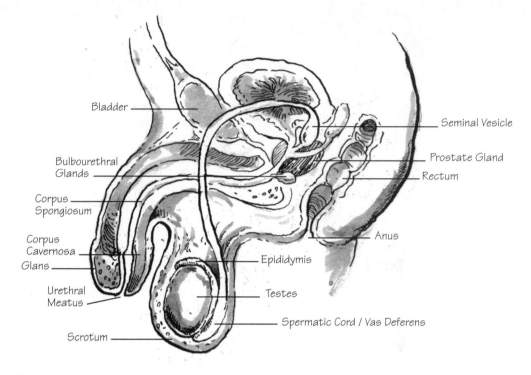

Bladder

Seminal Vesicle

Bulbourethral
Glands

Prostate Gland

Rectum

Corpus
Spongiosum

Corpus
Cavernosa

Glans

Anus

Epididymis

Urethral
Meatus

Testes

Spermatic Cord / Vas Deferens

Scrotum

Female internal reproductive anatomy

base of the penis that attach it to the body. Most of the penis is composed of three long cylinders of tissue: two *corpora cavernosa* (singular: *corpus cavernosum*) and the *corpus spongiosum,* through which the urethra runs.

Erection occurs because of blood; during arousal, blood flows into the penis and fills up the bodies of tissue in the penis. The corpora cavernosa run along the top of the penis, and the corpus spongiosum runs around the urethra. When the corpora cavernosa and the corpus spongiosum are filled with blood, they get stiff and the penis becomes both hard and erect, leveraged by the extension of those structures a little into the body.

The urethra is a tube about eight inches long that runs the length of the penis and connects to several internal organs: the bladder (where urine is stored), the testes, and the

ejaculatory ducts. Like the female urethra, the male urethra is one-way only (so if you're curious if you can insert something in there, yes, you might be able to, but in most scenarios, it'd likely set you up for a romantic date with the ER). The urethra ends at the urethral opening.

Get the Ball Rolling

The *testicles, testes,* or "balls" hang below the penis, in a sac of skin and muscle called the *scrotum.* There are two testes, but just one scrotum. It's divided in half by a wall of tissue, and you can see where that division happens from the outside via the *raphe,* which runs down the center of the scrotum. The testes produce sperm and the hormone testosterone.

s.e.x.

The testes are outside the body because the ideal temperature for the sperm inside them is slightly lower than body temperature. The size of the testicles varies among men: some may be the size of olives, others as big as small plums. They're *incredibly* sensitive to touch and pressure.

The scrotum's muscles are used to pull the testes closer to the body in order to protect or warm them (this is why when it's cold the scrotum can shrivel up); when the muscles relax, the testes hang a good deal lower, and the scrotum often looks longer.

Sperm is formed in the testes, and then

the ejaculation situation

What's the difference between sperm, semen, and ejaculate?

Ejaculate is another word for semen. Semen—the fluid that comes from the penis during ejaculation—contains sperm. Semen and sperm are not one and the same. Sperm, between 50 and 130 million in a given ejaculation, are only a small part of what is within ejaculate. Sperm are only about 2 to 5 percent of the volume of the semen ejaculated; the rest is composed of fluids produced by the prostate gland and the *bulbourethral* or *Cowper's glands,* as well as fluids produced by the vas deferens and the seminal vesicles themselves. The prostate produces fluids that are about 30 percent of the total volume of semen. These are added to the semen mixture at various points along the way before the semen is ejaculated. Most ejaculations are about one teaspoon of fluid, but that can vary a lot from person to person, or from day to day.

When does ejaculation happen?

Ejaculation and orgasm aren't the same thing, but they are often related. While ejaculation usually happens after orgasm, orgasm can occur without ejaculation. Although men get erections from infancy on, ejaculation doesn't occur until *after* puberty has begun, and some men may not even begin to ejaculate until they are in their late teens.

It's okay for men not to ejaculate during masturbation or partnered sex activities, either because they haven't begun ejaculating yet or because, for whatever reason, it just doesn't happen at a given time. As well, no amount of ejaculate is better than another, nor is "dribbling" rather than "shooting" anything to be embarrassed about—how much or with what force someone ejaculates varies based on levels of semen from day to day. To date, there have yet to be any Olympic competitions for ejaculating, so as long as a guy is physically comfortable and everything feels fine, chances are everything *is* fine.

What's healthy and what's not?

Semen/ejaculate tends to be whitish, milky, or somewhat translucent. It may sometimes also have a slightly yellowish tint (because it can contain some urine, by virtue of using the same road, the urethra, to travel through). Urination or ejaculation should not cause any discomfort.

If urination or ejaculation does cause pain or discomfort, if other discharges are coming from the penis, or if urine or ejaculate is discolored or contains any blood, however, it's time to see the doctor.

S.e.x.

moves into the *epididymis* to mature. Composed of a bundle of squiggly tubes, the epidydimis is a small organ that lies against the top of the testicle. When a man is going to ejaculate, sperm are moved from the epididymis into the *vas deferens,* the continuation of the epidydimis that takes sperm up and out of the scrotum area and into other ducts so they can be ejaculated. New sperm are constantly created and moved to the epidydimis. Sperm that don't get ejaculated stay there for around four to six weeks before they die and are reabsorbed into the body. This is why it's impossible—even if you never ejaculated in your whole life—to have "excess" sperm build up in your body.

The epididymis and testicles are anchored to the body by what is called the *spermatic cord*. The spermatic cord is a bundle of nerves and blood vessels that serve the testicle and epididymis, plus the vas deferens.

The vas deferens leads into the body, through a canal toward the bladder—which is also connected to the urethra—and into the seminal vesicles, where sperm get mixed up with some of the other ingredients of semen.

The bulbourethral glands, or Cowper's glands, are two pea-sized glands connected to the side of the urethra. They produce a liquid sort of mucus called *pre-ejaculate,* or *precum,* that occurs when a man becomes sexually aroused, usually with an erection. It may be emitted more than once during arousal, and many men don't feel it or become aware when it is present, especially during intercourse or other partnered sex activities when the tip of the penis can't be seen. It's a fluid intended to neutralize any acid (from urine) that might be inside the urethra. Since sperm do not thrive under acidic conditions, pre-ejaculate helps to make the conditions in the urethra favorable

for sperm to survive. The same fluid is also a component of semen itself.

Just above the bulbourethral glands is the *prostate gland*. A chestnut-shaped gland about one and a half inches around that surrounds a small part of the urethra, it's below the bladder and toward the rectum, the canal between the bowel and the anus. The seminal vesicles empty into the urethra at this location.

We all get hormonal.

 MEN don't have a monthly fertility cycle *just* like women do, but there ARE two different arenas of constant hormonal changes in the male reproductive system. Men experience hormonal changes daily–testosterone levels are highest in the morning, and decrease through the day, in cycles of every twenty-four hours. In additional cycles of every seventy-two days, men also have the hormones FSH and LH at work, just as women do; in men, these regulate the production of sperm. So, if you have the idea that only women can be "hormonal," or go through mood changes because of their reproductive systems, think again!

The prostate is sensitive to touch, so plenty of men enjoy prostate stimulus during sexual activity. Some people call it the "P-spot." Because of its location, it is stimulated by anal sex or stimulation or deep massage of the anus or perineum. The female equivalent to the prostate are the Skene's glands.

Once fluids from the prostate have been added to the mix of fluids and sperm that has traveled to this point, semen is ready to be ejaculated. Ejaculation occurs through the urethra, usually as a result of sexual arousal and stimulation, with the aid of contractions that continue all along the path that the sperm and fluid take in order to leave the body.

During ejaculation, a muscular gate called the *urinary sphincter,* which is located at the opening of the bladder, closes so that urine, even if it's present in the bladder, isn't released during ejaculation. During urination, that gate is voluntarily opened.

Blue Balls

. . . aren't about balls at all. Nor are "blue balls," correctly known as *vasocongestion,* exclusive to men. Women can and do experience a similar sensation.

During sexual arousal (as explained on page 55), the genitals fill up with blood. When we orgasm and/or ejaculate, the swelling from vasocongestion subsides and usually goes away. If we do **not** orgasm or ejaculate after sexual stimulation and arousal—and sometimes even when we do—vasocongestion can stick around for a bit, and can cause pain or discomfort, which we'll feel in the genitals.

In men, the primary source of discomfort when arousal is not followed by ejaculation is vasocongestive pressure in the penis, testicles, and surrounding areas. (When women experience vasocongestion, it's more a general pelvic pain or throbbing than the more specific pain men feel.) In many ways, vasocongestion is like having a tension headache in your genitals: blood pressure is increased, but the blood vessels that the blood must flow through are constricted. When high blood pressure and high blood volume meet narrowed blood vessels—like trying to force the flow of a kitchen faucet through a soda straw—it's uncomfortable and can be downright painful. The reason men may feel vasocongestion most profoundly in the testes is that the testes are so sensitive.

Taking care of vasocongestion is pretty simple. You can either masturbate to orgasm, take a pain reliever, use a cold or warm compress, get a little rest, or get some simple physical activity to redirect your blood flow.

Word up: If you've got a sexual partner, no matter your gender, your vasocongestion is not their responsibility. In other words, no one else can "give" you a "case of blue balls," and no one else should be manipulated or pushed into doing something to relieve it.

did you know . . . ?

As different as the male and female genitals are, for a while, when we were all embryos, our genitals were identical, regardless of our sex. Only after the tenth week of development, due to levels of hormones based on our chromosomal structure, fetal genitals turn into either the head of the penis or a clitoris, the genital folds turn into either testes or the inner labia, and the genital swellings become the scrotum or outer labia.

S.E.X.

▪ TOO LOOSE/TOO TIGHT! ▪ TOO LONG/TOO SHORT! TOO LARGE/TOO SMALL! Or, What Goldilocks and the Three Bears Have to Do with Your Genitals

FOR THE GALS:

Too Loose!/Too Tight!

The vaginal canal and vaginal opening are a whole lot like your mouth and your throat. In the same way that you can hold your mouth closed tightly, or open it wide, your vagina can do the same: it's elastic! There is no one size of any given vaginal opening or canal; how "loose" or "tight" it is depends mostly on how relaxed or aroused you are at any given time. So, throw away ideas that you need to find ways to "loosen" or "tighten" yourself up, because those are basically fictions.

If, during masturbation or partnered sex, you or a partner feel you are "too tight," relax (and tell them to, also). Stressing out is only going to make it worse. Take the time you need to chill out, to become aroused by activities that don't involve the vaginal opening and canal (like snuggling, massage, kissing, oral sex, stimulus to the clitoris, et cetera) before you attempt vaginal entry, either with a penis, fingers, or toys. You can also always opt out of any kind of vaginal sex entirely when it's just not feeling good. Sex of any sort really, truly, should not usually be painful.

Someone saying you're "too loose"? Maybe that person's previous experience has been with women who weren't aroused (which, in the case of young adults, isn't that unusual). How many female friends do you know who are EXPECTING penetra-

tion to be painful? Expecting pain is going to cause fear and anxiety, which will prevent full arousal. Since many people think that penetration is supposed to be painful at first, a lot of them don't know how to wait for full arousal or make penetration comfortable (for more on that, see chapter 8). So, if a partner is saying you're "too loose," either they're simply experiencing a relaxed, aroused partner for the first time, or they're blowing smoke—either because they think it's the thing to say, or they were expecting to feel trapped in a vise, which is not how penetration should feel for either partner.

If you like, you can do Kegel exercises to strengthen the muscles of the pelvic floor (men have them, too), which can be felt within the vaginal canal. You've likely done Kegels already: when you're finished urinating, know how you squeeze your muscles a bit to force out those last few drops of urine? That's a Kegel. Often, women are advised to do them after childbirth because pregnancy can weaken the pelvic floor, and many women have found that Kegel exercises heighten orgasmic and sexual response, as well as increasing bladder control. So, squeeze away, rhythmically, whenever and wherever you like—no one else can see you doing them. Keep in mind that young women, no matter their sexual history, really do not have to worry about being "too loose," but if doing something that's good for you anyway makes you feel more confident, knock yourself out.

Too Long!/Too Dark!

A lot of folks have the idea that there are "ideal" inner labia, and that what is ideal is any length or size that is diminutive and hidden. Some people may make lewd jokes or comments about various types of labia, or insult labia of a certain size or shape. It's not too surprising; we live in a culture that is often very ashamed about genitals and sexuality, especially female genitals and sexuality, so it's no big shocker that the "ideal" is genitals that are as hidden from view as possible. Think about how imbalanced that is: Men are sent the message that their penises should be larger than life, women that their genitals should be small, shy, and nearly invisible. Pretty whack, isn't it? And not at all based in reality: The reality is that fully functional, operative, and beautiful genitals—male and female alike—are diverse, just like everything else.

Like any other body part, labia minora come in a wide variety of shapes, sizes, textures, and colors. All of these variations are okay, and it's unlikely any of them are anything other than natural. Some young women worry that they've altered their labia by pulling at them, or via masturbation, but that's pretty unlikely, unless they've been stretched very extremely, such as with heavy genital piercings.

OF LATE, and in line with drastic increases in breast augmentation, some women have become convinced they need labiaplasty, cosmetic (for appearance, not function) surgery to "improve" the appearance of the labia. Rarely, there may be women whose labia are so extended that they cause pain or discomfort during sex, or even just walking around. For those women, considering surgery is not completely out of line. But for everyone else? Don't let doctors or advertisements convince you that parts of your body are abnormal or less than ideal! Labiaplasties can be dangerous. Cosmetic surgery, like any surgery, is costly and poses health risks. Cutting or shortening the labia,

when it's not necessary, may heighten the risk of infections, and may also cut or shorten your own sexual response and sensitivity, since the labia are full of sensory nerve endings, like other parts of your sexual anatomy. For more on not being duped by a culture that capitalizes on bad body image, see chapter 3.

Gynecologists have seen a whole lot of vulvas and labia in their day, of every imaginable shape, size, and hue. So, if you are seriously concerned or convinced that yours are abnormal or problematic, ask your gynecologist to take a look and give you an honest assessment. Chances are good that what you think is totally abnormal is completely normal. It's pretty easy to feel insecure about parts we hardly ever get a chance to see. (For others looking at our parts, such as male partners, it's pretty easy to think something looks "weird" when it's totally unfamiliar—chances are good that any guy who sees your genitals up close and personal and says they look funny is seeing female genitals that close for the first time.) There are a few books available that do show real diversity of external female genitals, such as Joani Blank's *Femalia*.

Pornography or pinup is often a poor place to look for "normal" genitals, because adaptations have usually been made. Not only are actors and models in porn chosen to meet whatever "fashion" or size of genitalia fits fantasy fodder (which is usually exaggerated in one way or another), but every sort of shaving, waxing, tucking, primping, photo editing, retouching, and lighting, and often surgical adaptations have also been employed to glorify genital appearance. Chances are good that if your own genitals were primped, photographed,

S.e.x.

and retouched professionally, you might not even recognize them yourself!

In the same vein, what peers have to say about what's "normal" in genital appearance usually only comes from their own very limited viewing of other genitals, from their viewing of genitals in photographs, or from what they've heard about what's "normal" from someone else. Too, a lot of times when someone proclaims another person's genitals are abnormal, it's coming from a place of insecurity about their own.

When it comes to figuring out what's normal in terms of genitals, appearance and function aren't the same thing. What's most worthy of concern is the latter, not the former, and if your genitals are functional, chances are pretty darn good that they're normal as far as appearance goes, too.

FOR THE GUYS:

Too Big!/Too Small!

Let's be honest: How often do we hear male complaints about penises being too big? Not very often.

Most of the worries we hear are about penises being too small, and often, those concerns are about vaginal intercourse, or about male partners who might compare sizes. Here's a tip: It may seem like a pretty remarkable coincidence, but the average vaginal canal is about the exact same length as the average penis. Go figure. Moreover, the vaginal canal (as well as the rectum, mouth or hands) contracts to hold the size of whatever is put in it, the first third of the vagina is usually the most sensitive, AND the most sensitive part of the female sexual anatomy isn't the vagina at all, but the clitoris. So being worried that a particular penis size won't satisfy a partner is generally unfounded, since

NO specific size or shape of penis is likely to produce instant satisfaction or orgasm via intercourse, or just by being there. And if your sexual partners are male, more times than not, less is more when it comes to what's most comfortable in the mouth or anus.

Concerns that you'll be able to get less sexual sensation or satisfaction due to the size or shape of your penis are also misplaced: sensation and arousal have nothing to do with size. Four-inch-long penises can experience and create just as many pleasurable sensations as those that are seven inches; a bigger penis isn't "better," any more than being taller is "better." We're all just different—no big whoop.

If you have an e-mail account, you probably get daunting amounts of spam daily telling you about this device or that one, these pills or those, all of which can increase your penis size: the whole lot of it is rubbish. And a lot of what you might hear about women preferring a larger penis size is the same sort of parroting you hear about men only liking larger breasts or blond hair. What people publicly state as their preferences often has a lot more to do with what they *think* they should be saying, than with what they actually feel, know, or prefer.

The truth is that, sometimes, a given person may want greater or lesser penetration, with either male OR female partners. If a woman has a male lover with a larger penis, at times she may prefer vaginal play with just a finger or two, instead. If she has a partner with a smaller penis, sometimes she may want greater vaginal stimulation with a sex toy, or manual sex with a few fingers—and that shouldn't be a big deal. Sometimes, oral or manual sex may feel better to a man than vaginal or anal penetration: it's the same sort of thing. When we drop the false idea that our genitals are supposed to be some sort of one-size-fits-all tool for satisfaction, rather than just one of many parts of our bodies that we can feel and give pleasure with, in numerous ways, it's easy to get a lot more comfortable with normal size and shape variations.

(Not) on the Straight and Narrow

It's common for a penis to have *some* curvature when erect. If you discover that you have any pain or discomfort when you become erect, or that the curvature of your penis is profound (basically, if you're looking at something like a 90 degree angle), then speak to your doctor. But otherwise, some penises curve up, some down, some to the left or to the right, and some don't seem to at all: all those variations are normal. In terms of partnered sex, mouths, vaginas, and rectums are all flexible, and have curves of their own. So, while two particular people may find they're a more exceptional fit in some ways or positions than others, curvature is in no way a problem.

If any of these vast and normal variations were all that problematic when it came to partnered sex, we'd have a lot less sex going on, and a lot fewer people on the planet. Don't sweat it.

Cut/Uncut

There is nothing wrong, dirty, or yucky about having an intact foreskin; at birth, all penises have one, and the majority of men worldwide are uncircumcised. Uncut men have to make a few adaptations: You need to pull back your foreskin and clean it gently when you bathe, and you need to use a condom a little differently. You may also need to be on the lookout a little more cautiously for yeast or fungal infections. But none of that is any big deal.

A circumcised penis is also fine and functional, if that's what you've got. Cut men have less sexual sensitivity of their penises than uncut men do, but that needn't be a major trauma: the whole body is involved in sexual activity and sensation, not just our genitals, and MOST sexual arousal and satisfaction actually lie in our brains and nervous systems. And there really isn't one sort of penis that is more prone to STIs. Some data on uncircumcised penises has shown that uncut men may be at greater risk for some infections, but some data on circumcised penises shows that cut men may be at greater risk for others. Foreskin or no, the only truly effective way to reduce the risk of STIs is by practicing safer sex (see chapter 9) or abstaining from partnered sex.

While in some countries and areas the look of an uncut penis may be unfamiliar to some, it is what is most common in others.

Ultimately, you have whichever you have. And while some doctors will perform elective adult male circumcisions, that procedure carries a WHOLE lot of risks and downsides, and it's not recommended.

Sometimes, just like partners who find being up close and personal with vulvas for the first few times unusual or daunting, some sexual partners may feel or act awkward around a certain type of penis. While it's hard not to take someone's fascination, curiosity, or even amazement about something so personal personally, it's helpful to recognize that that's pretty normal.

A FEW SHORT WORDS ON THE SHORT AND CURLIES

Because we're mammals, all of our bodies, male and female, are naturally covered with hair—and that includes our genital areas. On both men and women, hair grows

s.e.x.

naturally around the genitals, down to and around the anus and thighs, and over the pubic mound. As with genital size, pubic hair is generally accepted on men, and yet popular culture, mass media, and fashion often dictate that women should or must remove or modify that hair—even to the point that certain patterns and shapes are considered preferable or fashionable. Once more, the message is that the female genitals, just as they are, aren't acceptable and should be diminished. Hogwash!

As with the hair on your head, you can do whatever you want with your pubic hair. And just like the hair on your head, pubic hair is totally acceptable in any length, thickness, or color. If you don't want to mess with it at all, you don't have to. If you want to try shaving or waxing it, you can; like any hair, it will grow right back.

if you're going to remove your pubic hair:

- Shaving or waxing just before sexual activity can increase STD and STI risks, because of small cuts or scrapes, so best to shave or wax a day or two before, rather than just prior.
- Be careful: You really don't want to cut or nick your inner labia or testicles. When pubic hair is shaved, it's also normal to get more ingrown hairs, red bumps, and itching. You can exfoliate daily with a loofah or the like, and keep the area moisturized, to help reduce irritation.
- Same goes with waxing or sugaring: Genital tissue is delicate. So, if you're waxing yourself, be sure not to apply the wax on genital tissue, only on the EXTERNAL genitals: thighs, the mons, the outer labia, and for guys, the area around the base of the penis—not the penis itself or testes. Because waxing and sugaring the genitals can be tricky, you might prefer to have a professional do your waxing, at least at first.
- Shaving doesn't actually darken body hair. Body hair that grows back after shaving appears darker and more coarse, because it's been cut and hasn't been exposed to sun, water, salt, and air for years. So before you shave anywhere, just consider that the fine, lighter body hair you may have will likely not be that fine or light again once you start shaving it.

WHAT'S "NORMAL" DOWN THERE?

Most people in their teens haven't seen a whole lot of developed genitals of their own sex up close. At best, maybe you and your best friends have looked at one another's, maybe you've spied a brief glimpse in the locker room, seen your parents genitals, and, if you have same-sex partners, you've possibly seen the genitals of a partner or two. There are plenty of books out there with illustrations of genitalia, but sometimes it's hard to apply what pen and ink have created to what's there in the flesh.

Ultimately, when we say that genitals come in a seriously diverse array of shapes, sizes, colors, and textures for all genders, it's not a bunch of malarkey meant to comfort and quiet you. It's a fact.

We often confuse the word "normal" with the word "ideal." Normal doesn't mean this or that idea of what is perfect at a given time, it simply means what is most common. What's normal is diversity!

s.e.x.

the problem with perfect:
body image

OR, WHY APPEARANCE ISN'T ALL IT APPEARS

START A REVOLUTION: Love your body!

When you've got a healthy, holistic, and realistic body image, you're more likely to take good care of your body. You're more likely to be aware of when you're sick and when you are in good health. You're more likely to truly *like* living in your body—however it looks. When we've got good body image brewin,' we often feel more positive, powerful, confident, and capable. Positive body image allows us to have greater self-esteem, because we're better able to see that our bodies and what they look like are just one part of who we are. Positive body image can also help us make smarter choices when it comes to sex, to feel more able to set and maintain our limits and boundaries and more able to fully enjoy the sex we're having.

"Body image" describes how you view your own body, in function, health, experience, and appearance. "Self-esteem" describes what level of regard, respect, and value you have for yourself—not just your body, but the whole person who lives in it. Those two things are often linked, especially in young adults, and all the more in a culture that fixates on physical appearance. "Lookism" or "looksism" describes discrimination based on physical appearance, or the fixation of a person, group, or culture on physical appearance.

Too often, we and everyone around us place more value on how we look than on who we *are* and what we can *do:* appearances are often given more weight and attention than character, ideas, and accomplishments.

That isn't to say we have to ignore appearances or how others look at them and appreciate them. In our teens and twenties, when there's often so much added focus from peers and parents on how we look, that'd be nearly impossible to do, even if we wanted to. People are amazing critters, bodies are beautiful to look at, and visual sexual attraction and appearance are parts of our physical nature—but only *part.* Our bodies enable us to do everything we do each day: to go to work or school, to build cities, make art, and create cultural movements, to enjoy a stack of steaming pancakes or a swim in the sea, to nurture families and friends, to live out our whole lives, enjoying and accomplishing all the things we do.

Your body can seek out, nurture, and enjoy pleasure, alone and with partners. Your body is your partner in emotional intimacy. Your body can even create new life, new bodies. You'll also experience pain, discomfort, and illness in your body during your lifetime. At some point, you may be dissatisfied with your body for far more pressing and challenging reasons than because your thighs aren't thin enough or your muscles lean enough. You may be unhappy because you've experienced a serious injury or illness, because you have a disability, or because you can't feel pleasure the way you'd like, or give it to someone else.

Maybe you've already managed the fantastic accomplishment of having a positive body image; maybe you're not there yet. Maybe you feel as if you're drowning in insecurity, can't see how you'll ever get out of it, and think that if you hear the phrase "positive body image" one more time, you'll scream. Wherever you are on the spectrum—even you screamers—listen up.

▪ TEN BODACIOUS WAYS ▪ TO BOOST BODY IMAGE

1. **Make the real the ideal.** Less than 5 percent of the entire population looks like most models and athletes do (and without lighting, makeup, retouching, and such, even models don't always look like models). Collect photos of people you admire for all sorts of reasons; make your collection realistic and well rounded. For every photo of one model, celebrity, or pro athlete, add photos of nineteen other people who AREN'T models—friends and family, writers, musicians, teachers, scientists, activists, folks whose smiles or wrinkles are as interesting as their backsides—because **that's** a realistic and truly inspiring collection. Creating a realistic collage is an easy visual way to get a better idea of what a real range of whole-person beauty is, rather than the surface-level beauty the media often try to sell us.

2. **Exercise your enjoyment.** Engage in exercise that offers you more than thinner thighs or six-pack abs. Exercise is about staying healthy, enjoying the physical and emotional feelings it provides; about becoming stronger, more flexible and resilient; about learning new skills and accomplishing personal goals. It should be fun and should feel *good.* Don't try to force

s.e.x.

yourself to do exercise that feels like drudgery or a beauty contest. Consider self-defense or martial arts classes. Try yoga or boating. Pick a team sport. Indulge in a nice, long stretch each day. Go hiking, biking, swimming, or horseback riding in places where your exercise also lets you enjoy a beautiful day or a new place to hang out.

3. **See every body.** *Spend time in places with body diversity.* Shoe stores don't have just one shoe that's universally better than all the rest; there are different kinds of shoes for all sorts of activities, aesthetics, and preferences, and they come in a dizzying array of different materials, styles, sizes, shapes, and colors. Human bodies are the same way.

   Community centers, grocery stores, public parks, and swimming pools are all good places to see diversity. When we're regularly exposed to only one town, one age group, one social class, or one locker room, it can be too easy to forget how incredibly different we all are. Just as it's not sage to assume that the whole world is like your hometown, it's smart to keep in mind that our idea about how bodies look is often pretty limited.

4. **Be a body image guerrilla!** If you pick up magazines with articles or images that make you feel bad about yourself, or that support negative body image, use your voice. Almost every magazine includes inserts for subscriptions, which require no postage to send. Get out a pen and write what you're feeling on those cards, then toss them in the mail. Write an article for

your school or college paper about media lies and myths about bodies, health, dieting, or beauty. How about starting a no-makeup or plain-sweatsuits-only day once a month in your dorm or workplace?

Start at home by changing what you expose yourself to and how you process it. Recycle your fashion, muscle, or beauty mags or catalogs, or use them for kindling in your campfire. Reduce the number of hours you spend watching TV. For just one day, count how may times you look in mirrors, fuss with your hair or clothes, or think or talk about appearance-related things; just becoming aware of how much time and energy these things take can deliver a pretty loud wake-up call. Sit down and figure out how much money you spend each month on makeup, hair products or styling, clothing, gyms, and diet foods or books, and work to cut that amount in half—save the money you don't spend on that stuff for something you really want to do for your *whole* self.

5. **Ditch the dissing.** Most of us aren't even aware of how often we judge other people by how they look. We may call others fat, ugly, cheap, skinny, doggy, skanky, gross, what have you, so much that we don't think anything of it. Start paying attention. Think about WHY you judge people the way you do. When you call someone fat, even out of their earshot, is it because you're concerned about their health, or because it makes you feel less insecure about *your* body? Does dissing them give you a break from dissing

S.e.x.

yourself? If you talk about a guy having a small penis, or a girl having a "loose" vagina—likely without any idea of what their bodies are like, or without accurate ideas about sexual anatomy in the first place—how does that benefit you?

The same goes for tuning out and turning off *your* body image bullies. Often, other people who diss your body or get in a snit about it are doing it for the same lousy reasons you do: out of fear and insecurity. It's not always easy to be direct about an insult, but it usually feels better than sucking it up or pretending it doesn't hurt. So, if Mom says you look a little chubby or teases you about your size, remind her that what she says is hurtful, and that there are better ways she could express any concern she might have. If a friend or peer dogs your appearance, let them know that you're not interested in being a target for their insecurities. If you're getting harassed or teased at school, fight back productively, by filing a report with the faculty, or participating in or starting up grass-roots actions against school harassment.

6. **Look deeper: looks aren't everything.** A poll from the Eating Disorders Awareness and Prevention Center in Seattle found that teen girls were more scared of being fat than they were of a nuclear war or of losing their parents. Yipes!

It's hard to have a positive self-image and good self-esteem when you don't feel important or accomplished, even if you feel fantastic about the way you look. Put yourself in environments where you can *do* something and be someone you're seriously proud of. Volunteer to help build low-income housing for the homeless (bonus: it's also a great workout). Help with a community garden, or with landscaping at a community center, school, or domestic abuse shelter. Be a Big Sister or Big Brother, or tutor a kid in need. Help coach a Little League team. Join a letter-writing campaign for women and men in other countries who are fighting for their right to education, jobs, or freedom.

Remember, too, that you have many relationships of value in your life, not just sexual or romantic ones—friends, family, teachers, and mentors, and those to whom *you* are the mentor or role model. The array of feelings people have for you are all important, not just feelings of sexual attraction or aesthetic appeal.

7. **Dare to bare.** According to a study done by facial cleanser company Albolene, 73 percent of American women wear makeup, and 42 percent report that they never leave home without it. Makeup and grooming can be fun, but feeling that hairstyling, shaving, or clothes that accentuate this or hide that are *required* is an express bus on the road to poor body image and self-esteem. (Guys, this goes for you, too, even though men typically use far fewer products, and are often encouraged not to use them.) Ditch the stuff sometimes. Go places—not just hanging out at home—without makeup,

without straightening or styling your hair. Wear clothes that are comfortable, without spending time worrying about what statement they make or if they're in style right now. If you are in a sexual partnership, get comfortable being together now and then without a metric buttload of preparation first: the shaving or waxing, the makeup, the clothing. You don't have to look like you've been living on a deserted island for a year, and I'm not advocating that you shouldn't shower, wash your face, brush your teeth and hair, or wear clean clothes.

But sometimes, let the bare basics be all you do. You'll be amazed at how many people *don't* see a profound difference, and it's a cool thing to get comfortable really looking like *you,* turning off the messages that say you have to look like anyone else—and saving all that cash, too!

8. **Self-validate.** Remember that neither partners nor friends can magically deliver positive, lasting self-esteem. When someone you find attractive or are in love with tells you you're beautiful, sexy, or hot, of course you get a boost—but it can't usually make you feel those things about yourself *by* yourself. By basing your body- and self-image on what others think, you put other people in charge of your own self-worth. That can be particularly easy to do in your teens and twenties, when you're still in the process of some heavy-duty personal development, and when the pressures on you to conform and fit in are so intense. But, if you base your self-image on what a partner says, what are you going to do when that partner's gone, when their opinions change, or even when they're having a hard day and focused on things besides what you look like?

9. **Do unto others.** Imagine how you might feel if, a couple of times during the day, someone walked up to you and said, "Hey, you've got a beautiful smile," or "That was a *great* presentation you just gave," or "That skirt you made is really cool. How did you do it?" or "I love your laugh." Start the chain. And that doesn't just mean compliments about appearance, either; give others credit for their *accomplishments,* too. Not only can that be a serious day-maker for someone else, you'll find that doing it makes you feel more positive about yourself, too.

10. **Make friends with your doctor.** If you have body concerns; if you feel you need to diet, be at the gym twice a day, or go ballistic with weight training or protein powders; if you wonder if your body parts are normal, or if you just feel like crap about your body—your doctor or nurse is a great person to talk to. He or she can let you know what you really DO need to be doing for your body, as well as what's realistic for your body and your age. Doctors and nurses see a myriad of bodies every day, up close and personal, so they tend to have a good bead on what real bodies look like, and they're concerned with health above appearance, making them excellent people to talk to about body image and body concerns.

s.e.x.

THE PROBLEM WITH PERFECT: BODY IMAGE

don't make a mate a mirror

WHEN WE have sex partners, poor body- or self-image can make it harder to talk honestly about sex, to insist on things that keep us safe: limits and boundaries, safer sex practices, birth control. When we're insecure about our appearance or our worth, we may feel we owe favors to someone who finds us beautiful or interesting. We may find it hard to say no or ask for things we need, because we feel they are giving so much just by accepting us, when we can't accept ourselves. We may tolerate or agree to sexual activity or partnership we don't want because we think we can't do better, and believe that something will always feel better than nothing. Our character judgment of partners may be skewed by virtue of our messed-up self-judgment.

If you're going to enter into sexual partnership, it should be real *partnership,* not sexual performance or self-validation. When you seek a partner out, will it be because you want a mutually beneficial relationship, or because you need someone around to make you feel better about yourself? Are you willing to have relationships that are less beneficial and enjoyable to all partners because so much effort needs to go into securing *your* self-esteem? Some people seek out sexual partnership to try to fill a void in terms of self-esteem or positive body image, and then discover—alas—that the sex or boyfriend/girlfriend doesn't fill that void. They then get even more depressed and self-loathing, thinking something must be wrong with them, and screwing up their relationships in the process.

Whoever you're with, whether they're a friend, the Juliet to your Romeo, or the man of your dreams, you should be able to feel like yourself, act like yourself, look like yourself, and have sex like yourself: Be yourself FOR yourself. It shouldn't feel like an audition; you already got the part.

Most of us are going to spend decent parts of our lives on our own, without sexual partners or spouses, living by ourselves, being by ourselves. It's important to learn that we can stand alone; that we can love and accept our bodies, whether or not anyone else shows attraction to them at any given time; that we can love and accept ourselves, even during the days, weeks, or months when no one says anything good about us, even when we get negative feedback. We need to value ourselves when we're not in relationships or sexual partnerships; we need things we enjoy doing, be they work or hobbies we need a sense of body love that isn't just about how our bodies look, but about how they feel and what they enable us to do each day.

That'd be that "self" part of self-esteem, self-love, and self-worth.

▪ DISORDERED EATING ▪ AND EATING DISORDERS

A majority of American teens and young men and women have been or are on diets, and "diets" usually means fad diets, skipping meals, vomiting after eating, or using diet pills or weight-gain supplements. Polls from sources like *People* magazine have shown that well over 80 percent of young women are unhappy or dissatisfied with their looks or bodies. In 2003, the Centers for Disease Control surveyed fifteen thousand high-school students in the United States about eating habits. They found that over 44 percent of them (59.3 percent of females and 29.1 percent of males) were trying to lose weight. Many young people start dieting as early as the age of eight or nine. Obesity rates are increasing in young and grown adults, even though the majority of them are also dieting. You do the math.

Many young adults believe that if they could only be the "right" size or shape, they'd feel better about themselves, even though there's plenty of evidence to support that, realistically, even overweight people often find that losing weight alone doesn't fix poor self-esteem or body image.

Disordered eating can range from mild to severe. Skipping meals now and then, trying a diet, or binging on ice cream post-breakup would be considered mild. For some, occasional disordered eating becomes a serious eating disorder (ED)—such as anorexia (starvation), bulimia (binging and purging), or binge eating—which can jeopardize one's health and well-being, even one's life.

All types of disordered eating have side effects, long and short term, benign and severe. EDs carry serious risks such as malnutrition, heart failure, bowel problems, permanent damage to the throat, permanent gall bladder or reproductive damage, or diabetes, to name just a few, as well as serious emotional and psychological effects.

Fad diets, starvation, binging, and purging can mean permanently, irreversibly screwing up your body and your health. And if you permanently screw up your metabolism, all the dieting and starving in the world isn't going to fix it; you will usually end up less healthy, and *less* able to influence your size and shape than you are now.

WHO'S AT RISK OF DISORDERED EATING, BODY IMAGE, OR SELF-IMAGE PROBLEMS?

More than five million people in the United States are currently affected by eating disorders, and around 90 percent of those are young women, some still in elementary school. While the onset of most eating disorders has typically been around the age of thirteen or fourteen, disordered eating is now starting in many young women before puberty even hits. At least 10–15 percent of people with eating disorders die because of them. When some people say they're dying to be thin, they aren't kidding.

Some issues can increase risks of developing an ED. Low self-esteem is a biggie, as is depression or anxiety. During adolescence, it's easy to feel out of control and also easy to feel controlled. Teens can be at an increased risk

did you know . . . ?

During our teen years, to be as healthy as we can and to develop properly, we need to eat more calories than in any other phase of life. The average teen gal needs about 2,200 calories each day; the average teen guy 2,500. And if you're consuming most of those via fresh, whole, healthy foods, while keeping moderately active and managing your stresses, you are setting yourself up with the best foundation possible for sound short- and long-term health and good looks.

s.e.x.

when their parents, friends, or communities are exerting a lot of control on appearances, such as how someone dresses; are not allowing for healthy and normal social opportunities, freedoms, and responsibilities; or are pushing for particular goals, such as college, marriage, or certain professions. Research has shown that young women whose mothers or sisters are eating-disordered or diet-obsessed are at a greater risk for developing EDs. Plenty of parents don't realize how much their own eating is disordered, and how those behaviors affect their kids. Many teens are under extreme social, academic, and familial stress that is dismissed or isn't recognized, and those stresses can increase ED risks.

The bottom line is that EDs are serious illnesses caused by a complex mix of factors; EDs are much more than "a diet gone too far" and often have very serious physical and psychological repercussions.

WHILE disordered eating is primarily present in women, men aren't immune to EDs, either. For both sexes, some coaches or trainers support or enforce disordered eating. Plenty of men—especially gay men, men in some types of sports, and young men who are "late bloomers"—deal with an overemphasis on appearance and body perfection just as many women do. Young men may binge eat, overdo protein supplements or other weight-gain formulas to achieve a larger size, or engage in steroid use. And some young men *are* also anorexic or bulimic; both disorders are currently on the rise among young men.

If you think you might have an ED or be on the road to one, talk to your doctor or counselor. It's always okay to err on the side of caution, so even if you're not sure, ask. It's a whole lot easier to prevent an ED than to get past it once you've gotten into those patterns.

If you have a friend you suspect may have an eating disorder, seek out capable help. It's often impossible to help someone else through an ED alone, and time isn't on your side: the longer someone with an ED goes without getting effective help, the more sick they become, and the tougher recovery is. Even the well-intentioned ways people try to help often feed the problem. For instance, saying, "You're so skinny!" to an anorexic only validates the illness. Most eating-disordered people work very hard to hide their behaviors, so it may not be possible to get them to admit that they even have an ED. The better road to take—for yourself and/or a friend—is to talk to a trusted counselor, doctor, or parent and let them know what you suspect. For more information on dealing with an eating disorder, your own or that of someone you care about, see the Resources section.

· THE IDEAL SPIEL ·

We're constantly surrounded by messages about sexual appeal and performance, promoting often unattainable and unrealistic ideals. Women are supposed to be easily and multiply orgasmic—usually from vaginal intercourse. Depending on who is sending the message, women are either supposed to be "sexy" and yet NOT be sexu*al,* or be readily sexually available, but only in a way that fits the desires of men or male culture. Sometimes that message is flip-flopped, idealizing the woman who withholds sex until it is exchanged for something else (such as marriage or other material advantages). That might seem better, but it still supports the idea that a woman's worth is tied to her sexual value and commodity.

Men are supposed to be superhumanly potent and virile, and their sexuality means nada but their penises: we've got a million bunk penis-enhancing devices to fix the "problem" that is normal human physiology, and Viagra for what the devices don't fix. There's constant static that for men bigger—with height, muscle mass and penises—is always better. Of course, the "bigger is better" school bars those who are bigger because of being fat.

You're no dummy. The littlest bit of self-awareness will clue you in as to what is realistic for you and what isn't, what's authentic and what's hype, what's real and what's ideal. Even if some folks can't figure it out—or choose to misrepresent reality for their own purposes—you've got a little voice in there (and maybe even a nice, big loud one) telling you what the real deal is. Trust it.

We're all bound to have moments of insecurity about sexuality, about how others perceive us sexually, about our performance in bed, about our sexual normality. It is okay to enter into solo or partnered sex without being the most confident person in the universe, and moreover, most people go through a lot of insecurity, especially at first, feeling nervous and having doubts about themselves. But the better we feel about ourselves and our bodies, the better the sex and the sexual relationships will be.

If you're having issues with sexual self-esteem with a partner, take a look at your overall self-esteem. If you're worried about your body or your sexual performance with a partner, talk it out with them, with friends, with family or mentors you value. Getting those feelings out into the open and hearing about other people's perspectives and experiences can be a big help. Pace yourself however you need to: you might find that, in general, or sometimes, you're just not in the right frame of mind about yourself to be with a partner. If your insecurities are about partnered sex, go as slowly as you need to. If you don't feel right about showing your body to someone else, give yourself the privacy you require, whether that means dressing modestly or waiting to have a partner see all or any of you in your birthday suit. If you feel that you just can't measure up to some ideal—yours or a partner's—give yourself time for whatever reality check you need. Listen to yourself. If what you hear yourself saying is a big, nasty pile of negativity, put your energy into changing the channel. If what you hear is the good stuff, turn up the volume and tune in!

▪ WHOLE BODY/WHOLE SEXY ▪

What's "sexy"? *Anything* that elicits sexual feelings in a person. So, when you see, smell, or experience something that makes you go "Mrrow!" and gives you a tingle downstairs, you've just found something sexy.

Take a partner or potential partner out of the equation for a minute, then take what you or others *see* out of the picture as well. Your sexuality, your body, and your mind aren't just visual, you've got other senses to work with that are just as much a part of you and your sexuality as your eyes and your appearance.

For instance, when you're eating, what foods make you feel sexy? How does letting chocolate melt on your tongue make you feel? How about eating a ripe, sticky, messy

s.e.x.

mango? What smells make your head spin? Spicy cinnamon, rich vanilla, a fresh-squeezed orange, salty sea air, fresh-mowed grass, peonies or roses, sweat, just-washed hair? Your sense of smell not only remembers scents from times you have felt sexy or had a great sensual or sexual experience, it can also enjoy scents that are evocative and heady. How about how things feel under your fingers, or on any other tactile part of your body—warm sand, the soft down of hair on the back of your neck, cool paper, silk or cotton, coarse brick, a soft pillow, the inside of the lips, the warmth of thighs? When you've just worked your muscles from exercise, when you've had a great massage, when you're in a hot bath or waking from a nap, how do those things feel to you? How are tastes different then? So much of what really turns us on is multi-sense experience, and engaging as many of those senses as possible not only enhances the sex we may be having, it allows us to savor our bodies completely, not just how they look.

And when you *are* looking, open your eyes! On both your own body and that of a partner there are so many parts to explore and appreciate, beyond the parts our culture sexualizes. What parts of your own body, when you touch them, expose them, or put them in the limelight, make you feel sexy? Beyond what you think looks best, what feels best when touched, what parts are most sensitive, what parts do you like to touch with? What parts feel most uniquely you?

Our bodies certainly have more value and function than merely being sexual. But when they ARE sexual—by ourselves or with others—and when we bring all of our senses to the table and serve 'em what's sexy by our own standards, we can create a sexuality that is authentically our own, one that not only wards off bad body image, but celebrates our bodies to the fullest.

▪ VIVA LA REVOLUCIÓN! ▪

Whether or not you feel 100 percent good about your body right now, revolutionary body image is about as-is *acceptance,* not about perfection.

So many people are doing everything they can to alter their bodies and their appearance, in hopes that those changes will bring about acceptance. Not only will most never be able to make those changes—our appearance, our shape, and our size are determined almost entirely by our genetics—but often those who can STILL do not fully accept and enjoy their bodies, no matter how "perfect." Some people who "succeed" at weight-loss programs or have cosmetic surgeries discover, sadly, that they still feel crummy about themselves, because they also (or may only) need to work on accepting themselves full-stop, not on "fixing" their tummies or thighs. Your body is not a home-improvement project, nor does it exist apart from your mind; mind and body are an inseparable whole.

Nobody's trying to be cute by saying that loving your body can start a revolution. I think it really can, especially if a whole lot of us can get there. Anybody with half a lick of sense understands that it can be really hard to love and accept your body, especially when everywhere we turn, a million voices are telling us to do the opposite.

But all those negative messages we take in on a daily, even hourly, basis can only be so pervasive because of all the dollars—*our* dollars—that pay for them, and all the energy we put into them. What would happen if we all ditched the piles of beauty mags, blew off the diet industry, told the makers of all the miracle creams and pills to shove it, scoffed at the cosmetic surgeons, and kept our dollars out of the hands of everyone who capitalizes on the appeal and power of the superficial image? What if we put our money, our voices, and our real feelings about ourselves out there? What if we refused to let the mass media (and those stinky little voices in our own heads) dictate what we should look like? The whole system that helps keep us down might fall the heck apart.

How you live your life makes a big difference. Rather, *that* you live your life. In a nutshell, life's too darn short to waste most of it worrying about how we look. It's easier to get our knickers in a perpetual knot about this stuff when we don't feel accomplished, able, or happy with our choices. So, LIVE it. Do things that are actually important to you and that have real value. Follow your heart, your mind, and your bliss. When and if you have sex partners, or even have sex by yourself, with yourself, honor your body and revel in *all* your senses. Spend more time enjoying and experiencing all of your body than you do critiquing it or seeking approval for it. Smile a lot. Be an original. Have an *amazing* life. After all, most of us probably want our headstones to say more than, *"Beloved Spouse, Fat-Free, Great Abs, Perfect Hair."*

Loving your body—both in sexual situations and outside of them—and accepting your whole self unconditionally, in all your stages and phases, shapes and sizes, is powerful. That's totally *revolutionary.* And even if we all never quite get 100 percent there, just being, becoming, and owning YOU, being happy as you are and as you look, is powerful and life-changing, for you and for everyone around you.

s.e.x.

4

all by myself:
solo sex, arousal,
orgasm, and fantasy

▪ SOLO SEX (MASTURBATION) ▪

Self-love. Solo sex. Ménage à moi. Jacking off, jilling off, whacking off, beating off. Paddling the pink canoe, pocket pinball, teasing the kitty, testing the plumbing, fingerbating, jerkin' the gherkin, spanking the monkey, soaking the whisker biscuit, surfing the channel, the sticky page rhumba.

No matter what you call it—or how goofy what you call it is—masturbation is one of the few things that almost everyone does or has done at some point. In many surveys and studies, as many as 95 percent of men and 90 percent of women report that they masturbate or have done so. Many of us masturbated before we even remember doing so: infants and very young children commonly fondle their genitals. That early stimulus is very different from adult sexuality—much like thumb-sucking, it is largely about comfort—but while motives and execution may differ, it's masturbation all the same.

The short story is that not only is there nothing wrong with masturbation, it's even good for you. Most doctors and medical organizations, counselors, sex therapists, and sex educators agree: for your own sense of well-being, relaxation, and health; your sexuality with or without partners (for example, figuring out the right times for sex), developing a means for sexual communication, getting familiar with your own sexual response cycle and preferences, and finding out where all your parts really are and how they work, masturbation is the bomb.

false and true

MASTURBATION will not:

- Cause blindness, headaches, or vision problems
- Cause hair to grow on your palms or give you zits
- Make your genitals shrink or grow (beyond the temporary changes brought on by sexual arousal), or change their color, texture, or appearance
- Stunt your general growth or the development of your sexual organs, or make you more or less fertile
- Become chemically addictive
- Cause injury or harm (when done safely—obviously, sticking a penis in a vacuum hose, or using an electric vibrator in a bathtub isn't real swift)
- "Stretch" a woman's genitals
- Release "stored up" sperm or sexual fluids. You don't need to masturbate in order to get rid of "excess" semen or sperm, any more than you need to bleed out "excess" blood, because there is no such thing.

MASTURBATION can:

- Relieve menstrual cramps and muscle tension, and be a source of full body/mind relaxation
- Increase circulation (and even help fight genital infections AND acne by doing so)
- Increase the ability to be orgasmic
- Enhance sex with partners, physically and emotionally, and help build important knowledge for clear sexual communication
- Alleviate depression or anxiety by releasing endorphins
- Help improve sexual self-esteem and body image
- Possibly help prevent certain reproductive cancers, such as prostate cancer

• AROUSAL AND ORGASM: •
Human Sexual Response
Coming and Going

We can claim few absolutes when it comes to sex, but it's safe to say that there are very few people who don't enjoy orgasm. Most people enjoy being sexually aroused, though not at all times—it can be pretty awkward when it happens during class, for instance. When feelings of arousal are new to you, the situation might feel a bit emotionally or socially uncomfortable. If you don't understand how arousal works, some aspects of it might make you feel embarrassed or even a little frightened—of conflicted or unwanted desires, of an erection you can't control, of vaginal lubrication or the normal swelling that occurs during arousal, or of the elevated pulse or lightheadedness that can happen.

Human sexual response is not as simple as the media tend to present it, but it is easy

S.e.x.

enough to wrap your head around, and it is important. The whole process is just that: a process and a continuum, ALL of which should be pleasurable and satisfying, not just orgasm. Orgasm can't occur without all the preceding parts of the human sexual response cycle, and wouldn't feel all that amazing if it could.

Think about it this way: sex for the sole purpose of orgasm is akin to running like a maniac to catch a bus when you're late; having any sort of sex for the whole banana—arousal, intimacy, pleasure in your whole body and, yes, often orgasm—is more like going out for a long, slow jog on a beautiful, sunny day, just because. Thing is, too many people think of sex as a gender-specific set of directions that are a progression toward orgasm. A lot of people believe there are particular things that everyone will automatically enjoy, things that will satisfy every person every time (and, usually, the things they pick are simply those that work for themselves, that worked for a previous partner, or that someone else or the media told them always work). Sorry, Charlie, but while we're all human, we don't all function the same way sexually when it comes to arousal and orgasm—not by a serious long shot.

Yet, there *are* certain physical, hormonal, and psychological mechanics and basics of arousal and orgasm that we all share, and understanding *those* gives you an awesome foundation for effectively and enjoyably exploring and discovering all the good stuff.

THE BASICS OF SEXUAL RESPONSE

Any given sexual response cycle for all sexes involves some or all of five different stages (whose basics were first defined by ground-breaking sex researchers Masters and Johnson): *sexual desire, arousal, the plateau phase, orgasm,* and *resolution.* None of these stages is superior to others, and *all* should be pleasurable. For each of them, the stage preceding is usually vital to moving on to the next one. They follow on a continuum, just as we have to learn to stand up before we can walk (though we certainly can halt the whole process at any point; not going through all the stages isn't harmful to anyone's health). Someone who doesn't feel sexual desire in the first place is really unlikely to have an orgasm. Here are the five stages in detail:

1. **Sexual desire** is the strong feeling, emotional and physical, of wishing or wanting to participate in any sexual activity. It's a powerful attraction to something or someone. When a person says "I want sex" or "I feel horny," they are expressing sexual desire. Desire for sexual activity is exactly like being hungry in order to eat: if you aren't hungry, eating doesn't feel very good. Desire is a matter of having a sexual appetite. If you or a partner doesn't have a BIG feeling of sexual desire, sex often isn't going to feel good. We achieve desire any number of ways, but it is generally not just physical or chemical; it's also verbal, visual, and intellectual, based in our emotions, personality, life experiences, and individual preferences, wants, and needs.

2. **Arousal** is a state of sexual excitement that sends chemical messages to the brain, creating physical changes and sensations in the whole body. When we're aroused, our blood pressure rises, our heart gets all fluttery,

our breathing quickens, our skin may become flushed, and our body becomes more sensitive and receptive to touch. A touch just on the neck or face may suddenly feel way more intense than it did when we were unaroused. We can be aroused by physical stimuli as well as by intellectual, emotional, or hormonal stimuli. For instance, we might become aroused by being kissed or touched, but we can also be aroused just by our own thoughts and imagination.

We don't all experience or interpret the same things as "sexual." What is sexy and arousing differs from person to person based on our individual personalities, our sexual history and fantasies, our particular body sensitivities, and what we were raised to interpret as sexually or sensually exciting.

But when we are aroused, we all have some fairly similar physical responses. One of the primary physical responses to arousal is *vasocongestion,* the increased flow of blood to the genital area (and/or breasts and nipples), causing those areas to become swollen with blood. This is how a woman's nipples and man's penis become erect, and the testicles may elevate as well.

In women the clitoris and inner and outer labia become puffy, stiffer, and somewhat enlarged, and at the same time, the female sexual response cycle usually includes vaginal secretions, or a feeling of "wetness." That's not only normal, it's a bonus during sexual activities that involve the genitals, because lubrication (sometimes called "vaginal sweating") makes any sort of sex a lot more comfortable and enjoyable. As arousal continues in women, the uppermost third of the vaginal canal also expands a bit, which can result in an "open" feeling inside the vagina. Women may also experience a slight enlargement of the breasts when sexually excited.

Persistent Sexual Arousal Syndrome

Recently, it's come to light that a few people, usually women, have sexual arousal to a level that isn't pleasurable at all. There's a rare condition called persistent sexual arousal syndrome, in which some people—generally past puberty—experience constant and persistent genital arousal (for hours, days, or even weeks on end) or spontaneous orgasm, without any real feelings of sexual desire, to the degree that normal daily life becomes difficult or impossible. Orgasm rarely relieves these symptoms. The causes of this syndrome are still unclear, but some suspects include hormone or circulatory imbalances, psychosexual problems or issues, and reactions to certain medications. Current treatments include antidepressants, hormone therapy, or numbing agents. It's normal, during puberty, to often be a little more sexually fixated or more easily aroused than you might be in adult life. But if those feelings seem incredibly extreme to you or sound like the above, talk to your doctor.

3. If we continue to be all hot and bothered, and continue sexual stimulation, our arousal may progress to a **plateau phase**, where sexual arousal continues and elevates. Many people experience this phase as a feeling of being "on the edge." Our bodies may feel hypersensitive; we will get flushed and feel our heartbeat more strongly. Vasocongestion continues and increases. In women the uterus elevates and the cervix pulls backward, the vaginal opening and canal loosen, and the glands in and around the vagina produce more lubrication. Men usually secrete pre-ejaculate during this phase.

4. **Orgasm** (AKA the Big O, cumming, coming, getting off) is a culmination of sexual arousal that begins during and follows the plateau phase. Male orgasm involves involuntary contractions of the pelvis, prostate gland, vas deferens, and seminal vesicles, which usually cause the ejaculation of semen (ejaculation and orgasm are often related events, but don't always both happen). Women experience a series of involuntary muscle contractions around the vagina and pelvis that may or may not produce an ejaculate and/or extra vaginal secretions. In both men and women, through the

multiple orgasm

SOMEONE is fibbing about their sex life if they tell you they had forty-seven orgasms in an hour, because that's just not the way the sexual response cycle works. It's possible for a really intense orgasm, or an extended state of arousal, to *feel* that way, but not for that to actually happen. Somewhere down the line, great status was placed on experiencing multiple orgasm. But even people who experience multiples may not always want to. Sometimes, one orgasm is satisfying all by itself, and more than one isn't appealing. Sometimes, after a single orgasm, the genitals or other body parts may feel so hypersensitive, or we may feel so relaxed or wiped out, that more sexual stimulation isn't wanted or even comfortable. For those who do want more, and can be multiply orgasmic, we're generally talking about a couple to several orgasms in a given—and usually extensive—bout of sexual activity: not forty-seven.

Multiple Orgasm in Women
Multiple orgasm is generally divided into two types: sequential multiples and serial multiples.

Sequential Multiples are a series of climaxes that come close together (two to ten minutes apart), but are separate, with an interruption or pause in arousal between them. This type may occur when, for instance, a woman has an orgasm from one activity, such as oral sex, then another from a different activity following it, such as vaginal intercourse.

Serial multiples are orgasms that occur one right after the other, with seconds in between and no lapse or rerun of the arousal cycle. This type can happen with a single sexual activity, such as constant clitoral stimulus, or with G-spot concentrated vaginal penetration with fingers, a penis, or a sex toy.

The difference in how those two different types feel is a bit like this: Driving on a road with speed bumps every block or so is like sequential multiple orgasm—there are rests in between the big bumps. If, on the other hand, you're driving on a dirt road, or a block full of lots of potholes, that's a whole lot more like serial multiple orgasm—lots of smaller up and down bumps in very quick succession. It's really one orgasm with a lot of little peaks.

Multiple orgasm in women is generally achieved the same way a single orgasm is: without rushing or a single-minded goal of making it happen, with attentiveness to the whole of the genitals and body—not just the vaginal canal—and with information and knowledge that the woman has gained through masturbation and other sexual experience (most women who can reach orgasm with partners can also do so via masturbation, and most women who experience orgasm generally report having it first happen with masturbation).

Multiple orgasm in men

Multiple orgasm is rarer in men than women, because men require a *refractory* period between sexual response cycles to continue genital sex: a period of time that varies from a few minutes to a couple of hours, before they can begin the sexual response cycle in full again. In younger men, it's likely to take less time, so some young men may find that, in some situations, they may experience a second orgasm within a time frame similar to their female partners or peers. It's also not uncommon for men experiencing multiples to orgasm without ejaculation at some point.

Some men use techniques for experiencing multiple orgasm, such as holding back ejaculation after an initial orgasm, reducing amounts of penile stimulation during arousal to little or even none, focusing on their whole bodies during sex—not just their genitals—or simply slowing down the whole works with relaxed breathing and the like.

whole body there is an increase in muscle tension and relaxation, especially around the pelvis. Orgasms generally only last a few seconds, though it often feels like longer, and they involve anything from a few to around twenty contractions (the longest recorded single orgasm to date apparently lasted forty-three seconds with twenty-five contractions). Male orgasm, on average, is a few seconds shorter than female orgasm.

It's tricky to describe what an orgasm feels like. Not only does it differ from person to person, it often feels different for any *one* person from day to day, sexual experience to sexual experience. Orgasm can feel like a tickle or a hiccup, but can also feel like a very heavy head rush or wave of dizziness through the whole body, a bit like riding a roller coaster. Some orgasms feel earth-shattering and intense, but some just feel nice or relaxing. Having an orgasm is a bit like being a balloon: your body fills up with pressure, then releases that pressure when it gets to its fullest point, much as a balloon does when it pops. Only you can know if you've had one or not, because no one else can be in your body to tell. However, a partner may sometimes be able

s.e.x.

to feel your internal contractions when a part of their body is inside or wrapped around yours.

5. The last stage, called the **resolution stage**, is a relaxation of the muscles as well as a psychological relaxation and a sense of all-things-right-with-the-world that usually occurs following orgasm, due in part to hormones produced by orgasm (mostly endorphins and dopamine). All the blood that has been pooling in the genitals and other sensitive body parts will recirculate through the body again slowly, and the genitals will return to their normal "resting" state in a little bit. It's normal to feel a bit lightheaded, lethargic, or sleepy afterward (it's not just men who fall asleep after sex). The resolution stage can also happen without orgasm; if we simply stop being sexually aroused, our bodies will gradually return themselves to their normal, nonaroused state. It is perfectly okay for this to happen, and it cannot hurt you in any way: no one is harmed by not having an orgasm.

EJACULATION

For both men and women, ejaculation and orgasm are not the same thing.

While they are related, and ejaculation during sex often occurs just after orgasm (mainly in men), ejaculation is not to be confused with orgasm, or taken as "proof" of orgasm. At this point in time, it's believed that less than half of all women do ejaculate, and even for those who do, it is unlikely to occur with every sexual activity, or all the time. So male partners, perhaps looking for women to "cum" like they do, need to understand not only that female ejaculation is really not comparable, but that it is a lot less common.

Men, however, do ejaculate regularly with sexual activity and orgasm, barring certain conditions. However, some men may not ejaculate with orgasm, either purposefully or just because it doesn't happen that time (due to certain phases of development being delayed, or having come once already, or simple nervousness).

Female Ejaculation

Some women may experience a whole lot more fluid than they're used to—often *before* or upon orgasm, and usually with some form of continual G-spot stimulation or intense vulval stimulus, either with a penis, hands, or another object. Study on female ejaculation is still spotty, but here's what we do currently know: Female ejaculation is normal, and likely happens to at least 40 percent of women. Female ejaculate tends to be thin and clear or slightly milky, depending on the individual and the phase of the fertility cycle. It has been clinically analyzed in studies, and has been found to contain sugars and proteins also found in male ejaculate, leading researchers to believe that the Skene's glands are most likely responsible for the fluid. The size of that gland varies between women, which may help explain why the same stimulus causes some women to ejaculate, but not others. While it is possible that female ejaculate contains some urine, as it comes through the urethra, ejaculate is definitely not urine.

Most female orgasm happens without ejaculation. Being able to ejaculate doesn't mean someone is a better lover or has achieved some higher level of sexual *did you know . . . ?*

Believe it or not, orgasm is possible without any genital stimulation at all. Since a lot of what's happening physiologically during the sexual response cycle is a whole body experience—occurring in the brain and nervous system more than anywhere else—that isn't all that surprising. People with little or no genital sensation, due to injuries or disabilities, can still experience orgasm. People can experience orgasm by having other places on their bodies touched and stimulated, without genital contact. Some people can even experience orgasm purely through their own imagination; if you've ever experienced orgasm while dreaming, you've been one of those people.

awareness. It isn't a goal to try to reach, just something that may or may not happen, and that can feel kinda swell. It's also nothing to be embarrassed about; female ejaculation is just as natural and normal as male ejaculation, even though it's less common. If you do ejaculate, you'll get used to it over time. You may want to let partners know in advance that you do ejaculate sometimes—especially if you feel self-conscious about it—and/or lay a towel down during activities when ejaculation often occurs for you.

▪ HOW DO YOU MASTURBATE? ▪

How any one person masturbates at a given time is based on their mood, and on their individual psychological, emotional, and physiological makeup. All these variables affect what arouses people, brings about orgasm, and sexually satisfies them. So, while for one man, rubbing his penis briskly in his lotion-covered palms may get him off, another may enjoy a long soak in the tub followed by a slow and gentle massage. The same goes for women. And what a given person likes can differ from day to day.

Masturbation may not just be about genital stimulation. Plenty of people also incorporate touching or stimulating other parts of their bodies: breasts, nipples or chests, thighs, hands or feet, parts of their faces—you name it, somebody's touched it while masturbating. Some people experiment with certain sexual practices alone, rather than with (or before sharing with) partners, by using new sex toys or certain types of role-play or sexual fantasy.

For many people, it's common to combine activities like the above, rather than just doing one thing, or stimulating one particular area. You may also find it takes a while to find what really works for you, or that something that was satisfying once isn't so satisfying anymore, and want to mix it up a bit.

What's a good way to get started with masturbation? Start with a space where you'll have some privacy, where you feel comfortable, and where you don't have to worry about being walked in on or interrupted. While some people do approach masturbation in a perfunctory way, the truth is that it's like any sort of sex: it's far more compelling and enjoyable when you're aroused.

s.e.x.

ALL BY MYSELF: SOLO SEX, AROUSAL, ORGASM, AND FANTASY

some common ways
men and women masturbate genitally

MEN may stimulate the penis, scrotum, perineum, and/or anus:

- With hands and fingers (usually with a lubricant or lotion), such as by stroking, rubbing, or slapping the shaft and base of the penis
- By penetrating hands or an object with the penis, such as a sex toy made for that purpose, or household objects like fruit skins, socks, or warm towels, or via penetration with suction, such as with a penis pump
- With vibration or pulsation to the penis, scrotum, anus, or general genital area, either via vibrators or small vibrating objects, by sitting or leaning on larger vibrating items, or with water
- With vibration, massage, or penetration of the anus with hands or objects

WOMEN may stimulate the entire vulva, or some portions, including the clitoris, inner or outer labia, the vaginal opening or canal and/or the perineum or anus:

- With fingers, rubbing, pinching, massaging, or tapping the external genitals (such as the clitoris or labia) and/or penetrating the internal genitals, such as the vagina or rectum
- With general stimulus to the whole genital area, such as by squeezing thighs together rhythmically, by "humping" a pillow, or by sitting or leaning on a vibrating object, such as a washing machine
- With objects or items for vibration, such as by applying a water source (like a shower or water jet), vibrator, or massager to the clitoris or vulva as a whole
- With objects for vaginal penetration (and usually with lubricant), such as dildos or other safe and similar objects

Most of us have fantasies about what we'd like someone else to do with us, and that's as fine a place to start as any. While, no, you can't really kiss yourself, you can massage your lips with your fingers, for instance, or run your hands over the sensitive areas of your neck, nipples, legs, or arms. Remember, your whole body is full of nerve endings and sensory receptors, so the genitals aren't the only sexual spaces you've got, not by a long shot. Take your time: When you're masturbating, you are your own lover, so treat yourself, and your body, just the way you'd like a lover to treat you.

When and if you do want to move the action to your genitals, keep in mind that this is all about you—what feels good to you, what you want—not about what you've seen or heard works for someone else. So, while a lot of men might enjoy stroking the penis with their hands, others might find that rubbing their groin up against something feels good at a given time. Some women want to incorporate vaginal penetration, but others like to keep things clitoral. Because you don't have to negotiate with anyone about anything you do when you masturbate, what you do is 100 percent up to you and completely about what you want and enjoy.

HOW DO YOU TELL IF YOU'VE HAD AN ORGASM? WHAT IF YOU JUST CAN'T HAVE ONE, EVER?

Nobody can tell you whether you've had an orgasm or not. There are scientific tests that can be done to measure contractions, and these have been used for studies on orgasm, but it's not as if you can just waltz into the doctor's office and ask to be tested for being orgasmic. A lot of people will tell you that if you have had an orgasm, you "just know," but sometimes, it is hard to tell, and there isn't any absolute certainty, especially with women.

If you're not sure when you've had an orgasm, or if you've had one at all yet, give it time: you will get to know in fairly short order. Over time, you'll even start to recognize those orgasms that happen sometimes that are really subtle. As well, throughout your life, you'll probably discover that even when you are well aware what orgasm feels like, there will be times when you're not quite sure if you've had one or not, because sometimes the sexual response cycle is both so fluid and so enjoyable as a whole, that the differences in sensation can be subtle and murky.

Nearly everyone DOES have the capability to be orgasmic. Don't let media depiction or others' descriptions of orgasm influence your own discoveries; what we see in movies or what friends tell us tends to be elevated or exaggerated. Some young people who think they haven't experienced orgasm probably have at some point—it's just that their expectations of what it should

feel like or look like aren't in line with reality. So, yes, that little ripple, incredibly vague and small head rush, or slight shudder you get certainly CAN be orgasm, and some orgasms are just like that.

And not everyone masturbates to orgasm. It may be that you just haven't figured out how orgasm works for you yet. Orgasm may not be your motivation at all at a given time; you may just want to explore your genitals or your sexual feelings, or provide yourself some private comfort time. Whatever the situation, that's perfectly fine. If you just can't reach orgasm right now, don't freak out. Nobody's counting or clocking us. We don't need to know, beyond a doubt, if we've had an orgasm or not every single time; we don't need to have an orgasm every time we engage in solo or partnered sex. What's important is that we're feeling good with what we're doing, that we can provide or ask for as much sexual activity as we want, stopping whenever we'd like, regardless of whether or not we've had an orgasm. That's really the crucial point when we say sex isn't about orgasm: When you're really enjoying sex, you aren't focused on reaching or counting orgasms, or on orgasms as stop and go points. It's about the whole cycle, the whole experience, and orgasm is only one, enjoyable part.

Point is, like most forms of sex, masturbation isn't necessarily all about orgasm. It's about whatever you want it to be about, because you don't need to serve anyone's wants or needs but your own.

BUZZ KILLS

Even people who know what pleases them and are enjoying sex can have problems becoming fully aroused and/or achieving orgasm. More times than not, it isn't merely about what anyone is doing wrong physically, but about how they feel inside, and how those feelings come into play during sex. If we feel that sex is dirty, wrong, sinful, or unhealthy, or if we're nervous, anxious, scared, concerned about performance, or emotionally uncomfortable in general, it is going to be nearly impossible to enjoy ourselves and experience pleasure. If we feel unable to tell partners what we like or dislike, or how we'd like them to do something, we may be inhibited from feeling the pleasure we seek physically, and we may feel stifled emotionally as well. Relationships can suffer from the lack of sexual communication.

Other inhibitors to arousal and/or orgasm include general stress; tiredness or poor health; going without safer sex or reliable birth control methods (and thus worrying about those risks); rushing; worry about discovery (either immediately, such as by someone walking in on you, or long-term, such as by parents discovering that you're sexually active); feeling pressured by a partner, yourself, peers, or a situation to be aroused or achieve orgasm; past or current sexual trauma or abuse; some medications (like antidepressants or hormonal birth control); and the biggest one of all: psyching yourself out by trying way too hard to be aroused or achieve orgasm.

If you're having very serious and persistent problems with sexual arousal or orgasm, you can talk to your doctor or therapist. Existing sexually transmitted infections, hormonal imbalances, circulation or nervous system problems or disorders, diabtetes, general poor physical or mental health or illness, or the use of alcohol, certain drugs, and medications can be inhibitors that often can be corrected or subdued. But most of the

 There's a term for psych-out, and that's *spectatoring*. Sometimes, it's hard not to. We're led to believe that anyone who doesn't reach orgasm, all the time or often, isn't having good sex, isn't in touch with their bodies, or doesn't have a good lover—but none of those things may be so. Culturally speaking, we want easy ways to quantify and validate things, so the assumption and assertion that good sex = orgasm isn't all that surprising. Plus, there are times when we just *really* crave an orgasm.

But when it comes to arousal and orgasm, "mind over matter" is a key phrase to bear in mind. If you're over-thinking it, obsessing on it, or weighing the whole works down by placing ultimate importance on it, it's far less likely to happen than if you just chill out and enjoy yourself. The easiest way not to spectator is simply to do your best to become aware, and remain aware, that arousal happens in most people without really trying, and that orgasm—at least some of the time—is just as inevitable and natural, especially when we can have a relaxed attitude about it.

time, barriers to physical sexual enjoyment and sexual response for younger people are NOT physical, but emotional and intellectual. So, if you have a bill of good sexual and general health and your doc hasn't found any problems; if you feel that you're making sound sexual choices for yourself overall, at the right pace for you, then chances are you

s.e.x.

might need to look a little bit deeper. If you suspect common culprits such as poor self-image or body image, hidden relationship problems, depression or anxiety, sexual shame, or past or current sexual trauma or abuse, seek out support to address them via a counselor, therapist, or support group.

Even without buzz kills like the above, we just can't always reach orgasm or become aroused every time we want to. That's the way it goes. Our bodies are complex systems in which our genitals don't work independently. Cut yourself a break when that happens, whether it happens to you or to a partner. Do something else you enjoy, sexually or otherwise. If it's the physical release you're after, go engage in some strenuous physical activity or sport—the feeling of release from extensive exercise or hard physical work is hormonally, physically, and even emotionally very similar. Honor what your body is trying to tell you it needs and wants. Just as it's not a good idea to eat when you aren't hungry, it's not a good idea to have sex when you're not fully interested, or when your body isn't up to it.

KEEPING IT SAFE

While masturbation is the safest sex there is, there are a few safety issues to bear in mind. Your genitals can be delicate, and taking risks with them isn't a good idea. So, anything that might cut, scrape, or burn you, or anything that might cause electrocution or create very harsh suction is something to avoid. A good rule of thumb is that if it looks like it might hurt a lot, it probably will, and if it starts to hurt when you do it, stop.

Bacteria are a concern with masturbation. Washing your hands before you masturbate with them is always a good idea; our hands pick up loads of germs during a normal day, and these can cause genital infections. In regard to toys or objects used during masturbation, if they can't be boiled to sanitize them, it's always best to cover them up with a condom or other latex barrier to avoid bacterial infections.

ISN'T IT A SIN?

Some religions address sexual issues specifically, others do not. In some, masturbation or some forms of it may be considered problematic, while in others it is fully accepted and even celebrated. Many religions don't have a concept like sin at all; many spiritual traditions don't address masturbation at all. If you want to know what your tradition's stance is, talk to your religious leader, ask your parents (if you share their religion), or do a little research. Ultimately, in all aspects of your sexuality, you'll have to figure out how to reconcile your personal ethics and beliefs with your sexual practices. And that can be a little tricky if you're also at the point in your life where you're still figuring out what your own personal or religious beliefs are.

BUT ONLY LOSERS MASTURBATE!

Then most of us are losers! There are some whack attitudes out there about masturbation: that people who masturbate do so because they are sexually desperate, don't like the sex they have with their partners, can't get dates, or are just plain losers. In general, a sexually satisfied person—and most people who are happily masturbating are—is not a loser. People with partners masturbate, people without partners masturbate. In fact, many people who masturbate regularly enjoy sex more fully with others, and they're less likely to shack up with the first person available, no matter how unsuitable, because they don't know how to achieve sexual satisfaction by themselves.

Masturbation and partnered sex aren't interchangeable. They're interrelated sometimes, but ultimately different, and one can't substitute for the other. That's why a lot of people who have current sex partners, with whom they're satisfied, still enjoy masturbation; it fills different wants and needs altogether. (And it is absolutely fine to masturbate when you have a partner—if your partner has a problem with that, have a talk about it. Some partners even masturbate together!) Often, masturbation can easily fulfill the physical needs and desires we have for sexual gratification. Obviously, partnered sex carries a whole bunch of risks, consequences, and complexities that solo sex doesn't. But most of all, emotionally and intellectually, masturbation and partnered sex are pretty different. When masturbation just isn't cutting the proverbial mustard, that's likely either because we just haven't found what works physically yet, or, more likely, because we're craving more companionship and intimacy. When sexual partnership doesn't feel right, it's likely because the privacy, safety, and self-centeredness (in the good way) of masturbation is more up our alley at a given time.

HOW MUCH IS TOO MUCH?

It's normal, when you first get into masturbating, especially during puberty, to perhaps want to spend a lot of time doing it, just like when you find a band you really love, and want to listen to their latest CD over and over in an endless loop. For some,

it might start to feel a little compulsive or out of control—maybe you find yourself masturbating in places that aren't really private, or find that your masturbation habits are starting to interrupt or intrude upon other parts of your life.

Generally, it's a pretty simple formula: Is masturbation keeping you from doing other things you enjoy, like being with friends or partners, participating in sports, hobbies, goals, or interests? Is it interfering with your responsibilities (schoolwork, family duties, chores, or a job)? Is it infringing upon your health (keeping you up nights, keeping you from eating properly), causing any sort of injury (such as sore, swollen, raw, blistered, or chafed skin), or creating emotional conflict for you? If it's doing any of those things, then it's time to cut back. If it's not, and it feels good to you, don't sweat it.

AND YOUR FIRST SEX PARTNER IS . . . ?

We hear a whole lot about who should be our first sex partner. We're often told it should be someone we love and who loves us back, someone committed to us long-term, perhaps even someone we plan to spend the rest of our lives with.

And it should be. That person is YOU. You, all by yourself, have all of those qualities and abilities, more than any other person.

Claiming and recognizing yourself as your first and foremost sex partner is powerful. No one else is ever going to be able to get to know your body well unless you do. It equips you with tools you'll need for a healthy sexuality and balanced relationships for the rest of your life: the ability to determine when it's the right time for you to have solo sex and when it's right to take a partner. Getting to know your own body and sexual identity through self-evaluation, through masturbation, enables you to find out a great deal of what you like and dislike sexually and physically, to see and feel what your genitals and the rest of your body are like in a healthy state, to discover how your individual sexual response works, to explore your orientation and gender identity, to explore your fantasies, and to gauge your sexual expectations realistically.

That isn't to say that if you haven't started regularly masturbating before sexual partnership began for you that it's too late, because it isn't. It doesn't mean that if masturbation doesn't interest you, you're immature or that you'll necessarily have lousy partnered sex. Rather, the point is simply that masturbation is a great way for a lot of people to explore their sexual selves in a very safe, open setting.

It's not called self-love for nothing, you know.

▪ FANTASY FODDER: ▪
Sexual Fantasy

Nearly everyone has sexual fantasies. We might have them when we're bored to tears during algebra, when we're masturbating, or even when we're having sex with a partner. We may keep them locked in our own heads or share them. We may bring out a favorite sexual fantasy to play in our heads during any kind of sex, or may even find some of our sexual fantasies troublesome and try to lock them away. Most people, however, enjoy their sexual fantasies, and find them arousing, exciting, and inspiring.

Sexual fantasy might be about engaging in certain activities, such as anal sex or group sex; about sex in certain situations or places, such as at a concert or in a doctor's office; about sexual partnership with certain people, such as with a crush, a friend, an ex or current partner, or a celebrity. Some sexual fantasies may be very visual or tangible, playing out like movies or very realistic dreams, and others may be more like intangible feelings or senses.

Fantasy is extrapolated FROM reality. But it isn't reality, isn't often likely to become reality, and isn't usually even based in a whole lotta reality. Sexual fantasy is no different. Fantasy comes from our ideas about, ideals of, or experiences in reality, but fantasy is fantasy and reality is reality. They're separate, and that's what's often so exciting about fantasy in the first place.

We all have different needs and desires, and those can change by the moment. Someone who one day is aroused by the fantasy of a romantic and gentle lover may the next day fantasize about being roughly restrained—and both of these things are okie-dokie as fantasies, even if they might make you uncomfortable or even bored to visualize as reality. They're your fantasies, not your actions: to think is NOT to do.

It's typical to assume that sexual fantasy is our mind telling us what we want in sexual reality, but that's not always so, and not always realistic. Our fantasies may sometimes give us clues about things like specific sexual desires, sexual orientation, sexual ideals, people we're attracted to, or issues or scenarios we're grappling with, curious about, or wanting to explore. Our fantasies may also ensure our safety; we can explore, via our imagination, sexual scenarios that would, in reality, be unsafe or harmful. Fantasy may also help us to realize and work out sexual conflicts, guilt, shame, or unmet or unspoken desires creatively. All in all? Our fantasies are often a good thing, just as they are, with no need to make them real unless we want to, and the setting is right.

WHICH FANTASIES ARE OKAY, AND WHICH AREN'T?

Ultimately? ALL fantasy is usually okay, because it's in our heads, just as it's okay to *think* you'd like to slap someone, when you're mad at them. It's slapping them that wouldn't be okay, not thinking about it. Some people find that their sexual fantasy takes them places they feel weird about visiting—people have sexual fantasies about things like group sex, casual sex, or sex with a partner of a different gender than they want to be with in real life, even though the idea of doing these things for real may be totally unappealing to them. They may fantasize about being with someone incredibly inappropriate or dangerous, about being raped or raping someone, about sex with a family member, or about sexually manipulating someone. No matter what your fantasy, it's not a problem as long as you understand the difference between fantasy and reality.

It may happen that you have fantasies that truly trouble you or that just don't mesh with your ethics or politics; to a rape victim, for example, pervasive rape fantasies can very disturbing and upsetting. Someone very freaked out about homosexuality may feel tormented by constant same-sex fantasy. The normal and intuitive response to disturbing or uncomfortable fantasies is to try to shut them out of the mind altogether, but that approach usually doesn't work, and can even make them more persistent. So, the better tack to take is to talk to a counselor or therapist, even if it feels very embarrassing. In many ways, persistent disturbing fantasies are a lot like persistent disturbing nightmares or dreams: you may just need help finding out what the source of them is, and working through those issues.

Aside from those types of situations, your fantasies are probably fine just as they are, especially if they feel fine, and there's no need to sweat them, put a whole lot of effort into trying to analyze them, or try to make them realities; you can let sleeping dogs (or bustling threesomes, or amorous teachers, or shiny celebrities) lie (or frolic, or orgasm wildly, or plead to give you more).

• PORNOGRAPHY: •
One Big, Tricky, Sticky Issue

The whole issue of pornography is so incredibly loaded, controversial, and personal that even the terms used for it are murky, and the definition of pornography changes constantly. Just thirty years ago, many current music videos, movies, television shows, romance novels—and even some medical photographs intended to educate doctors, or a book like this one—might have been considered to be pornographic or obscene (and, in some circles, they still are). Many works once thought to be obscene or called pornographic are now considered great works of art or literature.

For as long as entertainment and media have existed, there's been sex in entertainment and media, and media have been expressly created for sexual entertainment or arousal, otherwise known as *pornography*. While modern media like the printing press, video, photography, and the Internet have made pornography more widespread than ever before, sexual art and literature have been discovered from ancient civilizations like Pompeii and Herculaneum, and in texts that are thousands of years old, such as the *Kama Sutra*. The term *pornography*—which literally means "to write of prostitutes," from the Greek words *porne* and *graphien*—was coined when Pompeii was first excavated and such material was found. In other words, porn is literally as old as dirt.

Porn and sexuality in media shouldn't be surprising. Human beings have always created art, literature, and other materials from their life experiences and imagination: sex and sexual fantasy are often integral parts of our lives and collective imagination.

What is or isn't pornography is sometimes murky. In our modern context, the word pornography means any material that is used to, or intended to arouse sexual desire in people. That means that, for a given person, pornography could be anything from a XXX video to Elizabethan love poetry. While many people use the word pornography to refer only to explicit visual material, pornography can also be textual or performed, and is not limited to videos or in photographs; sculptures, paintings, and illustrations can also be intended or used as pornography. Pornography may be explicit, but it may also be subtle. It may or may not contain explicit sexual language or depict sex acts graphically.

The word *obscene* often comes into play when talking about porn; that's a term used to label anything as lewd, crass, or simply objectionable to an assumed set of cultural values.

Sometimes, some sexually arousing media or material is called *erotica*. Often, this type of material is less sexually or visually explicit than, for instance, what we know as *hardcore* porn, or it may aim to be more subtle. Some people define erotica as suggestive,

and porn as directive. Some people use the word erotica when they really mean pornography, because it's more socially acceptable in some circles to peruse erotica than porn. Or, people will call something erotica if it's a kind of sexual or arousing material they enjoy and accept, but if it's not, they call it pornography or filth or smut, and argue that it is indecent or wrong for everyone.

Whether or not something is considered pornographic can also depend on context. For instance, few people would consider the literary works of William Shakespeare or Charlotte Brontë to be pornography, even though their work does contain passages of sexual description that may be arousing. An explicit sex scene in a film or book that is not primarily about sex isn't likely to be considered pornography by many people. Depictions of rape in films like *Last Exit to Brooklyn, The Accused,* or *Things behind the Sun*—intended to show the horror of rape—may contain "sex" or nudity, just as medical photographs may depict breasts or genitals, but those things aren't usually considered pornography because their intent is clearly not to sexually arouse.

So, who seeks out, reads, looks at, "uses," and buys or creates pornography? Men and women alike, of all different ages and social strata, though it's typical for men to purchase far more commercial pornography, and in much greater volume, than women. A Forrester Research report from 2001, for instance, states that 77 percent of online visitors to adult content sites—the largest pornography market now—are male.

Some people use porn during masturbation, as an aid to arousal or to inspire sexual fantasy. Others may use it to experience arousal or feed fantasy that they will bring to partnered sex later. They may or may not share or use the material with their partner. Some may use it to explore their own feelings about sexuality; others may just look at it out of curiosity. Those who use pornography may or may not have sexual partners at the time. They may only peruse porn alone, or during masturbation, or may use it with partners. The porn they enjoy may or may not contain depictions of people who look or act like their partners. Some people enjoy porn that closely resembles or mimics their sexual reality or their actual wants; others prefer porn that is very divorced from their real sexual lives.

Because sexuality is so individual, how people react to sexual material is also very personal. What arouses one person may leave another person cold, or even be offensive, emotionally distressing, or a big turn-off. What you enjoy one day or at one time in your life may be very different from what you enjoy at another time, and it's also normal for your feelings about pornography to change over time.

PORN PROBLEMS

Rarely in pornography are you going to see a couple disagreeing on whether or not to have sex at all, plainly discussing what kinds of sexual activities to engage in, negotiating safer sex and birth control, or just hanging out and snuggling before, during, or after sex. It's unusual to see pornography in which anyone isn't made up, has stubble on their legs, is wearing their ratty laundry-day undies, isn't in the mood, clearly has a bad head cold, or isn't okay with sexual language a partner uses. We're never going to hear an actress say to an actor in porn, "Hey,

don't call my vulva a pussy, okay? You know that really creeps me out. In fact, I don't think I can have sex with you now—let's just go watch a movie instead."

Pornography is fiction, and much of it is based on a given set of sexual ideals or fantasies. Even photos or videos of "natural" models or "regular" people usually have plenty of fictional elements: lighting is chosen, extensive editing or retouching occurs, and sexual behavior is often tailored to please viewers rather than the actors, to ensure they make money. The majority of material produced as pornography, like most mass media, portrays pretty unrealistic body types and appearances: many actresses (and more rarely, actors) in pornography, like many in mainstream films, have had cosmetic surgeries. It's incredibly rare to see actors in pornography who don't reach (or fake) orgasm, who have orgasms that are quiet or subtle, or who aren't turned on by (or are turned off by) typical "porny" stuff—yet all of these reactions are normal and common in real-life sex. People who don't realize that, or who expect their partners to live up to porn's fictions, ideals, and fantasies, are in for a rude awakening. Even porn stars couldn't live up to those expectations in their real lives.

DOES PORN CONTRIBUTE TO RAPE AND ABUSE?

How rape and porn may be related is an area of study that is still relatively new, and is a tricky thing to try to suss out.

Plenty of porn *does* contain violence or coercion that is put forth as sexy; some even pokes fun at rape. Some studies show pretty strong evidence that such pornography can blur the boundaries between consensual sex rape, for some people. In an experiment conducted by Neil Malamuth and James Check in 1985, for example, one group of students saw a pornographic scene in which a woman was portrayed as sexually aroused by rape, and a second group was exposed to control materials. Then, all subjects were shown a second, nonpornographic rape portrayal. The researchers found that the students who had watched the porn rape scene were significantly more likely than the second group to perceive the rape victim in the realistic portrayal as suffering less trauma, and to believe that women in general enjoy rape.

The evidence is not always easy to interpret, however, and there are many corollaries: most porn users are male, most rapists are male. While there have been studies that show that high percentages of rapists or abusers use porn, those numbers are basically the same as the percentages of men in general who purchase and use pornography. Global rape rates have gone up slightly in line with the greater availability of pornography, but rape was already very pervasive well before porn was so widely used and produced, so that increase may or may not be related to pornography.

Sometimes pornography is very clearly exploitive. Porn actors and actresses—unlike directors, producers, and distributors—often take physical, emotional, and social risks for their roles, but they usually receive the least compensation for their work. Porn often reinforces the same unhealthy or unattainable body ideals we find elsewhere in the media. The approach and language used in a lot of pornography can be violent, bigoted, sexist, and one-dimensional. Some pornographic material contains fantasy scenarios in which resistance from one person is shown to turn into an enthusiastic sex session—without any discussion about consent. Depictions of abuses of power or nonconsensually inflicted pain are common. A viewer or reader can be exposed to sexualized or sexual abuse, hate speech, violence, and brutality.

Sadly, we see plenty of that in all sorts of media—it's hardly exclusive to porn. But whether it's in porn, video games, or other media, if we immerse ourselves in the culture and celebration of violence, it can influence how we think and feel. Since arousal and sexuality are so core to us, we can be a lot more suggestible when we have sexual feelings going on, whether that's with a partner or with media. We're all affected by our surroundings in some way. How and how much we're affected varies.

What we can clearly say, however, is that a lot of the media designed to get us turned on presents people (or one sex) as objects, as sexual beings or sexual commodities, and this can obviously encourage people to view them in that way. While most people can differentiate between fantasy and reality, many cannot.

There are no easy answers to this one, but no matter how we feel about it, or what conclusions we draw, it is important to ask the questions. It's always a good idea to be mindful about what we make part of our sexual lives, and to think and question our choices—including the media we use and purchase—even when our culture tells us something is a no-brainer. (For more information on evaluating pornography, see the Resources section.)

IS IT OKAY TO LIKE PORNOGRAPHY? IS IT OKAY TO DISLIKE IT?

As you probably know from your own experience, a lot of people have very strong

s.e.x.

opinions about pornography, whether they like it or dislike it, support it or do not, and for all kinds of reasons. For some, it's an ethical or political issue, for others a more personal or interpersonal matter (or both), and for others still, it just boils down to whether they sexually enjoy it or not.

If you're old enough to purchase pornography legally, only you can make that call for yourself, and like any other sexual choice, you should make that call an informed one that's as right for you and everyone around you as possible. You get to decide what kinds of porn, erotica, or other sexual material, if any, are or aren't okay for you and with you, in your life and in your partnerships. Only you can decide if and how you use it, and what, if any, type of porn is supportive of your heart and mind, well-being, relationships, and sexuality. As with most other aspects of sexuality, you also get to change your mind or adapt your thinking and habits at any time.

multiple choice: gender, orientation, and sexual identity

TWO BIG FACETS of sexuality and sexual and personal identity for most people are gender—how we self-identify or identify others based on sex or ideas about sex—and sexual orientation—who attracts us, whom we partner with, based on sex and gender (or not, if we choose).

Gender and orientation are hardly rocket science. But making sense of them—and the roles and status based on them—and finding your place within them can sure get complicated. Ideas about them vary widely, yet are pervasive and often very limited. However we interpret these issues, they are a big deal in our world and identity, and so they play parts in everyone's relationships and personal identity.

▪ GENDERPALOOZA! ▪
A Sex and Gender Primer

You already know what sex is: the classification of a person (or plant or animal) based on whether their anatomy and chromosomes are what we identify as male or female, from a biological and physiological perspective. When you were born, it was sex that brought a doctor or midwife to holler out, "It's a girl!" or "It's a boy!"

It's typically assumed that sex and gender are the same. They're not.

So, what the heck is gender? Gender is a man-made set of concepts and ideas about how men and women are supposed to look, act, and interrelate, based on their sex. Gender isn't anatomical: it's intellectual, psychological, and social (and even optional); it's about presentation, identity, roles, and status based on ideas about sex and what it means to different people and groups. Like sex, gender is often presented to us as binary: as being only one thing or the other, without any overlap or gray area in between. When we talk about sex, we're talking about what is male and what is female; when we talk about gender, we're talking about what is considered masculine and what feminine. If our doctors or midwives were to call out our gender at birth, rather than our sex, they would be shouting "Heels!" or "Sneakers!"

Say "female" or "feminine" and a given group of people are likely to define the term pretty similarly, in terms of appearance and behavior, just as they would if you said "male" or "masculine." But the fact is that those categories differ with incredible variance, globally and individually. In many ways, the spectrum of gender is much like the spectrum of sexual orientation. Very few people are at the outer edges of the continuum of what is traditionally or currently defined as "male" or "female"—most of us are somewhere in the middle, with a variety of qualities, in terms of our appearance, emotions, behaviors, interests, goals, and strengths. Whether we live in one area or another, go to this country or that one, live in this or that period of history, have this set of rights or that, or identify ourselves this way or that way, our chromosomes under a microscope, or our genitals and reproductive systems, will always look the same. On the other hand, what our gender roles and status are, and how we identify and perform our gender, can be radically different, depending on whether we're living in ancient Greece or modern-day New York City, whether our sex grants us the right to vote, work, or get a fair trial, and what strengths and weaknesses, privileges or punishments, we or those around us may attribute and assign to our sex. Gender assignment is someone deciding that we're masculine or feminine—or *gendernormative* ("normal" for what our sex is)—not based on what's between our legs, but based on how we dress or speak, what our job is, what our interests are, or even something as meaningless as what our favorite colors are.

It'd be tough to find someone who hasn't been exposed to gender roles and status. Maybe growing up you heard that "real" boys weren't supposed to play with dolls, or that "good" girls weren't supposed to sit without crossing their legs. Maybe you've experienced how much emphasis is put on a woman's appearance or on a man's net worth. You may have gotten the message that only weak men cry or only hysterical women yell, that women are "natural" caretakers and men are "natural" providers or fighters. Perhaps you've heard snide remarks about male nurses or female construction workers. In your family or community, certain duties may be assigned to members of your household based only on gender. You may notice that women are often presented by the media and advertisers as being concerned primarily with romance, family, and appearance, men with sex, money, and sports. Those stereotypes are all about gender roles.

If you've studied history, you've seen how women have had to fight for the exact same rights men have, such as voting and fair pay. If you are aware of global issues, you know

s.e.x.

how many women worldwide are still viewed as property or are required to be submissive and/or subservient. These facts are about gender status.

When it comes to sexual behavior, gender expectations, relationships, roles, status, and identity often loom large. Many people decide who they will and will not date, or sexually partner with, based on gender as well as sex. Often, "feminine" men are assumed to be gay, "macho" men assumed to be heterosexual; "masculine" women are often assumed to be lesbian, and "femme" women heterosexual, even though none of those assumptions may be correct. Sex and gender are required components of the concept of sexual orientation: what sex and gender we are or identify with, and the sex(es) or gender(s) of those we are sexually and romantically attracted to.

Gender—both how we identify with it and how others identity us through the lens of gender—also often plays a part in the way we'll have any sort of sex, how we present our sexuality to others, how we feel comfortable or uncomfortable in our sexual behavior and attitudes, and how we might expect the dynamics of our sexual relationships to work. This is obvious in opposite-sex relationships, where there are so many assumed norms and roles between men and women: about who should be doing the asking out, taking sexual leadership, claiming sexual responsibility, setting sexual limits and boundaries, and being "outwardly" sexual. Gender can even determine the "right" way of having sex at all, such as ideas that it's not "manly" for men to enjoy receptive anal sex, or not "feminine" for women to ask for sexual activities to bring them to orgasm, after their male partner has had his. Gay people, relationships, and communities are not automatically immune from typical gender roles, either: lesbians have often—some voluntarily, but some involuntarily—been divided by appearance and behavior into binary butch and femme categories, mirroring traditional male and female gender roles. "Butch" is also often used among gay men to define a traditional gender role, as are terms like daddy or twink, top and bottom. Often, we hear people asking about a given same-sex relationship, "Who's the man?" when there's no man in the room at all.

While many young adults now see themselves as being more flexible when it comes to gender than their parents or grandparents, some studies and a lot of behaviors have shown that, despite what we might think, many "traditional" or stereotypical gender roles and norms are still assumed. A Kaiser

did you know . . . ?

Not all cultures and communities see or treat gender as binary. In many Native American tribes, a gender called two-spirit (a person considered neither male nor female, determined by identity, not by their genitals) was known and respected. In India, a "third sex" called *hijra* is recognized. *Xanith* is an Arabic term that recognizes persons whose gender identity is not in accord with their biological sex.

Family Foundation study from 2002 found that most teens think asking someone out initially, making the first move sexually, and providing condoms are male behavior, and that saying no to sex, setting and enforcing sexual limits, and bringing up or providing birth control are female roles. Most teens in the study agreed that it's a good thing, based only on gender, for young women to abstain from sexual activity or be a virgin, but didn't feel the same way about young men.

But many of us have, at one time or another, experienced what is called *gender dysphoria:* discomfort with our sex and/or gender identity and the gender norms and roles out and about in the world. You may have found that certain clothing picked out for you by parents conflicted with your gender identity—not all girls like ruffles; some boys prefer sparkly shoes to sneakers. As a young boy, you may have wanted a doll and been told that wasn't okay, or perhaps as a young adult male, you find that ideas like sexual initiation (or uncontrollable libido or sexual dominance) don't fit your own gender identity. Growing up biologically female, you may have found that your world changed radically during puberty, when you had more visible "markers" of being female, and were perhaps told that activities you once enjoyed were no longer appropriate for you. You may have once been comfortable with more stereotypical gender identities, but now feel a new discomfort. For instance, someone who felt that traditional gender roles fit them fine may feel differently the first time they face job discrimination based on their sex or gender. Sexual relationship problems may crop up when people are faced with the assumption that only women need to take responsibility for birth control

or safer sex, or that men should be the only ones to initiate sexual encounters. You may even feel funny about being gendernormative, because you have a hard time figuring out if you're really being you, or just identifying with what you've been told you're supposed to be.

It's not exactly accurate to say you can pick your gender roles and status. You may be able to in your own home, or in a given relationship or community, but out and about in the world we don't always get a whole lot of choice. How others perceive us based on how we appear, what our gender is thought to be, dictates much of our status and our roles. Few of us can completely escape or ignore those expectations. For instance, women can't just decide they're going to be paid as much as men for the same work; men can't just decide that strict ideas about masculinity won't be applied to them. So, it's common for our gender identity—and how we present ourselves—to be largely or entirely determined by the overt and covert messages we're all bombarded with from a very early age, telling us how we should be valued (or value ourselves), act, and appear.

Some people assume that presentation is a given: You're born male or female, so you look a certain way or act a certain way, and any appearance or behavior outside expected norms is a deviation, instead of a variation. Many assume that you either accept or deny looking or acting "male" or "female," rather than recognize that gender roles and presentation are active—not passive—choices we all make, and that those distinctions are largely arbitrary. Those assumptions and assertions cause very real problems for many individuals and groups: everything from just being called Mr. instead of Ms., to the overt violence of hate crimes (such as rape or the murders of gay men). The collective cultural notion, for instance, that men are physically "stronger" than women has caused numerous social and interpersonal problems for men and women alike (as well as simply being untrue). The notion that biological—anatomical or genetic—sex must and automatically does "match" socially dictated gender identity creates a world of confusion, conflict, and imbalance for many of us, and for some, it creates emotional and interpersonal torment.

But you CAN choose a great deal of how *you* present your gender (how you behave, dress, groom and carry yourself) and how you identify (what you call yourself and what that means to you).

You can also cast a wider net and work to change the status of your gender as a whole, or challenge large-scale gender roles with activism, especially when you are of a sex or gender with greater agency. For instance, a man could speak out about how traditional ideas about masculinity have really messed with his life and his head, or work with an organization to prevent rape.

Challenging cultural gender roles, status, and assumptions isn't always easy or successful, even when we just want to change them in our house, our relationship, or our own head. But often, it's easier in the long term to live with the discomforts we experience when we reinvent or defy assigned gender roles than to try to live out roles that don't feel true to us, or that we can't or don't want to support.

You get to—and should—explore, challenge, and ultimately decide whatever gender identity suits *you* best, whether it's a good fit and match with existing gender roles or it isn't—and even if the rest of the world isn't ready for you yet. It's just like that glass slipper in Cinderella. If the shoe doesn't fit, don't wear it. You can still go to the ball, and insist on wearing whatever you want when you go.

As with most aspects of identity, as you continue into and through your adult life, you'll likely find that your personal gender identity and your feelings about gender change and grow, becoming more clear (and more murky!). With time and life experience, you will probably realize that gender isn't anything close to binary, but like most things, is a wide, diverse spectrum, a varied, veritable genderpalooza.

▪ WAY BEYOND BINARY: ▪ TG, TS, GQ, and Other Two-Letter Words

Plenty of people find that gender roles, status, and expected behaviors don't suit them and create problems, challenges, and even a world of frustration. But for some, those disconnects and conflicts are even more problematic or traumatic. Here are some terms that describe these serious gender issues:

▶ **Transgender (TG):** Those who experience their gender identity or expression in profound conflict with their biological sex. *Transgender* or *transgendered* is an umbrella term used for those with full-time gender dysphoria.

▶ **Transsexual (TS):** *Transsexual* is generally used to describe a transgender individual who is seeking out, or has

s.e.x.

sought out, therapies or surgery to change their biological sex, to "match" their gender identity (called *transitioning*). TS is often used to refer to someone who is postoperative—who has had sexual reassignment surgery (SRS)—but sometimes *transgender* and *transsexual* are used interchangeably.

▶ **MTF (male to female)** and **transwoman** are common terms used for transgendered or transsexual persons who are or were biologically male but identify as female, and **FTM (female to male)** or **transman** refers to biological women who identify as male. Some transgendered persons may not use those terms, preferring others–such as ze, zir, gender outlaw, tranny boy, tranny girl, two-spirit, or even, simply, man or woman—or terms that are self-invented.

▶ **Transvestite (TV)** or **cross-dresser:** A person who wears the clothing, or performs the mannerisms, of a sex or gender that differs from their own, usually for the purpose of sexual gratification, but sometimes for other reasons, such as dramatic performance, goals, or achievements they cannot attain presenting gendernormatively, or plain old comfort. Psychologically speaking, whereas transgender is classified as a gender disorder, transvestitism is not; it is classified as a sexual paraphilia (more commonly called a *fetish*). It is most common among men.

Many transgendered people are considered to cross-dress, but again, you have to take into account that when you're transgender, those "opposite sex" clothes aren't opposites to your gender identity.

Too, many women in history—such as Joan of Arc, seafarers Mary Read and Anne Bonney, and Buffalo soldier Cathay Williams—have cross-dressed to preserve their safety, or to engage in pursuits that were forbidden or dangerous to women.

▶ **Genderqueer (GQ):** Those who identify as genderqueer generally reject typical, binary systems of sex or gender outright, often express or seek to invent a gender identity for themselves, and/or participate in endeavors, behaviors, or activism that queer up traditional gender approaches.

▶ **Cisgender:** A term often used in the context of trans issues to refer to a person whose gender "matches" their biological sex. For example, someone sexed female at birth who also identifies her gender as female.

TRANS-LATION

Transgendered people are not all alike: we can't place certain appearance, behavioral, lifestyle, or sexual attributes on them as a group any more reliably than we can for biological men or women as a group. Transfolk may be any sexual orientation under the sun, and may be attracted to any gender, just like anyone else (as may their partners). Sure, transgendered people may work as drag kings or queens, but more are teachers, nurses, bankers, lawyers, truckers, baristas, librarians, hairstylists, or physicists. They may be single or have families; they may be parents. Some transgendered people are politically liberal or progressive; some are conservative. Some work to resist or reinvent traditional or currently enforced gender norms, roles, and status; others support them.

s.e.x.

SRS

SRS isn't something one can just walk in and have done; it is often very difficult to even qualify for. It's an extensive procedure that begins with long-term counseling and personal interviews about gender development and history, family background, general lifestyle, interpersonal relationships, and aspects of sexuality. If those issues don't appear to be problematic, hormone and other therapies can begin. Hormone therapy is continued and monitored for SRS patients for a couple of years, as is the person's experience of living 24/7 as "the opposite sex." That's sometimes called the Real Life Experience (RLE) or Real Life Test (RLT). While these standards and protocols are ever-changing, some SRS patients, during this time, have to prove to their therapist and clinicians that they truly ARE the opposite sex. Therefore, "passing"–that is, appearing to others as that opposite sex, as it is most commonly defined—even if that appearance and given traditional gender roles are not in alignment with a patient's own gender identity—is often paramount.

If surgery is wanted and okayed, genital and/or nongenital procedures may be performed. These may include surgery that changes the genitals and/or internal reproductive system, breast implants or reduction, facial surgery, voice surgery, and/or other cosmetic surgeries.

Not everyone who is transgendered will engage in hormone therapy or surgical procedures. People who identify as transgender may, in fact, not look any different than is usually expected of their biological sex. Drag kings and queens, cross-dressers, and intersexed people may also identify as transgender (or may not).

For those who seek to physically change their sex, the procedures vary. For some, this involves lifestyle, external appearance, and legal name changes; for others, that and more: psychotherapy and counseling, hormone therapies, and even sexual reassignment surgery for those who wish to fully transition, physically, to the body of a different sex.

TRANSPHOBIA, DISCRIMINATION, AND BIAS

Despite all the strides we've made, gender discrimination is still rampant for cisgendered people, especially women. So, it's no surprise that transgender individuals also often experience profound sex and gender discrimination. As with any bias, misunderstanding and lack of exposure often breed prejudice and contempt. A lot of people who talk about transgendered, transsexual, intersexed, or genderqueer persons negatively have never actually spent time with any of them, instead forming their opinions from the media, gossip, or subjective assumptions. Often, they feel threatened by anyone who questions or contradicts a system and understanding of gender they feel benefits them.

There are plenty of people who feel satisfied with sex and gender systems, roles, and norms just as they are. There are plenty who've never thought about it much at all. For those people, the idea of gender dysphoria may not make much sense. They

s.e.x.

may be unable to understand it, and may label gender dysphoria as a mental illness (as some schools of thought and medicine have done). Some may politically or philosophically object to concepts of transgender or genderqueer. Some may be transphobic—scared of and/or hateful toward those who are transgender or intergender—and perpetuate or even believe the myths that all transgendered persons are sexual deviants, are homosexual, are simply trendy people who want to change their bodies the way others change hairstyles. Many of us have heard, seen, or experienced similar intolerance for other groups—toward women or feminists, people of color, the poor or homeless, gay, lesbian, or bisexual people, senior citizens or youth.

There are others who argue validly that current gender roles, status, and norms, even the whole concept of gender, are oppressive and problematic, but who nevertheless dismiss transgendered people or disapprove of them. The problem with that position is that gender is applied to everyone. If behaviors, roles and status assigned purely on the basis of biological sex or gender are oppressive and problematic, then they are problematic for everyone, as they are applied to everyone, not just one group.

Families often have an incredibly hard time treating gender dysphoria compassionately, and accepting the choices of a gender dysphoric person. Schools and workplaces can be unaccepting, and what are simple acts for some of us—such as buying a pair of shoes, riding the bus, or using a public washroom—can force transgendered people to face biases great and small, more frequently than many of us can imagine.

All too often, there is no community that will truly support or include transgender.

Even queer or progressive communities often reject transgendered people, diminish their issues, or see some or all TG issues as in conflict with their own. That isolation compounds the emotional distress of transgender, transsexual, genderqueer, or intergender people massively.

If you are transgender, transsexual, intergender, genderqueer, or questioning, or if you are having problems or feeling distress about cross-dressing or transvestitism, seek out support. There are several excellent online communities for TG/IG folks (see the Resources section). There may be support groups in your area, and you may find that some queer communities or alternative gender communities are welcoming and supporting, even if some people within them don't fully understand your issues. You may find that some of your friends and family can provide support and back you up when you advocate for yourself.

GENDERMENDING

We're all lucky, in that some aspects of gender have become less binary, less limiting, and less strictly enforced than they have been throughout much of our known history. Gendernormativity is becoming more of a choice than a mandate for many. Even though, as a culture, our progress is a bit slow, people coming of age now are often given more latitude when it comes to gender identity—and what's expected due to biological sex—than the generations before. Just a few hundred years ago, for instance, women who did something as simple as wearing pants or cutting their hair short, or who made bigger strides, directly challenging higher male gender

s.e.x.

how to be transfriendly and subvert crummy gender and orientation stereotypes in five easy steps!

1. Try not to assume someone's gender identity or sexual orientation based solely on appearance or behavior. Call people what they want to be called, identify them as they want to be identified, and find that out by either asking or listening for their cues. Many women don't like being called ladies, or being addressed as "Miss," "Honey," or "Ma'am." Plenty of people who self-identify as fags or dykes aren't comfortable with just anyone calling them that, or with being identified that way in every setting. Some people don't dig gender or orientation identifiers at all, and just like to be called their names: "me" is a totally acceptable gender and sexual identity. When in doubt as to someone's gender, sexual orientation, or preferred identity, just ask politely.

2. Turn off the switch in your brain that makes you say things like "All men are jerks," or "Women just want money," "Only gay guys talk like that," or "She looks/acts/sounds like a boy." There are NO sex, orientation, or gender absolutes, and the less we fall for and support them, the less power they have to keep all of us down.

3. Quit staring and whispering. When someone looks or acts in a way that you think is in conflict with their sex, orientation, or gender, check yourself out. Think about WHY you think that way, where your ideas about gender or orientation come from, and if your attitude and definitions are really reasonable or fair to apply to everyone. Take a few minutes to wonder how much the criteria you're thinking about even matter. It's okay to be curious or confused and to ask respectful questions. What's not cool is making someone else feel unsafe, insulted, or demeaned because you're uncomfortable with your own lack of knowledge or understanding, inflexible in your ideas about gender or orientation, or insecure about your own identity.

4. Subvert the status quo. If there's something in your school that is unfairly closed to a given sex, orientation, gender, or gender identity; that is based on gender appearance or heteronormativity; that unreasonably excludes others on the basis of orientation, sex, or gender, question it. If, in your relationships, you have a partner who is holding you to an identity, role, or status that isn't okay with you, speak up. Challenge sex, gender, and orientation discrimination directly when need be, and gather your forces to do so. Write letters. Engage others in discussion and awareness. Be visible. Don't accept gender or orientation norms, roles, or status at face value (even if they are just fine for you). Question them.

5. Work on tolerance and compassion. You don't have to agree with someone, or personally understand where they're at, to be kind, humane, accepting, and fair. Imagine yourself walking a mile in another person's shoes—including the blisters you'd wind up with in their heels.

s.e.x.

status, could nearly always find themselves victims of intense violence, social isolation, or even execution.

We could certainly still stand a lot of improvements. Women are still greatly oppressed as a class, and men who challenge their gender roles or presentation are still often met with disdain, aggression, and violence. Many men are still being reared to instigate violence or aggression to uphold a gendered status quo. Many transgendered, transsexual, genderqueer, or cross-dressing people, of all genders, are isolated, cast out of homes and communities, abused, sexually and/or physically assaulted, and even murdered, for nothing but their gender identity and appearance.

A lot of us would be safer, happier, healthier, and more whole if rigid ideas about sex and gender weren't so prevalent. But for now, a great majority of people accept, support, and encourage a very limiting view of sex and gender, so gender identity tends to be pretty important, as does the sex we're born with or assigned. Our challenges based on those things may be great or small, but only a rare few of us will have none.

As with anything else, though, gender is only one part of you, a whole person with a million facets. How you identify, and what genitalia you were born with, can only be as important and relevant to YOU, alone, as you want it to be. Even if you can't identify and present the way you'd like to, when you're out and about, what goes on in your head is all yours; the relationships you're in and your roles within them are up to you; and the way you choose to define yourself—as well as the latitude you give others in their gender identities—is your choice.

▪ GAILY FORWARD, STRAIGHT AHEAD: ▪ Sexual Identity for Everyone

News flash: EVERYONE has a sexual orientation and a sexual identity, not just people who are homosexual, bisexual, or queer. Not just people who are sexually active. Everyone.

As with a lot of terms developed to describe an "other," "them," or any group of people outside a current or accepted norm, it's common to hear orientation terms used within or about queer culture, and more rare to hear them when talking about everyone else. That's a bummer because questioning, sorting out, and learning to manage our sexual orientation and identity can be a big help when it comes to our sexuality as a whole: by ourselves and with partners, in reality as well as in our ideals and fantasies. Since there is no "default" orientation, exploring and identifying our sexual orientation is pretty darn important.

First things first: let's sort out the lingo.

 THIS isn't The Gay Chapter: you know, the one that says it's okay to be gay and it really will all be okay, but maybe we should wait a while longer before we decide that we're not heterosexual. Any of us who are queer and who needed that chapter have already read it in most sex books before, and already know that people tell us it's okay. Heterosexuality is a sexual orientation. Bisexuality is also a sexual orientation. "I'm attracted to whom I'm attracted to, and I don't know or care why," is also a sexual orientation. Everyone has one, and none of them is a default. And in case you *haven't* read The Gay Chapter before? It's all okay.

Sexual orientation: This term describes the sex or sexes, gender or genders to which a certain person is sexually, emotionally, and/or romantically drawn; which genders or sexes a given person can be in love with and want to have any kind of sex with. There may be varying degrees of attraction—for instance, a person may be very physically attracted to men, but more emotionally attracted to women.

Heterosexual (attracted to the opposite sex and/or gender), *homosexual* (attracted to the same sex and/or gender), *bisexual* (attracted to both sexes and/or genders), and *pansexual* (attracted to all or any sexes and/or genders) are terms for sexual orientation. So are terms like gay, lesbian, bi, straight, and queer, though those terms can also be used to describe a greater sexual identity. The term "asexual" is currently in common use for those who feel there is no gender or sex to which they are attracted. Those who identify themselves as asexual may not yet be in the right developmental place to feel sexual attraction or arousal, may not have met anyone they're very attracted to yet, or really may simply not feel any sexual or romantic attraction to others.

Sexual preference: This is something like being sexually attracted to people who are tall, who have a certain style of dress, or a certain hair color. Sexual preferences can also refer to preferred sexual activities, such as a certain sexual position or a certain kind of sexual language. Sexual orientation as a whole—such as being homosexual—is *not* a sexual preference. But sometimes, "preference" can be used as a subsection of sexual orientation; for instance, someone who is bisexual may not be equally attracted to both genders, but may generally *prefer* to be sexually involved with one sex or gender.

Sexual "lifestyle": Lifestyle or "gay lifestyle" is a usually negative term used to suggest that people of any one orientation have a given way of living, or are represented by the most visible or fringe sector of that group. A person's lifestyle is expressed in their actions, choices, interests, and opinions, including everything from how they dress to what their political affiliations or level of activism is; naturally, lifestyle varies greatly among people of a given orientation, just as it varies among a given gender, race, or socioeconomic group. In a medical context, however, sexual lifestyle may refer to certain sexual behaviors or practices; for example, a doctor may ask about sexual lifestyle to gather information on STI risks.

Sexual identity: This is an umbrella term used by a person to sum up the general gist of their sexuality, in terms of how they identify and present themselves. It may include sexual orientation, politics, affiliations or interests, relationship models, status and experience, gender identity, sexual preferences—the whole enchilada. Queer, dyke, and straight are terms for sexual identity, as might be kinky, polyamorous, slut, asexual, vanilla, tutti-frutti, and so on. Because sexual identity is so personal, some people get creative and come up with combination phrases, such as "genderqueer granola dyke" or "heteroflexible kinky poly switch."

Sexual identity is fairly fluid. While some portions of our sexuality are at least partially fixed—like our basic sexual

s.e.x.

GLBT... Q...A...I... WTF?

GLBT (or LGBT) is a commonly seen acronym addressing sexual orientation, and sometimes it has even more letters tacked onto it.

G = Gay

L = Lesbian

B = Bisexual

T = Transgender or transsexual

Q = Questioning or queer

A = Asexual (someone who doesn't feel they are sexually or emotionally attracted to anyone at all) or ally (a heterosexual person who supports all orientations)

I = Intersex

P = Pansexual (attracted to all people of all sexes and genders)

O = Omnisexual (like pansexual) or other

orientation (whether we're attracted to men, women or both/all genders), parts of our gender identity, and some of our sexual or partnership preferences—many aspects of our sexual identity will develop, shift, and evolve throughout our lives. For instance, during one period of our lives, we may explore a certain type of sexual activity, like role-play. At the time we're doing that, it may become a prevalent part of who we feel we are. Later, we may lose interest in that, or decide that it really isn't the thing for us and isn't a part of our sexual ID. While we're single, our relationship status of being single or multi-partnered may not be a big part of our sexual identity, but if and when we become monogamously partnered or married, it may then become integral.

As well, sex and sexual relationships are only part of our lives. If every part of us is completely wrapped up in sex and sexual identity, we're likely to miss out on other equally enriching and fulfilling parts of our lives. So, while your sexual identity is often an integral part of who you are, and a very big deal while you're seeking out the whole of your self-identity so intensely, there's never any hurry to claim or label it, nor to carve it in stone and make your current sexual identity your *whole* identity.

▪ THE RAINBOW CONNECTION: ▪ The Spectrum of Sexual Orientation

The most common terms used to describe sexual orientation—heterosexual, homosexual, bisexual—are often limited. According to solid sex research, the majority of people have at least SOME sexual or romantic attraction or attachment to more than one sex or gender. Most may not actively date or be sexually engaged with more than one gender, and the majority will usually partner with the opposite sex, but very few people are completely heterosexual or homosexual, even though they may identify that way. Because we use those terms primarily to describe a person's *actions* and active sexual or romantic life, rather than their intentions or aspirations, and because, currently, all orientations are still not equally accepted, their application is murky.

The twentieth-century sex researcher Alfred Kinsey devised a tool called the

s.e.x.

Kinsey Scale, to express orientation more accurately:

0 Only heterosexual
1 Mainly heterosexual, with some homosexual attraction
2 Mainly heterosexual, with a good deal of homosexual attraction
3 Equally heterosexual and homosexual
4 Mainly homosexual, with a good deal of heterosexual attraction
5 Mainly homosexual, with some heterosexual attraction
6 Only homosexual

The scale takes into account not just actual relationships—or actual sexual activity—and the labels people choose for themselves, but crushes, sexual and romantic fantasies, and even dreams. With all that in mind, very few people would be classified as 0 or 6—what we'd typically class heterosexual or homosexual. The majority of people, based on Kinsey's findings and those of more recent research, are 2s, 3s, 4s, or 5s. That's why some people say that most people are bisexual or pansexual.

Most people don't identify as bisexual or pansexual, though, nor do the majority of people with attraction to the same sex date or sexually partner with those of the same sex. That may have a whole lot to do with the lack of support and acceptance in our culture for anything other than heterosexual relationships. Even though things have gotten a whole lot better over time, for many people, being out as at all queer is an emotional and practical challenge, and plenty of people who aren't exclusively heterosexual may never engage in anything other than opposite-sex relationships, out of nothing but fear or shame. But the scientific reasons for people's behavior are academic. What's relevant to you is what feels right, what the best fit is for you, and how you are comfortable identifying.

WHILE transgender (the T in GLBT) is often considered part of queer issues, it's a mistake to assume that transgendered individuals are automatically gay or lesbian. The range of sexual orientation that exists for the transgendered is the same as for those who find that their gender fits their biological sex, and that is usually based in gender, not sex. A transwoman—a woman sexed male at birth, but who identifies as female—who is attracted primarily to men generally identifies as heterosexual; a transman attracted to men usually identifies as homosexual.

Ultimately, what you call yourself, how you identify, and when and even if you identify is all your choice. The important thing is that you do what you can to make yourself comfortable and at peace with yourself; that you are honest with yourself and your friends, family, and/or partners; and that you realize you have as much time as you want or need to become and discover who you are.

TO BE OR NOT TO BE: IS SEXUAL ORIENTATION A CHOICE?

Sexuality research over the last fifty years or so tells us that no matter our orientation, it's likely at least partially hard-wired, in that some aspects of our sexual orientation are probably fixed pretty early in our lives to a certain degree, based on a combination of genetics, early familial, platonic, romantic, and

s.e.x.

consider this:

- In terms of crushes, of romantic and/or sexual attraction, what gender, if any, is predominant? Am I mostly attracted to men, women, or both?
- In my actual romantic relationships, which sex or gender, if there is one that's paramount, do I date or wish to date most often? In my actual sexual relationships, which gender, if there is only one, do I date or wish to date most often?
- Which sexes or genders have a starring role in my sexual fantasy life?
- Is the sexual activity of certain genders attractive or repellent (as in, I'm grossed out by it) to me?
- What is the orientation of my peer group like? Do I feel I fit in or stand out?
- How do I feel about those I date, hook up with, or partner with? Do I often feel bored, as if I'm just going through the motions, or just not excited by members of the gender or sex I typically date?
- What orientation feels most comfortable for me right now, in terms of how I identify publicly? Is it the same one that feels best with how I identify privately, only to myself?
- Have I ever suspected that my orientation may be different? Do I ever feel like an impostor?

Questions like these are helpful when considering your orientation. How you answer those questions now may be different than you might when you're older, even without sexual partnership experience. For instance, many people who are grossed out by the mere idea of same-sex sex discover that, over time, as they meet and get to know bisexuals, homosexuals, and pansexuals, their repulsion fades away, because it is often based on irrational prejudice or stereotypes (or self-loathing). As we grow, we also start questioning certain aspects of our culture or community—like gender roles, or the dynamics and beliefs of our peer groups—that often play a part in our feelings about orientation and sexuality. And while you don't need to "experiment" with sexual partners to get a pretty good bead on orientation, as you become involved in romantic and sexual relationships, those relationships will often clarify some aspects of your orientation and give you extra food for thought.

sexual relationships, and the environments in which we're reared. Orientation is also both fluid and based on active choices. We all make conscious choices about whom we take as sexual partners, what we call ourselves, and what communities we participate in.

The American Psychological Association states that "sexual orientation emerges for most people in early adolescence without any prior sexual experience." (In other words, most people do **not** have to experi-

ment with partners of various genders to discover their orientation.) The APA continues, "and some people report trying very hard over many years to change their sexual orientation from homosexual to heterosexual with no success. For these reasons, psychologists do not consider sexual orientation for most people to be a conscious choice that can be voluntarily changed." The APA also has made official statements that "conversion" therapies are unethical.

"it's just a phase. you'll grow out of it."

YOUNG adults *are* often in big stages of sexual development, physiologically, emotionally and in their relationships. The nature of development is that it is a process which takes time, rather than being complete from the get-go. It's always been common, for instance, to have crushes on best friends, or sexual fantasies about same-sex friends, and even to engage in same-sex activity during childhood and adolescence, no matter a person's orientation in the long run. It's typical for many people who are homosexual to have opposite-sex partners during their developmental years and sometimes beyond, especially given the pressures most of us experience to be heterosexual. It's also normal for some young adults to be less choosy about their sexual partners than most older people are.

In other words, many young adults sexually explore and experiment with partners (same-sex OR opposite-sex) they might not choose later, depending on things like availability, peer and community pressures, safety or privacy, sexual or personal compatibility, and basic care and respect.

Honest, consensual sexual experimentation—whether it's in your own head or out and about with others—when you're a teen or young adult is normal and helpful. There also isn't a thing wrong with whichever sexual orientation you feel belongs to you. People who are queer aren't necessarily more cool, sexually available, or enlightened; people who are straight aren't necessarily prudish or narrow-minded. Having attractions or relationships outside what turns out to be your orientation base doesn't mean you're flighty, nor does it mean those relationships aren't or weren't important.

There's a lot of argument about this issue. Some folks use the notion of choice in how we *enact* our orientation as a way to support certain personal or political agendas, stating, for instance, that if a queer person has the ability to choose to partner with whomever they like, they can choose to he heterosexual. That's false logic when we understand orientation as both attraction and action, obviously, but the argument gets made all the same. Approaches like that make looking into the why of orientation a loaded issue, and they can bias the way even academic or medical researchers look at sexual orientation.

Asking about choice in orientation is tricky, because we just don't have an absolute answer yet, and we may never have one. Ultimately, one can confidently say we have enough research and real-life knowledge and experience to know that orientation is a combination of both choice and wiring. It truly doesn't matter very much what the exact combination is.

What's important is that, whatever our orientation, the active choices we do make feel right and okay with us and with our partners.

When so many parts of your identity are in flux, it's understandable to be in a hurry to affix a label to your orientation, especially if ambiguity or false assumptions are causing you grief. But sexual orientation can't be rushed, nor is determining it something you need to "just get over with." It takes time, and it's common for many adults in their twenties, thirties, and even forties to be uncertain about theirs, or to experience gradual or even radical shifts in orientation. So, yeah, it's possible that what feels like your orientation at times may be a phase, but orientation is often phasal for everyone, young and old, gay

s.e.x.

and straight, and everything in between. But even when it is a phase, there's no "just": it's still meaningful, still relevant, and still 100 percent who you are.

WHAT DOES IT MEAN TO BE BISEXUAL OR PANSEXUAL?

For many, figuring out homosexuality and heterosexuality is pretty simple: homosexuals are primarily or solely attracted to the same sex, heterosexuals to the opposite sex. Bisexuality and pansexuality can feel more murky.

A bisexual is someone who can or does experience attraction to either sex or gender; a pansexual is someone who is or *can* be attracted to any gender or sex, though not necessarily both at the same time. In other words, like heterosexuals and homosexuals, bisexuals and pansexuals can be monogamous; most do not need or desire one partner of each or every gender at the same time, nor do they "miss" one gender or sex when they're with a partner of another. Also, many bisexuals and pansexuals do not have a 50/50 split of attraction between sexes: a bisexual person may, for example, be mostly attracted to women, but sometimes attracted to men.

Bisexual/pansexual people often have to deal with a lot of bogus misconceptions about their orientation. Some people may assume they are just greedy or indiscriminate, or even that they're so sexually out of control, they'll sleep with anyone. Heterosexual or homosexual people may be reluctant to date those who live in the middle, for fear that a bisexual/pansexual will be dissatisfied with one gender—even if their bisexual/pansexual partner is more interested in monogamy than they are. In many ways, bisexuality or pansexuality is the most complex, or least clear-cut, form of sexual orientation, so it's no wonder it perplexes so many.

If you do identify as bisexual or pansexual, it's good to be prepared to do a little mythbusting now and then, without taking it too personally. As with any sexual orientation or identity that isn't considered a norm, there isn't a lot of accurate public awareness out there, so every person who can have the patience to do some sincere

did you know . . . ?

Not only are bisexuality, pansexuality, and homosexuality natural in humans, they occur commonly in other mammals and animals as well, such as chimpanzees, guinea pigs, ducks, ostriches, cats, dogs, insects, gorillas, horses, sheep, monkeys, and a plethora of other creatures. It also is nothing new. Though through much of history many homosexuals and bisexuals have not been "out," most anthropologists and biologists agree that it has occurred in humans for just as long as heterosexuality.

Psychological and sexual research has shown clearly that orientation in and of itself is not a cause for emotional or social problems. More often, when such problems are associated with homosexuality or bisexuality they are rooted in the nonacceptance of those orientations, and taunting, scolding, or punishment because of the perceptions of them.

s.e.x.

and honest educating, even just among friends or family, can help to make those misconceptions and stereotypes fall away.

"BAD" WORDS

Certain terms for sexual orientation and identity vary in use and acceptance from place to place, from person to person. So, while for one person, self-identifying as a "fag" feels right, it may not to another. Even those who do self-ID with "fag" may not like *others* using the term to identify them; in other words, they may be hurt or insulted by being *called* a fag, especially in certain contexts.

Over time, it's common for some negative terms to be revisited or reclaimed, even those that were once considered insults. Terms like slut, queer, dyke, straight, or poof are good examples; many people now use them as positive self-identifiers. However YOU choose to identify yourself, whatever feels best to you, is fine. It's also fine to object to how another person identifies or describes you—though if you don't like others using the term you use for yourself, you may want to evaluate whether it's really the best ID for you.

Your sexuality is with you through your **whole** life, so take all the time you need to explore it on your own. You can look through Web sites about various orientations; attend youth groups for questioning, gay, lesbian, or bisexual teens; or see if your school has a Gay-Straight Alliance (GSA). You can talk to teens and adults of varied orientations to get an idea of how much diversity there is, and what living with a given sexual orientation might be like. Ultimately, you're the person you have to live

with every day. Trying to make yourself into something you aren't, or fighting who you feel you really are, may seem like the easier thing to do in the short run, but in the long run it's incredibly stressful and can have serious ill effects on self-esteem and all your relationships.

Homophobia

Homophobia, like any phobia, is an irrational fear or hatred, in this case, of people who are gay, lesbian, or bisexual/pansexual, or of the mere idea of such sexual orientations. Unfortunately, just like sexism, racism, and anti-Semitism, homophobia is still perpetuated by some public figures, by the media, by a lack of visibility, by generational prejudices. Homophobia is often the root of hate crimes against GLBT persons, or those assumed to be. Many hate crimes still go unreported and unpunished, or do not get media attention, which helps to perpetuate homophobia.

Homophobia is not exclusive to heterosexual people; some GLBT people have internalized levels of it themselves—about themselves or other portions of the queer community—which can lead to serious self-esteem problems and severe emotional distress or self-hatred. Those feelings often contribute to self-destructive behaviors like cutting, substance abuse, risky sexual behavior, or even suicide.

No matter who you are, or what stage of understanding your identity you're at, the

s.e.x.

real goal is to accept yourself as you are, and have your identity and actions—sexual and otherwise—come from that place. If you're sincere, open, honest, and caring, if you live with integrity, you're someone to be proud of, no matter your orientation.

• DON'T LET THE DOOR HIT YOU • ON THE WAY OUT
Or, How to Come Out of the Closet without Tripping over Your Baggage

While there are plenty of things about orientation and gender that apply to everyone, the process of coming out of the closet— voluntarily making your sexual orientation or gender identity public—is fairly unique to those of us who are homosexual or bisexual or differently gendered. Since it's most often (falsely) assumed that everyone is heterosexual and cisgendered, by default, heterosexuals and cisgendered folks usually don't need to raise any flags.

There's no time limit on when you need to come out: you get to take as long (or as little) as you need to feel comfortable. How "out" you are is also up to you: whatever level of private or public works best for you and/or your partners is just fine. Nobody has to cover themselves in pride pins, feather boas, or leather chaps to be out (but if you want to, knock yourself out). You may not even need to come out in any formal way; sometimes it's casual and incidental.

But at a certain point, life in the closet can do a real number on you and your partners. When you're with someone, being reluctant to even hold their hand in public can put a painful strain on a relationship, and feeling like a dirty secret doesn't help anyone's self-esteem.

straight or gendernormative, and about to skip this part?

PLEASE don't. Not only may you find that, over time, your orientation or sexual identity shifts, but GLBT people need allies. In many places in the world, it is still *really* hard to be out as gay, lesbian, bisexual, or transgendered. GLBT youth suicide rates, for instance, are two to three times higher than rates for heterosexual youth. GLBT rates of homelessness, abuse, and depression are also higher. So, even if this isn't about you, have a read and prepare yourself to be a great ally to a friend or family member who may need your support more than you'd suspect.

When it starts to become clear that a given orientation or gender ID is more than a curiosity or a passing crush, many people become nervous or scared, worried that they might not be "normal." Others strongly suspect or know for sure that they do have certain gender attractions or gender conflicts, but are afraid to say so, either because they feel they will be branded in some way, or simply because they fear being rejected by their friends, family, or community. For example, in the United States, during the 2004 elections, exit polls indicated that 4 percent of all voters self-identified as gay or lesbian, yet an overwhelming number of people in the world, despite solid evidence to the contrary, still think of homosexuality as an illness or perversion. Transgender is even less generally accepted, even among "alternative" or progressive communities. In the United States alone, there are still at

s.e.x.

least 1,500 sexuality-based hate crimes reported every year, with a great number of the perpetrators and victims under the age of twenty. In many schools, teachers and school administrations often fail to intervene when orientation-based abuse or harassment occurs, and in some, teachers and administration have even been responsible for the attacks themselves, toward students or GLBT staff. Being nervous or afraid to come out, especially for certain orientations and identities, is completely valid.

But when you come out in gradual steps, even when it's a rocky road, being out usually feels a whole lot better than being in ever did.

COMING OUT: A BASIC HOW-TO

Being a young adult is stressful enough as it is. While it's typical to hide some aspects of your sexual life or identity from some people (not telling parents you're sexually active, or not telling a friend what sexual activities you've engaged in), hiding very basic aspects of your sexual and personal identity can really limit your quality of life and the quality of your relationships. Here are some points to keep in mind:

▶ **Take the time you need to prepare.** Consider the positives and the negatives. Ready yourself for the sorts of questions you're likely to be asked, even the stupid ones. Expect friends and family to ask if you're sure you're queer, or how you know; how important it is to you; if someone else is pushing you to be out or be queer; how out you need to be in your town, school, or extended family; how you want to handle it; what you expect

from them; if you're dating—and if so, whom you're dating, and what you're doing with them sexually (don't be surprised by the infamous "How can two women have sex, anyway?" question). It's normal for people who are not queer or differently gendered to have basic, earnest questions about orientation or gender, so prepare yourself to be able to address them calmly, or refer friends and family to groups or resources for more information. Have a good idea of what you want and need from the person or people whom you're coming out to.

▶ **Start small.** Start with someone you have a pretty good idea will be supportive and accepting. (If you truly don't have even one such person in your life, then try starting with a support group, in person or online.) Testing the waters first is a good idea. For example, you might bring up a current event that involves GLBT issues, such as gay marriage or hate crime law. Talking about queer issues in a general—rather than personal—way can give you a good idea as to what someone's feelings are, and if they're a safe person to come out to.

If you get a good feeling about them, then you can move a bit further. A good opening for coming out is something like, "I have been going through something important for a long time. I want to share it with you, and it feels very necessary. I'm not sure if you'll understand, but I trust you, and I need your support and acceptance, even if you can't give it to me right away: I'm queer/bisexual/lesbian/gay/transgender."

s.e.x.

► **Expect surprises.** It can be a tough blow when someone you were sure was going to be behind you 100 percent turns out to have some reservations, or some prejudiced ideas. Soften it by communicating, over time, both by talking and by listening. If what they say to you is hurtful, let them know that. If they say things that simply aren't true, especially for you, correct them gently.

Most people with a bias developed it when they were pretty young, and got through life without having those attitudes challenged. Most prejudice is based on ignorance and lack of personal experience. If you have to deal with it, you may feel validly pissed at having to take responsibility for a situation you did nothing to create and one which does you harm. But try and think about that differently. An opportunity to teach, to work to undo prejudice and intolerance, is always a good opportunity, because even one person can foster change that has a ripple effect in the long run.

Once you've got an ally in your corner, figure out where you need to go next. If it's your parents you want to tell, first call on family members you know will be the most supportive. Choose neutral settings for coming out: places that are conducive to calm communication and aren't stressful. Family gatherings, holidays, public restaurants, or workplaces are not usually good choices. If you want to come out at school, see if you can start with a GSA (Gay-Straight Alliance), or form one with friends. The more support you have at every stage of the game, the better.

Chances are, there will be stops and starts. A friend or family member who is supportive at one point may backpedal or stall a bit with certain issues, or at certain times. Many good people have blind spots, hidden biases they aren't even aware of. They may find it hard to recognize these, or may become angry and resentful when your issues bring them to light.

Of course, sometimes the surprise we find is a nice one: there are plenty of times someone has come out cautiously to a parent or friend only to be told that they already knew all along and were completely down with it: they were just waiting for you to figure it out for yourself!

► **Be fair to your parents, even when they're hyperventilating.** For many, coming out to parents is the scariest part, and the fear of rejection is intense. But for the most part, parents are cool people who love the heck out of you. That doesn't mean it's always easy as pie to come out to them. Your parents may go through a wide range of emotions: some may cry, others may yell, others may get very noncommunicative for a bit, even very angry. Your parents may suggest therapy for you. Some parents feel that having a homosexual, bisexual, or transgender child means they were lousy parents, or that you're betraying them by being different. Some may hold typical misconceptions or strong beliefs, such as that homosexuality is sinful or unnatural. Some who aren't homophobic or transphobic, who are perfectly accepting of GLBT or are even queer themselves, may still have strong emotional reactions. Queer parents, for instance, may feel upset about a child coming out because they have faced a lot of discrimination, rejection, or violence in their lives, and are scared their child will have to deal with those things, too.

Your folks have been through a lot during your adolescence. They've watched you change in so many ways (and so quickly, from their perspective) that they sometimes have to sit down just to fend off motion sickness. So, even the most accepting, open-minded parents may not want to throw you a party the minute you come out to them, and they may choke on their carrots instead of saying "congratulations" when you announce your sexual or gender identity at the dinner table.

As it is, most parents have a tough time adjusting to, and keeping up with, their teens' sexual development, maturation, identity, and relationships. (You can probably understand that: to a lot of us, thinking about our parents having sex is at least slightly squicky.) If you've known about your orientation or identity all along, or had that niggling feeling, then being GLBT may not be a change for you at all—but your folks may not have seen this one coming.

So, when you lay it on your parents, be kind. Be patient. Be mature. Be compassionate. When you are, you're more likely to get the same treatment from them. Offer to answer any questions they might have, and be ready to listen, even if what they say isn't so great

to listen to. Make yourself available to talk about it. Let them know that you're okay with it if they're not elated right now. Give them the time they need to absorb it all before you hang a rainbow flag on the front lawn. In time, most parents really do come around.

closed doors

 IT will take some parents a much longer time to accept having a gay or bisexual kid. Some won't ever be okay with it. It's a harsh reality that really hurts. Sometimes bias and prejudice are unsurpassable, even in people we love. Some parents kick teens out of the house when they come out, cut off college-age kids financially, disown them, or ship their kids off to therapists or communities that claim to be able to "convert" GLBT people. If that happens to you, or you suspect it might, call on your support system of friends or extended family to help. Remember that parents are people, and like any other people, sometimes they're really messed up: Do what you can not to internalize their bias. It's the biased person who is always the problem, not the person whom the bias is against. If nonacceptance of your sexuality turns into any sort of abuse—physical, verbal, emotional, or sexual—handle it as abuse: get help and do what you need to get yourself in a safe space. If you suspect you may face abuse in coming out while still living at home, it may be safest to wait to come out until you're in a safer setting. For more on abuse, see chapter 10.

With parents who don't take it to the absolute extreme, but really aren't happy about it or accepting, you may find that at some point you have to agree not to discuss the issue, to keep the peace. If you find that that simply doesn't feel right, you may have to come up with some other solution.

S.e.x.

▶ **Think before you pull out that megaphone.** When you first come out, you may feel like you want to tell the whole world. It's exhilarating to feel that you can be honest and forthright about your sexual identity, with yourself and with others. Just be sure that you're doing it in the right places, and most importantly, *in safe places.*

For instance, going to a drunken party and loudly announcing that you like to feel up other girls and might enjoy group sex isn't so swift. Ditto for getting it on with someone who you know isn't aware of your biological sex, or for macking down with your boyfriend on a public bus at two in the morning. Sexual safety smarts apply to being queer just as much as they apply to straight people, and in many places, more so. When you broadcast anything sexual about yourself—be that your orientation or the practices you like to engage in—others may interpret that as an invitation to react or participate. And some people's idea of reacting is harassment or assault.

Not every place is the right place to be sexual or discuss sex, especially when your sexuality is controversial or titillating in the eyes of some, or even completely objectionable in the eyes of others. Be sure when you do choose to be out or sexual in public, that you're making safe choices. Be alert. Know the risks you are taking, and minimize them. If the place you're in doesn't feel to you like a safe place to be out in, you're probably right. (For more on hate crimes and sexual assault, and protecting yourself, see chapter 10.)

mentoring in the queer community

 IT'S unfortunate, but a lot of queer youth find that the only "in" to the queer community and to queer mentors or support is through dating or sex. Thing is, while sexual or romantic partners may love and care for you, they're not the best mentors when it comes to queer life and community, because they may be very temporary, their love is likely not very unconditional, and if you do seek out support via sex, you may find that it starts to leave a pretty bad taste in your mouth.

So, if you're seeking out queer community via a personals ad, for instance, make clear you're looking for FRIENDS, rather than lovers. Don't make a lover your whole support system. Remember that you're a whole person, and that your sexual orientation and identity are about more than the sex you're having: they're about you as a whole person.

If you're having a hard time finding queer community outside of dating or the club scene, broaden your horizons. Many cities have GLBT youth groups, on campus and off. Hook up with an activist community working with GLBT issues. The queer, questioning, or straight-but-supportive friends you don't date can also be great, nonsexual support, or people you can go with to places where you can all broaden your community. If you're having a really hard time of it, many counselors and therapists who are queer-friendly or transfriendly advertise in print and online publications for the queer community.

▶ **There's a difference between holding the door open for someone and pushing them through it.** Once you're out, past the toughest parts, and feeling all the relief of being

s.e.x.

out, you may want others you know to experience the same thing—even if you aren't entirely sure they're queer in the first place. Well-intentioned as that may be, it's never a good idea to pull someone kicking and screaming out the closet door.

You can talk to your maybe-definitely-in-the-closet friends about how great you feel right now, and about how much being out benefits you. You can share the things you did that helped make the process easier. Just be sure that you're also respecting their own pace and allowing them the same sort of time you needed to come out when you were ready to. When they're ready, they'll likely let you know, and then you can be the supportive, wonderful friend that you are, and tell them about all the mistakes you made coming out yourself. Maybe by then they'll be funny.

▶ **Celebrate yourself.** In the midst of all the complexities of getting used to your sexual identity, and amid all the mistakes you'll make, don't forget to take time out to really appreciate the good stuff. It takes guts to be honest about our sexual or gender identity when it's not easily accepted or considered the norm. It takes a lot to make yourself a little more vulnerable for the sake of living honestly, to have the patience and energy to work through all these issues with others while you're still getting to understand them yourself—but it's a truly great thing. While it's got its rough spots, it usually feels really good.

Do nice things for yourself. Have a coming out party with some close friends. Pamper yourself. Get a new haircut, buy some new books. Explore it all: write about what you're going through, talk to close friends you know are supportive, listen to music that makes you feel good about this.

Coming out isn't usually something we only have to do once in our lives,

---

did you know . . . ?

In 1977, when Harvey Milk became a city supervisor of San Francisco, he was the first out homosexual to be elected to public office in a large city in the United States. Milk knew that as an openly gay man in public office, his safety was precarious. Sadly, he was right: he was assassinated only a year later by a fellow official. However, Milk had prepared for his possible death, and recorded several tapes of his own words to share with the world should he not get the chance to pass them on himself. In those tapes, he said that if everyone who was gay, lesbian, or bisexual told their friends, family, coworkers, and fellow students the truth about who they were, then none of the stereotypes about queer people could stand in the light of reality. One of Milk's last recorded passages was, "If a bullet should enter my brain, let that bullet destroy every closet door in the country."

S.e.x.

it's a lifelong process. Since you'll be entering into new situations, new partnerships, new communities throughout your whole life, you'll probably have to make choices about coming out more than once, and go through it more than once.

As time goes by, as your support network grows, all that gets a lot easier, and your sexual identity through the years will usually become a more integral and effortless part of your entire personal identity. Even amid coming-out chaos, be sure to take care of and enjoy yourself and who you are. Sexuality is supposed to be about joy and about pleasure and about feeling good. Honor it—all parts of it—and you honor yourself.

on board
the relationship

IT'S PRETTY COMMON to assume that "relationship" means a heterosexual, monogamous, romantic and sexual relationship between two people, and that that sort of relationship is automatically the best or most important one we can have.

But *any* ongoing interaction we have with another person is a relationship. A platonic friendship is a relationship. We have relationships with our parents, siblings, teachers, bus drivers, boyfriends, girlfriends, and more casual sex partners. There need not even be another person involved for a relationship to exist: we also have relationships with our pets, and with the world we live in. How important any of the relationships we have are, no matter their type, and what place they have in our lives isn't assigned to us: it's individual.

When we enter into a sexual and/or romantic relationship with another person, we usually can't make many—if any—assumptions about what that word means and what the specifics of that relationship are, without discussing them with the person we're in a relationship *with*. The specifics of a relationship are things we need to think about, examine, discuss, and agree upon actively, not passively.

▪ "RELATIONSHIP" SHOULD BE A VERB ▪

Good sexual and/or romantic relationships take some effort, especially when it comes to communication, time management, and integration into all the other parts of your life. But ultimately, no relationship should take so much work to maintain that most of the time it isn't pretty easy to just enjoy yourself and the other person or people within it. Intimacy should feel good; it should be comfortable and beneficial to you and yours. Almost always, after you spend time with a partner—even in just thinking about your partner—you should feel cared for, happy, and rejuvenated, not physically or emotionally exhausted, stressed out, dissatisfied, or riddled with doubt or fear.

The reason to be in a romantic or sexual relationship is to be with, and get closer to, someone who makes you feel good, who is a friend as much as they are a lover, and who supports you, appreciates who you are, **as-is**, and vice-versa.

An intimate relationship being fun and joyful doesn't mean it's childish or not serious, nor does a relationship being a constant struggle or drama mean it must be true love (in fact, that's a good sign that it very much isn't). For people of any age, intimacy should be about celebrating, sharing, and enjoying your life with someone else—for however long it lasts, in whatever model works best for you.

▪ RELATIONSHIP MODELS: ▪
What Works for *You?*

When you're entering into a sexual or romantic relationship it's time to think about what's probably going to work best for you and yours. There is no one model or type of relationship that is best for everyone, no one label, no one set of rules and regulations, wants, and needs that fits all. Think it's a simple matter to define when someone is a boyfriend or a girlfriend? To get an idea of how different our ideas on that subject can be, check this out: Mediamark Research, Inc. found that in one large group,

while 38 percent of the girls said they had a boyfriend, only 29 percent of the guys said they had a girlfriend. That means that almost 10 percent of the girls had a "boyfriend" who didn't think he was one at all! It's not sound to just assume a relationship with someone based on arbitrary criteria: it's something we need to actively decide *with* our partners.

There's a lot of noise out there that healthy sex or love can ONLY happen within a certain context: within marriage, within heterosexuality, within a certain time frame, at a certain age, only if two people are "in love." However, healthy, beneficial sex and quality sexual relationships happen not in one specific framework, but in an environment that is tailored very specifically to best fit the people involved. Realistic expectations, a solid friendship, healthy boundaries, constant communication, and negotiation may be key, but trying to fit every person and every relationship into one ideal model is like everyone in town trying to fit into the same pair of jeans.

Active communication needs to be a constant in any relationship: you may find that, over time, the needs and wants of one or both of you have shifted, and you may need to discuss those things and renegotiate your agreements. Deciding on a relationship model, and on the specifics of your relationships and how you live in them, tends to be something ongoing, not something you choose and agree to for life. You don't have to feel the need to go on a first date with a monster checklist in your hand: you can start talking about it at a pace that feels comfortable to you both, when it becomes clear that you are going to spend more than one or two dates together. When you are in constant communication with a partner,

S.e.x.

what works for *you?*
Some things to think about to create a
relationship model that works for you and your partner:

- **Time together:** How much time, alone and with others, do you need from your partner? How much time do you have available to devote to the relationship yourself? What sorts of time are you looking for: private, with family and friends, at school, on the phone, on the Net?

- **Time apart:** What do you both need in terms of having enough time to manage all the parts of your life AND be sure you get plenty of time just to be by yourself, whether that's working on your artwork or just hanging out listening to music? How do you feel about your partner just dropping by, about what times are good for phone calls, and such?

- **You, them, and everybody else:** How do you want a partner to fit into all of your other relationships, with friends, family, the rest of your community? How much does each of you need in terms of family approval and inclusion? For instance, if you're queer, how do you both feel about being out or not with your family? What about disclosure to parents in terms of sex? How do you both feel about how much time you want to spend as a couple with all of your friends, and with your own friends without your partner? Are there any friends or family that do or might create conflicts you need to talk about (such as an ex who has since become a platonic friend)?

- **Fenced in:** Almost every sexual and romantic relationship has an invisible fence that defines what we want to be for us and our partners, and ONLY us and our partners. What are your limits and boundaries in terms of sexual activities? Are you comfortable with monogamy—only having each other as sexual/romantic partners—or a more open relationship? What level of openness is okay for you? Is flirting okay? Cybersex? Engaging in sexual activities with others? If so, what are your limits there, and how do you want to manage them? What are your partner's feelings: how do *they* define monogamy, an open relationship, or friends with benefits, and how does that mesh with your own needs and definitions?

- **Number one and number two:** What priority does a romantic or sexual relationship have for you? Do you and your partner(s) want or need it to come first, or after other priorities, like school, work, friends, family, sports, personal projects, or hobbies? What does each of you want when it comes to sex and the priority it has in your relationship? Are your wants and needs similar and compatible?

- **Grunt work:** How will you both shoulder responsibilities like birth control and safer sex, initiating and facilitating important discussions, managing joint plans with friends and family? Who pays for what? What joint responsibilities are both of you comfortable shouldering, now and later?

- **What's in a name:** What one calls a relationship or a partner can be a big deal. Is it important to you to be called the boyfriend or girlfriend, or not to be? Is your relationship casual

continues

s.e.x.

continued

or more formal? How do you want it to be? A lot of common relationship models have names like "friend with benefits," "boyfriend" or "partner" which may mean very different things to each of you. Do certain words or phrases carry special meaning or expectations for you, such as those (in)famous three little words: "I love you"?

- **End goals:** Some people enter relationships with certain expectations: sex, cohabitation, marriage, or lifelong partnership. If you and your partner have end goals, are you on the same page? If not, is there time and room for compromise, whether that means accepting this isn't a permanent relationship, one or both of you agreeing to adapt your end goals or just being willing to see how it goes over time to find out what's really best for this particular relationship?
- **Extra value:** How will you work practical issues related to values? For instance: If you or your partner doesn't believe in sex before marriage, how have you agreed to manage that? What ethics and values of yours are "dealbreakers"? Are there gender or relationship roles you feel you need, to make a relationship work? What expectations in terms of roles and values does your partner have for you? How can you manage and work out differences in values between you?
- **Emergency!** Do you know each other's individual styles of dealing with crisis? For instance, do you get quiet, withdrawn, or bottled up, while she's a yeller? How do you feel about privacy in crisis, in terms of what gets discussed with friends and what shouldn't? Communicating these things in advance, and working to find methods of crisis management that you both feel good about can help you to avoid a lot of misunderstandings and pain when you're already hurting or stressed out.

when you're fostering intimacy, a lot of this stuff will come up in casual conversation.

Relationships are active, not passive; over time, the nature of some relationships does change. Someone who has been a romantic or sexual partner for a while may start to feel more like a platonic friend, or vice-versa, or one portion of a relationship may become more or less important than another. Much of the time, people don't have great conflicts or feel devastated when a friendship or more casual relationship starts developing romantically or sexually; however, may people feel far differently when the opposite happens. That's not too surprising—our culture puts a lot of status on romantic relationships, often deeming them more important than other kinds of relationships. Plus, romantic and sexual relationships tend to be highly charged, and also include friendship and other aspects of intimate bonding and relating, so when those feelings start to fade or change, we may feel that we're losing something, rather than simply evolving and growing. It's entirely possible to move from a romantic relationship into a platonic friendship; often, it just takes time, some mental adjustments, and a person that we still care for and want to keep in our lives, even though it may be in a different way than we're used to.

Wheeeeee! NRE: New Relationship Energy

You're in a brand-new relationship, or have just met someone you're seriously into; you're head over heels. Just thinking about them makes you restless, anxious, dizzy, or giggly. You feel like you've found—and maybe you did!—the one person in the whole wide world who was made for you and you alone.

NRE feels fantastic, but it can do quite a number on your critical thinking. Very few of us can be particularly objective when we're head over heels or super-lusty. So, when making sexual and relationship choices in a brand new thing, you can rest assured that your judgment is bound to be a little wiggly.

When you're in that space, you need to use a little more caution than usual when making big decisions. Additional factors may also be at play: body or self-image issues, feeling pressured to be sexually active or have a sexual or romantic partner, fear of being alone, performance pressures, rebellion or conformity issues, and even simple curiosity.

Don't ditch your life when you're in a new relationship: keep up your platonic friendships and family relationships, and be sure you also get some quality time all by yourself, at least a couple of days or nights a week. Just add a little perspective, some limits and boundaries, and a wee bit of distance to the mix as needed. There's absolutely no reason you can't enjoy a new love and keep your head screwed on right at the same time.

▪ DATING: ▪
Different, Not a Dinosaur

Studies—and practical experience—are showing that fewer young adults are going out on dates now than ever before. According to the Child Trends DataBank, the percent of high-school seniors who report they never date rose from 14 percent in 1991 to 22 percent in 2001. And the frequency of dates has also declined: 34 percent of high-school seniors reported dating once a week or more in 1991, and ten years later, that figure was 29 percent. Of course, that may be because the definition of "dating" is changing: more often, dates now—especially at the start of relationships—are happening in groups, and more casually, instead of the formalized one-on-one dates your parents were likely used to. Too, right now, it's common for the start of more serious relationships to happen a bit more organically and fluidly, rather than with someone asking a partner to "go steady."

Dating isn't extinct, it's just changed over time. A basic definition for now might be: when a romantically unattached person has casual outings or spends time with one or various people in whom he or she has some romantic and/or sexual interest to discover if they both want to pursue those interests. Dating is, in a word, shopping: you're trying on different pairings and dynamics with different people before (or without) deciding if there's one that's just the right fit. When you're dating, you're not necessarily making a commitment yet to anyone; the aim is to test the waters, get to know people in different settings and social groups, and spend time with them to see if you'd LIKE to develop deeper romantic or sexual relationships with them over time. *Or not.* Dating

S.e.x.

can be everything from hanging out at a concert with a whole group of friends and your "date," or stepping it up a notch and going it alone with a date to dinner or lunch, on a beach day or hike, to a dance or other more formal social gathering, to a night spent in with a date, on your couch with a pile of movies. You may already know the person you're going on a date with, or you may find yourself on a "blind date," where friends or family have set you up with someone you're meeting for the first time. Someone in the process of dating may or may not be engaging in sexual activity with the people they're dating. Obviously, established couples can also have dates, even when they're past the stage of dat*ing*.

There's no rule in terms of sex or gender identity for who is supposed to ask whom out. Asking someone out on a date also doesn't have to be formal or require background music. It can be as simple as, "Hey, I'm going to the bowling alley with some friends later, and I'd like to spend some time with you, want to come with us?" or "Do you want to go to the movies or something together sometime? How about next Friday?" That doesn't mean you're not allowed to be nervous. But it really doesn't have to be a big, honking deal just to ask. Clichéd as it sounds, the worst someone can do is say no.

It's good protocol, when dating, to inform the people you're on dates with that you ARE dating, rather than making any sort of commitment just yet. They don't need to know the name and Social Security number of every single person you've recently dated or are dating, but informing them that you are considering others is polite and considerate. Everybody's got a different theory about the right time to say, "Hey, by the way, I don't know how you're

feeling, but right now, I'm still testing the waters here," so when to say that is really a matter of personal preference and just feeling things out as you go.

 What a lot of people do now, rather than more casual, gradual dating, is what we call **"serial monogamy,"** going from one serious partner to the next, without either spending some substantial single time in between, or spending more casual time with a person before making a commitment to them.

It's easy to get sucked into this sort of pattern, especially if we feel lonely, or feel like the only one of our friends who isn't part of a couple, or if our friends and family only approve of or recognize "serious" relationships. But hopping from serious relationship to serious relationship, without a breather or any downtime, can also skew our character judgment and make it harder for us to pay attention to negative patterns we keep ending up in. It can become difficult to keep the rest of our lives balanced with our romantic lives, allowing us less of the time we need to figure out what we really want in relationships.

Know how you're supposed to wait at least twenty minutes after eating before you go swimming? Apply a similar rule to big-time relationships, and you'll do just fine.

Let's face it: some dates are GREAT dates, some dates are total yawners where you and someone else find out you just don't connect, and some dates are just plain awful. (Even bad dates, believe it or not, can be fun in their own weird way. The guy with the bizarre pet ferret he brought in his jacket to the ballet or the girl who accidentally tripped the waiter by showing off her dance moves at the table make pretty excellent stories on a rainy day, after all.) Dates aren't synonymous with commitment, and how many dates you have with someone is up to you. If the first two dates are lackluster but something tells you to give it a bit more time, go ahead and give it another shot. If a date is so painfully bad you know you do NOT want to go there again, there's no need to. In those cases, a simple (albeit sometimes awkward) statement at the end of the date—at whatever point you decide is the end—that you just aren't feeling it will suffice.

Dating is also a good way to find out if you feel ready or able, at a given time, to pursue relationships at all. Sometimes, a few dates— or a conversation about stepping things up a notch that just doesn't feel right—can make clear that, at a given time, it's really not what you or the other person is up for.

better safe than sorry

 WHEN on dates with new people, or in new relationships, do be sure to also keep your safety in mind. Tell your folks, a sibling, or friend where you're going and with whom, when you go out with them for the first time or two, just to be on the safe side. The United States has the highest rate of date rape in the world, and date rape is especially pervasive among young adults. To find out how to protect yourself, see page 235.

On the other hand, at a certain point, you may discover that after a couple dates with someone your feelings ARE growing, and you DO want to pursue something deeper with them. You may even feel you want to stop dating others to focus on them. You both get to talk about and decide that as you go, in terms of what relationship model you want and what pace feels right to you both.

I say: reclaim dating. Call it hanging out if you want, or call it something else entirely. But it's usually a good thing—even for people who are shy or feel socially awkward, even when you wind up on a date with pocket-ferret-guy. And, ideally, gradual dating can be the best way to start ANY kind of romantic or sexual relationship.

INTERNET DATING

It's a misperception that relationships can't begin, exist, or be sustained on the Net. But it's also a misperception that you can have the *same sort* of relationships on the Net you can have in person.

Popular Internet dating venues such as chat rooms and messaging, as well as Internet personals, are a fine way to get to know someone, as long as you're following some basic safety practices. But they're a way to get to know only one aspect of someone. Think about it this way: If you only knew your friend or partner in a classroom, would you know them the same way you do when you also see them at home, alone and with friends, with your family and theirs, at work and at play?

Often, when we're on the computer talking to someone, it's in our leisure time. We get to take as long as we like to say something, and can even edit it as we go, something we can't do when speaking. Our

s.e.x.

writing skills may give the impression that the way we write is the way we are—when often, that isn't the case. If we get involved with someone we haven't met, we may find that it feels easier to get closer to them without the static of physical attraction, face-to-face talking, without having to see how a person meshes or doesn't with our friends and family. Overall, it can be really easy to sustain illusions about people in online relationships, more easy than it is to get out of touch with reality in in-person relationships.

basic internet safety

- Withhold very personal information for a while. Keep home addresses, school names, phone numbers, last names, and the like, to yourself. Once you've been talking to someone online for a few months, if you want to know them more, you may even want to set up a public meeting *before* you give out information that could result in stalking or other dangers. Often, we're able to get a better feel for who someone really is by being around them in person than online or even on the telephone.

- Don't **ever** meet anyone from the Net alone or in a private or unfamiliar place the first couple of times. Make sure you tell someone you can count on—a close friend, a family member—where you're going and at what time to expect you back. If you use a cell phone, make arrangements for that person to call you a half-hour into a meeting, to make sure everything is going okay. If a person you're meeting balks at the smart, cautious steps you're taking, that's often a big sign that their motives aren't safe. If you meet someone from online and pick up a

weird vibe, trust your instincts, and get outta there, even in a public place.

- Be honest. If you're sixteen, don't say you're nineteen. If you're male, don't say you're female. There is a person on the other computer you're communicating with, and purposefully deceiving them—or they deceiving you—for whatever reason, isn't okay or safe for anyone. Recognize that many people online are NOT honest, sometimes about very critical things, like their gender, age, or relationship status.

- Keep your radar up for weird or inappropriate questions. Someone asking you how you masturbate, or if you're a virgin, the first few times you talk to them, probably isn't on the up-and-up. Someone asking for personal photos or a blow-by-blow physical description is cruising, or even just looking for something to masturbate to, rather than trying to get to know you. Someone who tries a sneaky way to get you to give them information you're withholding—for instance, if you don't give them your phone number, but they then ask what school you go to, what street you live on, if you have a private line—is probably not trustworthy.

Safety issues aside, the prime catch phrase with Net relationships is: *Walk, don't run.*

Don't get too invested in those relationships before you meet that person and establish a relationship in the whole context of your life and theirs—not just a small sliver of it. Starting to talk about moving, engagement, or marriage, for instance, before you've even met someone is unrealistic and pretty kooky. This is real life here, not a Meg Ryan and Tom Hanks movie.

We may like to think that in-person physical attraction and chemistry are irrelevant, but more often than not, they're *very* relevant. The way we communicate together in person, the way the rhythms of our lives do or don't work together, and how a partner works with our friends and family are all very important, too.

It's ultimately best to consider the Net stuff dating until you meet the other person. If and when you take the step to in-person dating, mating, and relating, and that's all going well, that's the time to start getting more serious.

▪ WITHOUT A MAP: ▪
Alternative Relationships

"Standard" relationships—like being a monogamous boyfriend/girlfriend couple—have plenty of cultural support, media coverage, and in-person modeling. Even when we want to reconfigure them, shake them up, we have a lot of examples with which to contrast and compare.

But what about relationships that aren't as visible, or those that are considered wrong or unacceptable, even if they seem right as rain to us?

GLB RELATIONSHIPS

Despite myths to the contrary, queer relationships tend to go a whole lot like straight ones do. The absence of certain opposite-gender patterns and expectations, as well as living outside established norms, may bring about some differences, but overall, between two people, relationships are relationships are relationships.

But some special issues *can* come into play. If only one partner is out of the closet, things can get pretty tense. Baby steps are often helpful here, like coming out to one mutual friend at a time, or to the out partner's family first. People rushed out of the closet tend not to adjust well, and taking things at the right pace for them is very important. The other partner's needs need to come into play, too, though, and sometimes, simple affirmations or reminders that they are very much NOT a dirty secret are a big help and comfort.

U-hauling

One of the biggest mistakes some of us make when we're newly out is to rush into our first relationship so fast that it takes less time from a first date to picking out china patterns than it did to pull together that outfit we're wearing today.

It's very easy to get caught up in the rush not only of being out, but of being out WITH a partner for the first time. Your first same-sex partnership may very well feel like THE same-sex partnership, but what's the rush?

There is no special magic that makes same-sex relationships move any faster than opposite-sex ones, though often there may be an increased intensity due to the smallness of queer communities and the incredible relief at finding someone who shares your feelings. Take your time and get to know not just the person you're with, but your own identity before you start packing. Just as with any kind of relationship, if it's meant to be, it'll keep at a healthy, sane pace.

s.e.x.

People of all orientations may discover they have romantic or sexual feelings for friends, and that's tricky for anyone. But it can be doubly tricky for those who are queer: Not only is a risk being taken when it comes to stating feelings that may not be reciprocated, and that might jeopardize a friendship, but an additional risk is being taken in exposing an orientation that the friend and others may not know about, or may not react well to. It's also pretty hard to express romantic feelings for someone AND come out at the same time.

Young adult queer relationships often have another major issue, which is that it's common for at least one partner to be questioning, experimenting with someone, or to discover that their feelings about being queer are too uncomfortable for them to live with. Because of the cultural controversy around same-sex relationships, in some circles, having a same-sex partner is a rebellion, a novelty, a mark of cool or sexual adventurousness. In others, it's simply unacceptable. As in any other kind of relationship, people's motives can be other than they appear, or even other than they think they are.

Having a relationship go kaput because one partner discovers they just can't deal with being in the relationship can and does happen in ANY kind of relationship. But it can sting a bit more when you're queer, because it may feel like a rejection of *you*, your identity or your orientation, things you might still feel shaky about yourself. You may have also taken extra risks in having a same-sex relationship, such as being a bit more out than you were ready for, or burning bridges with friends or family who were unaccepting of the relationship.

A good way to retain perspective in queer relationships, especially given cultural stigmas, is to seek out support in your queer community. Double or group dates with other GLBT folks can be both fun and helpful. Being able to be out and hang out with other gays, lesbians, and bisexuals besides your partner can be a godsend. Anybody queer in our culture needs more community than just sexual partners: having others around you who aren't your sexual or emotional partners, and having plenty of time with your partner outside one room or on the phone can be a real lifesaver. Even your straight friends and family can sometimes be more help than you know: in any marginalized group, it's easy to get tunnel vision and forget that how things should go in queer relationships really isn't that different from how they should go in straight ones.

ACROSS THE LINES

We hear all the time that "opposites attract." In our culture, many things are set up or seen as opposites that really aren't: race, gender, appearance, religion, or economic or social status. The idea of what a "normal" relationship is sometimes integrates personal or cultural biases into those so-called norms; in a more enlightened world, there would be absolutely no reason for interracial relationships to be considered any different from those between people of the same race.

People of different races, sizes, or shapes aren't "opposites," though the environments they grew up in and live in, and the approaches people have to them can differ, sometimes vastly. Same goes for those who are wealthy and those who are poor, those who are loners and those who are popular, those who are atheist and those who are religious. Very few people want to date an exact replica of themselves, and very few people have control over whom they have feelings for. So, it's typical for people to date those who differ from them in any number of ways.

But when those differences are profound—or appear profound to others—it can cause some conflicts. Some friends, families, or communities may have overt or hidden biases, like racism, xenophobia, classism, fatphobia, or homophobia, that make relationships between certain groups taboo or problematic.

Bias is tough stuff. It tends to be learned really early in life, and is very, very hard for most people to unlearn, especially if that bias is supported by the people or culture around them. It's rarely overcome by arguments, by grandstanding, or by telling someone what an awful, intolerant bigot they are (even when they're being one). Many people with bias, intolerance, or bigotry have little choice but to learn to adapt right now, due to the law as well as the changing, merging world we live in. So, some folks' resistance may be stronger than ever, because they feel forced to adapt to new circumstances.

Bigotry is best unlearned by simple, slow exposure to whatever group or relationship someone has an issue with. In other words, if your family has an issue with your interracial relationship, avoiding them altogether or just yelling about it isn't as productive as slowly letting them get to know your partner in contexts that are less threatening to them, like a family dinner or a school picnic. Talking about issues of bias outside the context of your relationship, such as discussions of current events, can also be helpful, because those are less in-your-face. As with many types of less-accepted relationships, patience is also key: sometimes, time alone will take care of things. You might also find some extra help in support or activist groups that focus on tolerance.

The hard part is that some people aren't ever able to—or don't want to—unlearn bias at all. You may have to face the fact that your relationship will never be accepted by your family or current circle of friends. You may even decide that, given a certain level of bias, you can't maintain that relationship in a way that's healthy or beneficial for everyone. Or you may decide to distance yourself from those whose biases are putting up the roadblocks, or sever your relationships with them. That can be a very hard choice to make.

AGE-DISPARATE RELATIONSHIPS

You're fifteen, he's twenty-one. You're twenty, she's fourteen. You're seventeen, she's thirty-six. You're twenty-one, he's forty. You're looking at an age-disparate relationship, where both of you are dating outside—and in some cases, *way* outside—your general age group. Age-disparate relationships hold special challenges for people of all ages, but they're more challenging when they involve teens. For an adult, any sort of sex with a teen can carry very heavy legal consequences; for a teen, a relationship with an adult may involve serious power imbalances. For instance, a partner who is a legal adult has some rights and liberties—including reproductive rights—that a teen does not. Adults also often have more autonomy, mobility, and agency, as well as more life experience.

An older person may be dating someone for the same reasons anyone of any age dates anyone else. Or they may be dating someone younger for some pretty crappy reasons.

s.e.x.

They may realize that the younger person is less savvy than someone their own age, especially when they're in love: an older person has a level of hindsight when it comes to teen love and what it can feel like that a teen doesn't yet have. The appeal for the older person may be that they have more power in the relationship, that they can control things more easily than with a peer, or can get a younger partner to go along with behaviors, risks, or scenarios their peers would know better than to accept. The younger partner may not question things like risky sex, for instance, because they trust that someone older must know what they're doing.

A person may even be dating someone much younger for reasons that aren't horrible, but aren't that great, either, such as to impress friends, to feel younger, or to be able to back out of a relationship more easily. Younger people may also want to date someone much older because they'd really rather *not* be treated, in all respects, like an equal partner—which includes being fully accountable and making choices, rather than having someone else take all or most of the responsibility. Or, the younger partner might feel that dating someone older improves their social status, gives them a more distinct identity, or demonstrates greater independence or sexual maturity.

For more information on the legal aspects of age-disparate relationships and statutory rape, see page 144.

---

did you know . . . ?

Statutory rape is sex between an adult and a person under the legal age of consent, and there are some pretty unnerving realities about teens in relationships with legal adults. While there are exceptions, the rule is that these relationships are often detrimental for the younger partner. Jennifer Manlove, PhD, of Child Trends DataBank, shared the following facts at the 2005 Conference on Sexual Exploitation of Teens:

- Teen women in statutory rape situations more often keep relationships secret.
- Teen women with a legal adult partner have higher rates of drug and alcohol use.
- Teen men and women alike with older partners are more likely to drop out of high school, and less likely to use contraception and safer sex.
- Teen women in sexual relationships with legal adults are more likely to become pregnant and have a teen birth.
- The youngest teens are more likely than older teens to have first sex with a legal adult partner.

In addition, a Washington State study of 535 teen mothers revealed that the first pregnancies of 62 percent of the participants were preceded by experiences of molestation, rape, or attempted rape. The mean age of their offenders was 27.4 years.

s.e.x.

That isn't to say there aren't exceptions. Some young adults have had and do have healthy relationships with an older partner. Just as big differences in wealth, style, social status, or personality can be a conflict, but can also offer exciting variety and contrast, so can age differences, for some people. Some young adults may feel that they have more in common with partners of a different age than with partners their own age. For some people in age-disparate relationships, there's no strong draw to this age or that one: it's simply a matter of mutual attraction.

The biggest way to spot that what you've got going on ISN'T kosher is when the word "secret" becomes your mantra. The elder partner on the up-and-up in an age-disparate relationship is willing to face the hard challenges of that relationship and go at the same pace as with something more easily accepted, sometimes even a bit more slowly due to resistance or wariness on the part of family or community. If a partner is rushing sex (or manipulating you into rushing it); if they don't take the time to meet and spend time with your friends and family, while being open about the fact that you have a romantic relationship; if they can't be seen with you in certain settings, or if you're told outright to keep what's going on a big secret, then you're treading emotionally dangerous ground. Someone in a position of authority over you is an extra-big issue: coaches, teachers, the parents or adult family members of your friends are all people who really shouldn't be coming on to you, even if they do feel attracted, or know you are. As adults, they should be aware (and usually are, even if they deny it to teens) that there is a gross imbalance of power there—because there is, whether or not you want to see it. It's not romantic for someone to take advantage of their power due to their age or yours: it's exploitive.

A healthy age-disparate relationship shouldn't be all that different from a healthy same-age relationship. The adage that age doesn't matter is wrong: age DOES matter, and does create differences that often need to be managed and compensated for. And for someone older, age *should* matter; it should provide them with the perspective to know how to choose and manage their relationships decently, and the wisdom and patience to do so.

FWBS AND HOOKUPS

Some people want a sexual relationship, but not a romantic one, for any number of reasons. Friends with benefits (or an FWB) may occur because two friends have sexual attraction and desire and decide to pursue it; hookups or a one-night stand can happen for similar reasons. Sometimes FWB relationships or other more casual scenarios evolve into a romantic relationship, and sometimes they do not.

When an FWB or sexual friendship IS what both people truly want, it can be as healthy a relationship as any other, so long as both partners are communicating, being honest and respectful. Romance doesn't have to be present for care and respect to occur. Some people may even find these types of relationships are better for them because of all the assumptions and baggage romantic relationships can carry, or because they just don't have the time in their lives to truly nurture a more constant relationship. For some sets of people, a casual sexual relationship IS the one that suits their individual chemistry best.

s.e.x.

But there can be some pitfalls. If you're in an FWB because you want to get off, but don't want to have to deal with another whole person, you've knocked on the wrong door. Just because two people aren't boyfriend/girlfriend, in love, or making long-term commitments, that doesn't mean it's okay for one partner to disregard the other or be cavalier about their feelings.

Casual sex, hookups, and FWBs are also a bad idea when one partner is accepting something very different from what he or she really wants, or entering into the scenario with the hope that it'll become a different relationship entirely. They're also a bad idea for anyone who has trouble being really vigilant about safer sex and their sexual health; an FWB is not for someone who can't be pretty darned direct about those issues, as in "We are using a condom or we are not doing this at all."

Who's a good "candidate" for a healthy FWB or casual sex? Someone pretty independent, confident, and autonomous. Someone keenly aware of both their limits and their expectations. Someone able to be very savvy when it comes to sexual health, birth control (when applicable), safer sex, and laying down the law with a partner about those issues. Someone who really only WANTS a casual sex situation, not because it's all that's available, but because that's their ideal. And someone for whom the other person in the scenario also is all of the above.

OPEN RELATIONSHIPS

Monogamy—being with one sexual partner, only—isn't a rule in romantic or sexual relationships, it's a preference and a choice. Monogamy works for a whole lot of people just fine, and is what plenty of people want

and need. But for others, it may not work so well, or they simply may not want that model: they may prefer an open relationship or a polyamory.

 Polyamory is a term for having more than one partner at once, usually with at least one of the partnerships being a committed one. Polyamory isn't "cheating," nor is it simply "dating." It's about making a conscious choice to have more than one ongoing partner, with full disclosure to, and agreement from, everyone involved. Open relationships may involve more casual secondary relationships or hookups, perhaps even in the company of the other partner; polyamory usually involves more than one partnership, all of which involve some level of commitment.

For example, Jane has a committed sexual and romantic relationship with Jack, and sees him every few days, but sees Joe every couple of months for a sexual and romantic relationship as well. Both Joe and Jack know what the situation is and have agreed to whatever terms and conditions work best for all of them. Those conditions may involve amounts of time spent together, certain activities that are okay with one partner but not another, and/or different commitments to each. They should also include an insistence on safer sex religiously among all partners. There may be various levels of disclosure: some polyamorous people enjoy sharing all the intimate details of their other partnerships among partners; some poly partners don't want or need that much information.

Sometimes, poly may mean that everyone involved in a given poly partnership is sexually involved together, as in a threesome. That is less common than those partnerships existing somewhat separately.

Honesty and communication are the keywords here, to a degree that's difficult for a lot of people. Keeping communication channels open with one partner is a pretty big challenge as it is. Adding more partners to the mix—even only once, or very casually—doesn't just mean making more time for more partners; it means having the time and the ability to be honest and open with more than one partner. It also requires some pretty good negotiation skills. In a polyamorous or open relationship, everyone involved is going to have to come to agreements that work for all of them fairly, and because we all have different wants and needs, that can take a lot of work and get really frustrating sometimes.

Open relationships can be challenging for some, because it's common to experience jealousy or insecurity when others are sharing your partner's romantic or sexual attention. Problems can also arise when there are time or attention constraints; when someone in the entire relationship is not being honest, or has questionable motives; when lack of family or social acceptance becomes an issue; or when one partner just believe in their heart that monogamy really is the best option.

If you're thinking about an open relationship, start talking. And get good at listening—to everyone involved. You're going to need to be able to do a whole lot of it. If you, or anyone else involved, can't do that before the fact, or you'd rather avoid it

and just jump right in, you're walking into a minefield.

▪ THOSE THREE LITTLE WORDS ▪

Feeling and saying *"I love you"* is no small thing for a lot of us. Just three words—but so much can be read into them or meant by them, it's dizzying. One person may say them very casually, while to another they're sacred. What "I love you" means to you may be completely different from what it means to someone else. Some people aren't comfortable using those words at all, either because they feel they're so overused as to be meaningless, because they feel those words imply actions they're not comfortable with, or because they're just plain scared.

What's "real" love mean, anyway? Would that there were one answer to that question!

Overall, love means that you accept and respect someone for who they are, strengths and weaknesses *both,* not just for who you want them to be or what role you want them to play in your life. In many ways, "real love" is about friendship more than anything else. Love usually means you care very deeply for someone, not as *what* they are to you, but *who* they are to you, as-is. Real love usually comes without many conditions: the person we love doesn't have to look a certain way, be our boyfriend or girlfriend, or call us a certain number of times a week. Love means support, even when giving that support means a result that isn't so great, like supporting a partner in going to the college they want to go to most, even though it's two thousand miles away. It involves really caring for someone: not just when they're well, but when they're sick; not just when they're happy, but when

S.E.X.

they're upset, too. In many ways, love feels like being **home**—that place we feel is safe for us, where we don't have to worry about impressing anyone, or always saying exactly the right thing. It's giving as well as receiving, for both parties. When someone loves *you,* it should also involve all of these sorts of things.

It's sometimes easier to talk about what love isn't than what it is. Love isn't obsession, infatuation, or fixation. It isn't control, rescue, or ownership. It isn't validation of self-worth or self-image. It isn't a means to make someone stay with you or do something specific for you. It isn't a way to manipulate someone's emotions. It doesn't make us unbalanced or dizzy—that's how passion, new relationship energy, and being "in love" make us feel. More than anything, real love tends to make us feel whole and grounded.

It's normal to be nervous when you start to feel love developing: it may even make you want to withdraw a bit, because loving someone is big, scary stuff. If and when you want to say those three little words, the other person may not say them back, or may be overwhelmed, shocked and surprised that you've said them. They may not yet feel ready to say them, or they may even say "I love you, too," just because they don't want to hurt you, even if they aren't sure about their feelings yet. And someone who says it to you first might get any of those same reactions from you.

As with anything else that involves another person, all of that is okay: just talk it out. As partners, we don't always have to be in exactly the same place at the exact same time for our relationship to be healthy and beneficial; we both just need to feel okay about where we're both at. Talk about what

those words mean to you, and what you mean by them if and when you say them. You can even talk about why you don't like the L-word, about baggage you may have attached to it, about misuse of that word. Heck, you and yours can invent new words altogether for your feelings, if you like. Everyone communicates differently, so words may not even be the best way to show the love you feel. When people say you "just know" that you love or are loved, most of what they're talking about is actions, not words.

You can't screw up by really loving someone. You can get your heart broken, a relationship may not go as you'd like, or you might be disappointed, but these are all inherent dangers when we live like real people, not locked away in some small room by ourselves. Loving someone for real is pretty much always a good thing. Same goes for really being loved.

soulmates and forevers

IT FEELS wonderful to be involved with someone who says they'll always love us, forever and ever—and means it. Yet, most romantic relationships of our youth will not be the relationships we're in forty, twenty, ten years—or even one year—down the road. We're much more likely to find our longest partnerships when we're out of our teens and twenties: the average span of a young adult's first sexual or romantic relationship is less than six months. According to Mediamark Research, Inc., only around 12 percent of teenagers are currently in a relationship that has lasted more than one year. That reality does *not* make your feelings of eternal love any less important, nor do you need to be jaded about the whole works. But a little reality can go a long way, not just in terms of protecting your heart, but in terms of keeping your current relationship as excellent as it can be.

Appreciate and honor those feelings of forever, but do most of your planning for now and the not-too-distant future, and spend most of your time right here in the present. That way, not only can you have a relationship that's grounded, you can be sure you don't miss all the great things going on today that often get taken for granted when you're too busy daydreaming about tomorrow.

▪ THE TEST OF TIME: ▪
Long-Term Relationships

Most couples therapists and relationship experts consider the first six months of a relationship to be the period in which two people are getting to know each other; what comes afterward is considered long-term. These professionals usually work with older people, however; young-adult life tends to have a different pace and velocity. For teens and young adults, feelings are often more intense far earlier, and attachments form more quickly. To account for that, let's say that if you've been in a relationship for three or four months, you can consider yourself to be entering something long-term, by your clock.

Here are some things to expect, if you're going the distance.

WHAT'S TYPICAL IN LONG-TERM RELATIONSHIPS?

▶ **More vulnerability:** It's normal to start to feel more vulnerable, even more insecure, when a relationship has lasted a while. Your partner knows you better and you've likely shared a lot more with them than with someone you've only dated a short time.

▶ **Doubts about hanging in there:** There's nothing wrong with doubt or questioning a relationship. It's not a sign of disloyalty or betrayal, it's what people do who are trying to stay aware and keep evaluating things as they go. There's also nothing wrong with wondering if, maybe, you're missing out on other things because of a long-term relationship when you're young. Remember: there is no one type of relationship that is best for everyone, so if you start feeling that something long-term and serious isn't right for you, it's okay to switch gears.

What feels best to you is only up to you. Solid relationships where two people have mutual feelings for one another *are* hard to come by, and nurturing them does take an investment of time, patience, and energy. Few people in relationships of quality are going to be missing out on anything valuable, because little is more valuable. Dating is fun and great, and certainly, more experiences with more people give us greater perspective, but we can get that perspective from all types of relationships, not just romantic or sexual ones. So, if you've got a really good thing, and you know you want something long-term, don't take it for granted.

Obviously, if a long-term relationship is keeping you from achieving other goals, if it's causing conflict, if you just don't feel able to maintain it, or if you question it more than you actually enjoy it, it's worth considering terminating or changing the terms of the relationship. And if your friends and family are observing that this is the case with you, it's worth a listen. One aspect of long-term relationships is that, over time, a partner becomes more involved in your inner circle: your closest friends, your family. When they're a viable part of that core, you're both going to have to work with that integration, and give it more cooperative care and attention than you did when you were more casually dating.

If you are in something long-term and have family or friends who are skittish about it, or you are—talk it out. If they have specific concerns (such as your rushing into marriage, or relationship blind spots you seem to have), hear them out, tell your side, come to compromises if you can. Even if you don't agree with what's being said, hearing it can alert you to issues to watch out for, and working with everyone can strengthen *all* your relationships.

▶ **Less sex, or sex with a slightly different flavor than you might be used to:** It's common for the "honeymoon period" to fizzle a bit over time. As a couple settles into a relationship more, sexual activity can move away from the forefront, and that doesn't mean anything is terribly wrong. The heat and intensity may ebb because the newness is replaced with familiarity and a more diverse array of ways to share intimacy. Partners may likely have sex less often over time, or it may have peaks and valleys. But usually, in good relationships, while sex may become less frequent, the *quality* of that sex improves because you've had time to get to know one another, learn about each other's responses, likes and dislikes, wants and needs.

For people who wanted to wait for sex until they were in a long-term relationship, it may mean the beginning of sex for you, a whole new aspect of your relationship to get used to and work with.

If you and your long-term partner are still holding off on sexual activity, until marriage or just a far later date, you may find that waiting gets a little more challenging the longer you're together. If that's the case, revisit and reevaluate both your needs and wants in terms of celibacy. Make sure that is what you both still want, and if it isn't, talk about how to make your changing wants or values work between you. If you and/or your partner find that decreased sexual frequency or intensity is an issue for either or both of you, talk it out; reinvest yourself in the relationship and in the fun of refreshing its spark. Be creative: now you've got even more tools to do that, because you know one another even better.

▶ **Disagreements:** When you're just getting to know someone, it's normal to let a lot of things that bother you slide. You're still getting your feet wet, finding your comfort zones, and developing the trust and comfort to be able to really speak your mind.

So, if you find that you and yours argue a bit more than before, there's no need to leap to the conclusion that you've hit the skids. Certainly, if those arguments are ugly or become constant, or if you find you disagree on things that pose a very big problem— like birth control, life goals, or people near and dear to you—you've got a problem. But a few more conflicts or

s.e.x.

arguments, or ones that aren't resolved quite as easily with a kiss and a flower, are normal when two people stick around long enough to have things to disagree on, and the confidence to disagree.

▶ **Relationship Shifts and Tougher Breakups:** At some point, you may be looking at a relationship model change or a breakup. It's pretty obvious that the longer you're with someone, the tougher a change or a breakup often is. When they take longer to get to, they can take longer to get over. Inertia can be a huge factor in long-term relationships that aren't going so well. It may seem easier to learn to deal with a dysfunctional relationship than to go through a breakup, to be alone, to be dating, to cultivate new relationships. It usually isn't. When something is over, it's best to let it be over. Seek out a new way for both of you to be happy apart, or as something new, instead of going nuts trying to make something keep going that just isn't working or has run out of gas.

If something sudden and intense facilitates a breakup—like a partner's cheating, an accidental pregnancy, or a job or school transfer—you're probably going to need a good deal of time to grieve, and plenty of support from friends and family, throughout. However, sometimes a longer relationship does reach a natural end, in a way that's oddly pretty comfortable and easy.

LOOKING TOWARD THE FUTURE

It's typical for long-term couples to eventually live together, to get married, or to commit to one another in other ways available to them.

While for those of certain religions and/or cultural beliefs, living together before marriage isn't an option, baby steps are a good idea. Living on your own or with roommates for some time, for instance, before living with a romantic partner, is a very good idea, and everyone can do that.

If you do move in together, expect to be surprised. Couples who don't argue or fight at all may discover that sharing the same space or spending a lot more time together can create conflicts. When you see each other while rushing to get to work or class, when you're crabby and tired, when you're doing the dishes or laundry, it's often a different deal than only seeing each other at prearranged times. Having to bring everyday things into your relationship—like rent, bills, and who leaves their dirty underpants where—often takes some serious adjustments. That's not to say living together doesn't have its high points. It's great to wake up with your partner in the morning, fun to make dinners together and to share a home. But all of those things can take some serious getting used to, and couples who move in together may even discover that their great relationship isn't so great with that level of union (or that one or both partners would really prefer to live alone, even when they've got a great relationship).

Same goes for engagement, marriage, or commitment ceremonies. If you're looking toward marriage, talk about it with your partner in depth, with a keen eye toward ALL you'd be opting into—not just daily life and family stuff, but also legal and financial issues, as well as what you and yours really feel about certain aspects of marriage, such as gender inequity. Talk to friends and family, to community or religious guides or mentors. Long engagements are completely accepted, so if marriage to you is a major tenet of commitment, you can take the first step by becoming engaged, then take all the time you both really need to consider everything. If the person you're with really **IS** "The One," then there's no hurry, because they're not going anywhere.

What's the best recipe for marriage or cohabitation that stands the test of time, with both partners happy? **Don't rush it.** Don't agree to either arrangement because of pressure from anyone, including your partner, and don't try to push a partner into anything when they aren't ready or interested. Work to be aware of your own expectations, of what living together or being married really means to you, and why. Be realistic and be honest. If you feel your mind changing at any point in the process, pipe up and say something; don't keep it inside for fear of hurting your partner, or because NOT getting married or living together scares you. Be flexible with yourself and your partner: during all of our lives, we grow and change all the time, so learning to be flexible is a major key to having healthy relationships, in any situation.

▪ DYSFUNCTION JUNCTION: ▪
The Crummy Stuff

A lot of relationship problems aren't the end of the world, and can be managed and repaired, sometimes without even having to work all that hard. The biggest part of the battle isn't fixing problems, so much as it is recognizing that there ARE problems, and being willing to address them and work a

little to seek out healthier patterns of behavior. According the Mediamark, Inc. research, more than half of all young adults report that their relationship causes them stress, and it's likely a lot of that could be alleviated by just being able to recognize dysfunction when it's in the mix, and developing skills to manage it. Facing problems and working through them doesn't have to be awful: for many people, doing so strengthens their relationships with their partners and themselves.

The following isn't an all-inclusive list, by many means; there are whole sections of every bookstore with books on relationship issues. Rather, these are just some of the more typical, key problems that young adults report facing in relationships.

All by myself: We're often given the impression that it's better to be in a love relationship—any relationship—than not to be in one, and that just isn't so. Being single doesn't mean a person is undesirable or unattractive. In many cases, a single person simply isn't interested in relationships at a given time, or is waiting to meet someone whose needs and wants will really work with their own.

Entering into or staying in romantic or sexual relationships primarily to avoid being alone is a really bad idea. Not only is it hard to have good judgment when you're so freaking scared of being alone or sick of your own company, but it usually means you're using the other person to try to fix feelings that you need to work on yourself. It's also all too easy, when you're in a relationship and deathly afraid of being alone, to become very dependent and clingy, which can really tank even a good relationship. A study

s.e.x.

done by the Department of Psychology at Macquarie University in Australia found that, in relationships, both partners were equally dissatisfied when either partner suffered anxiety over abandonment or fear of being alone. Too, some experts have linked fear of abandonment with abusive behaviors: a partner afraid of being alone may be more inclined to try to control their partner, to ensure that they stick around.

If you're in a relationship, be sure to give time and energy to parts of your life that are just yours alone: your friendships, your hobbies, your goals and dreams. Try to balance the time you spend together with the time you spend alone. Or, just wait for intimate relationships until you feel pretty good about yourself and your life just as it is, so that you've got a self and a life to share in the first place, rather than seeking out partners to provide you with one.

For relationship's sake: Feeling funny because you're eighteen and have never been kissed and can't wait another second? Sexually frustrated? Does it seem like all your friends are in a relationship right now, and you'd better get one too? Are you with someone just because they're interested in you, even though you're not as interested in them? Feel the need to prove to parents, friends, or yourself that you're mature enough, attractive enough, to have a relationship, no matter with whom? Just plain bored?

Entering into or staying in a relationship just because you are primarily concerned with "having a relationship" is a really good way to ensure that at least one of you, and likely both, will feel like crap in pretty short order. The good stuff is always worth waiting for. If you feel the need to have some things in the interim, you can, and you can do it in ways that are fair and healthy. You can date more casually. If you feel sexually frustrated, you can masturbate. If you're lonely, you can make friendships and community connections based on interests other than love and sex.

how do you find a fantastic relationship, anyway?

- **Be open:** If you refuse to believe anyone else could like or love you as you are, and keep all your doors and windows firmly closed and locked, there's no way for anyone else to get in in the first place.
- **Be prepared to be surprised:** The people you really click with, with whom you have a major love connection, may very well not look or act like your "type," or be anything like you idealized, expected, or imagined. That's often part of the adventure!
- **Be self-aware:** Learn who you are, what you want and need, and where you're going in your own life—with or without partners. That will put you in a much better place for knowing the good stuff when you see it than focusing on how others see you, who THEY are, and what they might want from you.
- **Learn to love and accept yourself:** It sounds cheeseball, but if you don't earnestly care for yourself first, and love and accept who you are, nobody else is going to be able to do it very well, either. Bonus: If you're really being yourself all the time, then when someone does fall for you, you don't have to wonder if it's really you they're into.
- **Trust your instincts:** When you feel in your guts that something just isn't right,

s.e.x.

chances are it's not. When your instincts tell you that something *is* really right? It probably is. By all means, temper those feelings with logic, but pay attention to your instincts: they're often pretty smart.

■ **Stop looking so hard:** You're more likely to find quality relationships when you're living all of your life fully, rather than spending every waking moment fixated on hooking up or finding a partner. Desperation isn't generally attractive to healthy people, and someone who will really love you for who you are is going to be attracted to you when you're following all of your dreams, as an active participant in your own life, clearly able to drive the car of your life all by yourself.

■ **Take safe risks:** "Nothing ventured, nothing gained" is the order of the day. To get something started or kick things into high gear, someone has got to make a move at some point—asking someone on a date, getting a phone number, expressing love or care, even just saying hello.

■ **Know you're always worthy:** Everyone IS deserving of love and affection. Everyone. That includes you.

Liar, liar, pants on fire: Lies and omissions can cause big problems in relationships, whether you're not being fully honest about your feelings, seeing someone else when you're supposed to be monogamous, saying you feel sexually ready when you really aren't, or staying in a relationship that is itself based on a pack of lies.

Sometimes, you may have to or want to wait a little to disclose things to a partner—for instance, it often takes sexual abuse survivors a little while to feel comfortable sharing that history—but important information does need to be shared, so if you're waiting, be sure you're doing what you can to get there in fairly short order. Between partners, even when it's hard to tell the truth—when it may mean hurting a partner's feelings or putting the relationship at risk—you should always be working toward it by just spitting the tough stuff out or taking small steps to get to being fully honest in time. That may even include telling a partner you have something important to share, but are not quite ready yet.

Drama major: A lot of people confuse drama with love, affection, or real connection. The higher the level of drama gets—friends or parents disliking a partner, promises of marriage, a profound age difference, even emotional or physical abuse—the more a feeling of love or passion may be assumed, because the emotional stakes are raised. That's understandable; after all, writers have been using that exact same device to elevate their readers' emotions for thousands of years. But.

Often, people are simply reacting to those escalated circumstances, and the drama can keep young couples together, but stand in the way of real love or bonding. So, if the drama kicks in, try to recognize it and remember that then, more than ever, is NOT the time to leap in blindly, but to step back and really look at what's going on.

Traffic patterns: One partner may want to move things along a lot faster or slower than the other—things like sex, commitment, being publicly out as a couple or as queer. Sometimes the general pace of a relationship flows pretty easily on its

s.e.x.

own, but sometimes you wind up with stalls, speeders, or bottlenecking, and you may need to direct your relationship traffic with a little more effort and intention. Either partner has the right and the ability to turn on a green, yellow, or red light at any time. If you find you're feeling rushed or stalled, or that the pace of your relationship just isn't in your control, stop where you are and evaluate. Talk to your partner about how you're feeling, and what pace is more comfortable for you and why.

You might WANT to be sexually active with a partner, but feel emotionally unprepared, or know you can't afford birth control or sexual healthcare. A partner may want to be monogamous, but be worried about doing that too soon and then feeling fenced in instead of enjoying it. Outside factors may also affect pace: parents may have rules or restrictions that don't allow for serious dating or sex yet. Relationships don't exist in a vacuum, and for young adults, all your choices don't get to be fully your own yet, so you may have to manage and accept limitations and disruptions to your ideal relationship MPH.

Tug o'war: Feel like you have to earn a partner's time, attention, or love? Are you making a partner work pretty hard for things you should be giving easily? Don't feel fully worthy, or feel someone you're seeing isn't? Do things just feel unbalanced?

Everyone who gives love, care, respect, and affection is worthy and deserving of love, care, respect, and affection. No one has to earn it. If you're having to work your buns off to get attention or time from your partner, if you often feel you're begging or pleading with them for the things you need, or if, on the other hand, you feel really reluctant to give very basic things to a partner, that inequity needs be repaired or you need to get out of that relationship.

A relationship is a lot like a seesaw: if one person isn't carrying their weight, and is making the other do all the work, somebody's going to stay stuck on the ground and the other person stuck dangling midair. To make the seesaw worth riding, both people need to be doing the give and take evenly .

▪ ADVENTURES IN SPLITSVILLE: ▪ Breakups and How to Deal

Even when a breakup is the best option, or when one or both parties really want one, it's just not a whole lot of fun. But it is safe to say that nearly everyone is going to have to deal with at least one in their lifetime, and there are ways to do a little damage control to take care of yourself and your ex or soon-to-be ex.

WHEN IS IT TIME?

Have you gone round and round with a given issue or set of issues, tried everything to make it work, to no avail, or have you (one or both of you) just given up? Is your relationship clearly not mutual or balanced? Do you spend more time arguing, fighting, or in uncomfortable silences than feeling good and enjoying each other? Do you and/or your partner just feel done with the relationship, or do certain aspects of it just no longer feel "there"—is the sexual attraction

S.E.X.

healthy/unhealthy

WHAT'S in a healthy relationship? According to Access Excellence, a national education program affiliated with former U.S. Surgeon General C. Everett Koop, in a healthy, beneficial relationship, both of you are:

- Able to find healthy ways to work through disagreements together
- Able to make decisions together
- Able to share honest feelings freely and trust each other
- Able to understand yourself more, not just your partner
- Able to respect one another's feelings and opinions, even if you disagree
- Feeling comfortable, respected, loved, supported, safe, and secure

WHAT'S expressly *un*healthy?

- My partner or I set or would like to set all or most of the rules for our relationship.
- My partner is, or I am, often jealous or possessive.
- My partner follows me around, checks up on me a lot, or insists I check in constantly, even when it's difficult or impossible for me to do, or I do any of these things to them.
- My partner is very concerned with how I look, what I wear, who I spend time with (friends, family, coworkers), and how much time I spend with others, or I have these strong urges to control about them in these respects. My partner or I may okay some friends or family, but only those who have a blind loyalty to them or myself, or friends and family who are loyal to only one of us.
- I hide things that I think would upset or anger my partner (phone numbers, letters, photos), or they feel the need to do so with me.
- Either my partner or myself don't talk about parents' or friends' objections to or worries about our relationship, and/or I'm or they are afraid to disagree with each other—even about the small stuff—or talk about problems in the relationship.
- My partner yells, calls me names, puts me down, accuses me of things I have not done, or seems to always have something negative to say about me, my family, or friends, or I do so to them.
- I feel as if no matter what I do, it isn't enough to earn my partner's attention, approval, support, or love, or my partner feels that way about me.
- I or my partner is afraid to say no to sex in general, or to sexual activities one of us likes but the other does not, or to ask for things that one of us likes, wants, or needs sexually.
- Myself or my partner refuses to use birth control or safer sex practices.
- My partner threatens me, or has threatened me, my property, pets, friends, or family, or I have done so to my partner.
- My partner has, or I have, a bad temper, and/or major mood swings.
- My partner hits, throws, or breaks things when angry, and/or has pushed, hit, grabbed, restrained, or otherwise physically hurt me, or I have done such to them.

s.e.x.

■ I feel that my partner's anger is my fault, and/or feel that if I change or behave a certain way they will behave differently, or my partner feels this way about me.

■ I have, or my partner has, an exit plan for when it gets "really bad."

The behaviors above are often red flags of a dangerous or abusive relationship; if you find you nodded a "yes," to at least a couple of them—and certainly if you found even more—you have sound reasons to be concerned, or to start getting concerned, if you aren't already. Stuff like this often escalates and becomes constant. While emotional or verbal abuse may not escalate to physical or sexual abuse, those abuses are still harmful and unhealthy. And in many cases, emotional and/or verbal abuse does escalate to physical or sexual abuse.

For information on identifying and dealing with abuse, see chapter 10.

diminishing greatly, are romantic feelings fizzling, has your friendship has gone kablooie? If so, your breakup train is pulling into the station. And if a relationship has become physically, sexually, or emotionally abusive or manipulative, it is definitely time to head for the door and close it behind you.

Often, with well-balanced people we really care for and have been open with, a "breakup" isn't so much a dramatic split as a rearrangement. Someone who isn't working out as a lover usually can, with a little time, patience, and communication, become a cherished friend. Breaking up, when it's the right time, isn't the sign of a weak or uncaring person most of the time; in fact, it's generally a pretty clear sign of real caring, awareness, and respect.

HOW DO YOU DO IT?

When a breakup is looming on the horizon, talk about it, together. That may mean saying something like, "I know we (or you, or I) have been working on <insert big thing here>, but I'm starting to feel like we should talk about the option of splitting up, too." That way, you can both have some time to

consider that choice alone, then share what you're thinking and feeling as you go, making the whole process more gradual, rather than sudden. It's normal to take some time to think this through by yourself, or with your support system of friends before bringing it up to a partner, but once you ARE considering it in earnest, don't hold off too long before telling your boyfriend or girlfriend: there's a difference between a breakup and a trip to the dumps. Ideally, breakups should happen jointly and be a process, since they impact both people and both get to make choices.

There are some exceptions to that rule: If your partner is very dependent, codependent, emotionally unstable, or abusive, you may find that a gradual, cooperative approach doesn't work. If, for instance, you've tried to talk about a split with a partner again and again, and they just won't hear it, or they beg and plead and will not let go, you may just have to handle it on your own. Make clear you're done, and ignore phone calls for some time, or call on friends or family to help mediate. An abusive or volatile partner may be someone who isn't safe for you to discuss a break up with, or even split

s.e.x.

with, alone. You may need to split with little fanfare or warning, with safeguards in place—by breaking up in public, for example, letting your family know not to let them in your house later, or telling school or job authorities. And sometimes, after a very big fight, after something intense and unexpected like a partner cheating, betraying your trust, or doing something very unacceptable, breakups just happen.

THE MOURNING AFTER

There's no one way to process a breakup that works for everyone. Any sort of grieving is really personal and individual. Often, even two people who were together for years and had loads in common will process a breakup differently, and of course, it also depends on how a specific relationship and breakup went. Some people need lots of time alone, and others need extra time with family or friends. Usually after a breakup, we're whacked with a bevy of mixed feelings. You may find you miss your ex and are happy they're gone at the same time, that you're sad and sappy and pissed off all at once. Honoring and accepting those feelings—all of them—in constructive ways is pretty important. If you need to cry for a few days, do it. If you need to sit with friends and kvetch about every stinky thing your ex ever did, go for it. Expressing yourself in ways that work for you—via creative writing or playing music, for example—is often a great help. Try throwing yourself into things you usually enjoy and find satisfaction in, such as sports, research, work, chores, and hobbies.

Trying to push all of your feelings away is not dealing. Certainly, you can't be processing all of the time; there are other aspects

Boing, Boing, Boing: Rebounding

Most of us feel really lonely after a breakup. Too many of us, rather than working through that alone, with platonic friends and family, look to quell that loneliness by jumping headfirst into another relationship, when we've still got salt on our cheeks from the first one.

New relationships RIGHT after an old one has ended, or before we've had time to deal with the residual feelings from a breakup, are called *rebounds*. Rebounds have this funny tendency to work out pretty badly, for both people involved. The person rebounding usually discovers they picked someone inappropriate or just got involved before they were ready, and the other person ends up feeling used, or spending a large chunk of their time comforting their partner about their last relationship. Not cool.

People you meet right after a breakup, if they're a good match for you, will almost always still be around in a little while. Very few people can't accept, when you tell them so, that you're just not ready for a new relationship yet, because you have to get over the old one. It's best to wait until you are ready: you can then really give a new person and a new relationship your full attention and the right amount of emotional energy. Keep your eyes peeled for rebounding: if within a few weeks of a breakup you suddenly have a bona fide boyfriend or girlfriend again, you're bouncing, baby.

of your life that need your time and attention, and they may be comforting, to boot. But make sure you're taking at least SOME time to work through what you need to, and to just feel how you feel, without having to pretend you're happy or okay all the time.

post-breakup behavior that just isn't healthy

- You still show up at their house, dorm, or locker, even if they've made clear they aren't comfortable with that and need time apart.
- You threaten suicide or harm to yourself or them, their friends, family, or property, or you would sincerely like to see them harmed.
- You cannot, even a couple of weeks later, keep it together to do any of the things you normally enjoy, or to cope with your normal daily life and responsibilities.
- You engage in forms of self-harm, such as self-mutilation, drug or alcohol abuse, or knowingly risky sexual behavior. You truly do not feel that you can go on, weeks after the breakup, and are sincerely worried about your survival.
- You try to sabotage their friendships, dates, or other current relationships, or deliberately spread lies or half-truths about them to make them look bad.
- You feel you would take them back in two seconds, on ANY terms.
- You lie or manipulate them to try to get them to come back, or to keep them from breaking up with you, by feigning illness or pregnancy, for example, or threatening self-destructive behavior, using blackmail, making promises you know you can't keep, or agreeing to things that don't work for you (like agreeing to an FWB, when you really only want a serious relationship).

If any of this sounds like you, reach out to a friend, trusted adult, or family member; be honest, and ask for help dealing. Do NOT ask your ex to help you deal: that's not their responsibility or place. If you have an ex behaving this way, try talking to a trusted friend of theirs, kindly, and asking if they'd help your ex. If the ex is approaching you with any of this stuff, be firm, clear, and kind, without making future promises to placate them, as in: "I'm sorry, but you need to stop coming to my house now," or "I know you're hurting, but I can't help you with that. Why don't you talk to <*insert their close friend's name here*>, they're a better person to be there for you now than me." If all else fails, and you or an ex are just completely off the map in terms of healthy behavior, call in the reinforcements: parents and school counselors can be of great help in those sorts of situations.

Sometimes, breakups come after a very long time of knowing things are over or heading that way. So, when they finally do happen, you may already have processed your upset, or you may just feel relieved. If you had emotional investment in a relationship, but feel you have ZERO processing to do, it may just come later. But overall, there's no rule that, post-breakup, everyone has to be seriously depressed or upset.

After a breakup, it's also normal for friends or family to express that they're not sure about your feelings or how you're managing them. They may think you should move on more quickly, stop crying at a certain point, or even be more upset than you are. Sometimes, people will butt in that way because they care—for instance, if it just hurts them to see you so upset. They may also be projecting, assuming you should feel how they have after a breakup. Sometimes, even when you've only been in a

s.e.x.

relationship for a very short time, a breakup feels as huge as one in a much longer and deeper relationship, and that can be tough for others to understand.

close the gate when you leave

 CLOSURE is often important when something comes to an end, no matter how it has finished. So, it's normal for exes, either after a breakup or in the midst of one, to want to talk out all of their feelings as they tie things up, or afterward. That may include making plans and room for a friendship during or after, or saying things that were left unsaid. It may also include on or two last, long, knockdown, dragout fights. Or, some time after a breakup, you may just want to write a letter or have coffee with an ex and talk about things you've figured out, or residual issues you feel bad about or want to understand better. Often, those can be really productive conversations, sometimes leading to quality friendships. But in some situations, especially with really bad breakups, you may not be able to, or want to, get resolution with a partner; that's something you may need to do for yourself, or with the help of friends, family, or a counselor.

Of course, you'll probably want to shove most advice like this forcibly up a narrow crevice when you've just broken up, no matter how old you are. That's normal, too.

▪ "JUST" FRIENDS? ▪

In most cases, if you want to be friends with your ex, it's going to take a little time. It's normal for people to need a few weeks or months—sometimes longer—to themselves, with very little or no contact, to process.

After some time has passed, you just have to feel this stuff out together, as far as developing a friendship goes, and it's normal for it to be touch and go for a while, or for certain subjects or places to be off-limits (like, say, your bedrooms, or places associated with sexual or romantic experiences). You may hit snags now and then. If one or both of you starts to date, it may be difficult to hang out with an ex-now-friend when you see them being romantic with someone else, even though the friendship seemed to be going well before. As well, some issues that were problematic in your romantic relationship may continue to be issues in your friendship, and you may or may not be able to work them out any better than you did as partners.

A lot of people say or decide they want to be "just" friends, often as a consolation prize, as if a romantic or sexual relationship were automatically better than platonic friendship. Really, it's not, even if our culture presents it that way. All sorts of relationships are different, and what type they are doesn't dictate the quality of them. People who weren't very good together as lovers can turn out to have a far better relationship as friends. If you've known the person you were with for a while, you probably already DO have a friendship as part of your existing, albeit changing, relationship.

The cornerstone of any longlasting relationship *is* friendship, so learning to cultivate that, above all else—even with your exes, whether they end up as your best friends or just casual, friendly acquaintances—is really valuable.

to be, or not to be . . .
sexually active

WHAT WE'RE TALKING about over the next few chapters is *partnered sex*.

Since the definition of what that even *is* can be so varied and arbitrary, let's make it crystal: A partner is anyone, in any relationship model, with whom you actively and consensually engage in sexual activities. *Consensual* means you both initiate or say yes to these activities wholeheartedly and freely, without pressure, obligation, or ambivalence, and with a very good idea of what you're getting into. That includes the absolute allowance to stop or set new limits and boundaries at *any time,* without a battle. *Sex* means any number of things you might both actively engage in, which you both find sexually exciting, fulfilling, satisfying, or interesting.

Your potential or current partner might be your girlfriend or boyfriend, but he or she also might be your best friend, an acquaintance, a casual date, or a hookup. Sex might be a makeout session, fingering or a hand job, oral sex, vaginal intercourse, anal play, mutual masturbation, massage, cybersex, or phone sex—any of which, or all, may or may not have great importance or relevance to you; it may or may not be a "rite of passage" for you and yours the first time you do it.

No one but you can assign a given value or importance to what you do or whom you do it with, or define "sex" for you. What we can define clearly, is being sexually active and partnered sex.

Willingly engaging in intimate, sexual contact with someone else, often including genital contact, for the purpose of deriving sexual fulfillment, achieving satisfaction, or "answering" sexual urges for *both* of you, is partnered sex. Oral sex

What is "It" All About

"It" is common cultural shorthand for whatever sexual activity we've decided (or our peers, partners, culture, or community has decided) is *the* rite of sexual passage, or *the* activity that means, to us or others, that we have become sexually active. Often, "doing it" is assumed to mean heterosexual intercourse, and the first time one does "it" is almost always supposed to be a profound rite of passage and a Very Big Deal.

But. Not everyone is heterosexual. Not everyone is interested in having intercourse—for some people not right now, for others, not ever. And for plenty of people, the sexual activity or experience they felt was *their* rite of passage may not have been intercourse, or there may not have been one Big Partnered Sex Thing at all. There may have been several "its," and there may be more to come. Some people later realize that their big sexual rites of passage didn't happen in their teens—even if they were sexually active then. Some adults, even those who have been sexually active for years, are still *waiting* for that One Big Thing. Some feel that there really isn't one important or cornerstone partnered activity at all, but that their sexual rites of passage were about the first time they had an orgasm with masturbation; about how they felt about sex or their sexual selves; about a relationship they were or are in; or about doing things to sexually empower themselves, such as their first GYN or sexual healthcare exam, or the first time they laid out and stated all of their limits or boundaries confidently.

With anything this hazy, it often pays to redefine things as much as we can, to try to think about things in new ways and define them for ourselves. That's especially helpful with something as incredibly individual and personal as sex.

For now, let's not make a big deal out of "it."

IS sex. Anal sex IS sex. Manual sex IS sex. (Hint: That's why all those terms end in the word *sex*.) Engaging in those activities is sex, no matter the gender of your partners, no matter your age, no matter how (or if) you define common cultural concepts like virginity.

If you are involved in any of that contact, to any degree, or thinking about it, then it's time to think about all of the things sexual contact entails, so that you can make the choices that are best for **you**: taking into account sexual and reproductive health issues, risks and safety precautions, possible outcomes (both wanted and unwanted), relationship issues and models, your wants and needs, limits and boundaries, personal ethics and beliefs, happiness and satisfaction—and all that stuff for your partners, too.

Let's face it: many people don't give their sexual choices enough thought after whatever it was they considered their one big first. But that's hardly ideal, nor is it any way to have a healthy, safe, and satisfying sex life. Given the level of sexual dissatisfaction, lack of communication, ignorance, and all-around screwed-upness running amok when it comes to sex, it's pretty clear that

THE SEXUAL READINESS CHECKLIST

MATERIAL STUFF:

▶ I have a safer sex kit (see page 213), including several up-to-date, quality latex condoms and/or other latex barriers, latex-safe lubricant, and other needed items for the activity I want to engage in, and both my partner and I know how to use them.

▶ If engaging in activity with a pregnancy risk, I have a secondary method of birth control for use with condoms, if my partner or I want one (see chapter 11).

▶ I have the phone number for a local sexual health clinic, or the phone number of my own gynecologist or general physician.

▶ I have a savings account I can use myself at any time (preferably with a pad of a couple of hundred bucks), and I have a "sex budget" of at least thirty dollars per month to take care of birth control, safer sex items, and annual testing and sexual healthcare, including having to treat or manage a potential STI or pregnancy. I am either covered under a healthcare plan or service that can cover (if applicable) pregnancy, neonatal care, gynecological visits, STI testing, and birth control, via public healthcare or clinic care, and/or I have the funds or means to pay for these services, even if I need them quickly.

BODY AND HEALTH:

▶ I have already begun annual sexual and general healthcare and exams (page 183) and disease and infection screenings (page 205), and I am in good health. The same is true of my partner.

▶ I understand and am familiar with my own anatomy and my partner's basic anatomy (see chapter 2), as well as the basics of the sexual activity I want to participate in, STIs, and human reproduction (if your partner is of the opposite sex).

▶ I can tell when I am sexually aroused (page 55), and also when I am not; I have a good idea about what I need to be aroused, and can comfortably communicate when I just am not aroused. I feel my partner can say the same.

▶ I can relax and feel comfortable during sexual activities without great fear, anxiety, or shame.

▶ I can handle a mild level of physical pain or discomfort, and am ready to handle and manage any pain or discomfort my partner may experience.

▶ I feel confident that my partner and I are entering into a sexual situation that poses no serious physical or health risks, and that we both clearly understand what our risks may be and how to minimize them.

RELATIONSHIP REQUIREMENTS:

▶ I am able to set limits (to say no whenever I want to) and uphold them, and can trust my partner to easily respect them at all times, and vice-versa (see page 234).

- ▶ I can assess what I want for myself, and separate it from what my partner, friends, or family want, and feel my partner can do the same.
- ▶ I am able to trust my partner, and I know myself to be trustworthy.
- ▶ I feel I can tell my partner what I want and need sexually and emotionally, and when I do and do not like something, and I feel able to hear and respect them when they do the same.
- ▶ I can talk to my partner about sex comfortably, in or out of bed, and be honest and forthright, and feel they can do the same with me.
- ▶ I care about my partner's health, emotions, and general well-being, and act accordingly, and know that my partner cares about mine and is able to show that care in their actions and sexual behavior.
- ▶ My partner and I understand what consent is (see page 144), and I feel confident that we are able to give full informed consent to the activity or activities we're going to engage in.
- ▶ My partner and I have already discussed most of these issues together, in advance of sexual activity.

EMOTIONAL ITEMS:

- ▶ If my partner or I have any strong religious, cultural, ethical, or family beliefs or convictions that pose serious conflicts to sexual activity, we have evaluated, discussed, and resolved them.
- ▶ I feel I can take full responsibility for my own emotions, expectations, and actions, and know my partner can and will do the same, even if that is difficult or creates conflict.
- ▶ I can handle being disappointed, confused, or upset about sex, and am prepared to handle a partner's disappointment, confusion, or upset (see page 139).
- ▶ I have a trusted adult I can talk to about sex, and friends I can go to for emotional support, and know that my partner also has a strong support system.
- ▶ I can separate sex from love, and do not seek to have sex to use it to manipulate or harm myself, my partner, or anyone else. I feel my partner's motives are sound, safe, and realistic, as well.
- ▶ I am not currently in an abusive relationship (see page 120).
- ▶ I feel confident neither of us is entering into a sexual situation that is likely to be emotionally unsafe or harmful for either of us (see chapter 9).
- ▶ I feel my partner and I both understand that sexual activity may change our relationship for better or for worse, and we feel we can handle and accept whatever may (or may not) happen.
- ▶ I feel I can emotionally handle a possible pregnancy, disease, or infection, or rejection from my partner, and feel my partner can handle these things, as well.

that approach isn't working very well. Nearly everyone could use a renovation in terms of the way we think about our sexual choices and how we make them, no matter our age or level of experience.

Yes, the first few sexual choices you make are very important and worth taking time to consider. And, yes, here's hoping your first few times with any sexual activity will be great. But ALL the sexual choices you will make are important and worth taking time to consider, and ALL of your sexual experiences should be great (and the fact is, over time, they usually get greater, not the other way around). That's important, not just to protect you and yours from trauma or undesired outcomes, but to enable you and yours to have a sexual life that's better than "not bad," or "not risky," or "not painful," but is entirely *excellent,* on all levels. After all, if the best we could hope for from partnered sex were just to escape it unscathed physically or emotionally, there'd really be no point in engaging in it at all, since it's totally optional.

The goal for the sex you have isn't to avoid bad sex; the goal is for it *to be good.*

When you first decide to start being sexually active *is* a big decision, because stepping onto that path dictates ongoing and lifelong actions you'll need to be taking from that point on, like having annual STI screenings, keeping reliable birth control (if you have opposite-sex partners) and safer sex supplies on hand, entering into relationships, evaluating others as potential sex partners, understanding how being sexually active impacts your relationships, friends, family, and yourself, and even dealing with something as seemingly small as partnered

sex taking up more real estate in your brain.

new perspectives

 WHEN you're thinking about becoming sexually active, it can be helpful to talk to other people you trust and respect, who became sexually active around the same age, or in the same sort of environment or relationship as yours. While their experiences may not be identical to yours, just listening to others' feelings about their initial sexual experiences and choices is often helpful when making your own decisions: you can be reminded of some possible positive and negative outcomes, and find out different ways you might feel.

Teens and parents often have a disconnect when talking about this stuff. Often, neither party actually listens to the other about their experiences. Nobody has to agree; just listen, and ask to be listened to. Your folks are people, too, who went through the same things, and chances are good that somewhere between their experiences and your expectations is where the reality lives.

When you are at the point where you're making that choice, start with the Sexual Readiness Checklist. If just looking at that list makes you dizzy, now's probably a bad time to become sexually active. If you find yourself rationalizing why you don't need half the stuff on that list, or why it's unimportant, you're probably rushing or in some big denial about what partnered sex really requires. If you flipped right past it and feel you have no need to look at it at all, you are seriously kidding yourself, even if you already ARE sexually active. If, in going through the list, you find you already have most of those things in

s.e.x.

hand or in mind, you're probably in really good shape in terms of readiness.

Partnered sex is unique in that there rarely are missed opportunities. Because good sex happens when everything falls into place. It happens when we're in the right headspace for it, when we have the things we need, when we don't feel pressured or rushed to make a choice too quickly, when whatever sort of relationship we're in supports sound sexual and emotional health and well-being, when our wants and needs align pretty closely with our partner's.

▪ GREAT SEXPECTATIONS ▪

A day rarely passes when we're not exposed to at least one message about what sex is, what it's supposed to be, how great it is (or not), how important it is (or not), or how big a part of our lives it should or shouldn't be. Those messages are often biased, flavored by the person doling them out, intentionally or not. A friend going on about her sex life can exaggerate or report enjoyment that wasn't really there, to make herself or her partner look good or feel better—or because it wasn't great, and she's worried something is wrong with her. Someone preaching about the dangers of sex may inflate or misrepresent the risks, based on a moral agenda of their own, or based only on their own experiences of sex. A film may show us totally unrealistic sex or sexual relationships just because it suits the plot.

Expecting sex to be like what see in the movies or popular culture is unrealistic, and thinking it has magical capabilities is an error. In real life, it's quite a good deal different. Rarely in the movies, for instance, do we see a couple taking care of their sexual health with regular exams and testing, which a sexually active person NEEDS to do to keep themselves and their partners physically and emotionally well. Rarely in the movies do we see "quiet" orgasms, or sex that's neither awful nor heart-racing. Rarely in the movies or in popular literature do we see the full spectrum of a couple's or a person's sex life, and all the many, many issues that must be dealt with. Rarely do we see unhappy endings to sexual conflicts. Rarely do we see couples taking a long, slow time to wade through issues—instead, we usually see colossal fights, huge dramas, or stormy, wailing breakups. Rarely do we see normal-looking people with normal-looking bodies, people who have emotional needs and communicate realistically about sex. So, if you base your expectations on things like movies, books, porn, or friends' accounts of their relationships, you're bound to end up feeling confused, lost, or disappointed, and will likely find it hard to stay grounded in your very real relationships and sexuality and deal with them appropriately.

regrets, we've had a few.

A BIG worry many young people have about becoming sexually active is that it will be the wrong choice, with the wrong person, or at the wrong time. There *are* lots of people who regret their initial sexual choices. There are a lot of reasons why regret might come into play, from the obvious (something unexpected or traumatic happened) to the not-so-obvious (they feel regret because they assume another choice could have been better). Sometimes, those worries are based on age (Is this too young? Is that too old?), and while age can be part of the equation, often this, too, is an issue of what our expectations are. Some studies have shown that the younger a person is, the more unrealistic their sexual expectations are likely to be. If your expectations of sex are really inflated or unrealistic, it's not going to be too surprising that when you do have it, it won't measure up. And given that the sex we have later down the road is often better than our first experiences with sex, it's also not surprising that many people feel the sex they had later "should" have been the sex they first had.

Mindfulness and intuition are your pals in this choice. If your head or your gut says "not just yet," listen. If you feel that you have to hurry up and make a choice, remember that if you don't yet feel "Yes!" and not "Er . . . I guess so," the best decision is usually to wait for an opportunity that allows you to give it some real thought. But if it all feels really right right now—including all the stuff on your checklist, not just the stuff in your heart or between your legs—it probably *is* time.

It's not uncommon for our expectations of partnered sex to end up having little or no resemblance to what we actually experience. Those surprises can run the gamut: there will probably be things we expected to be better, and things we enjoyed more than we expected to. You may even find that what happens *does* meet your expectations to the letter. We're all unique, our expectations are all unique, and so is the sex we have.

GET REAL:
UNREALISTIC EXPECTATIONS AND SCENARIOS

While partnered sex has a lot to offer, there are some things sex really can't do for us:

- ▶ Sex cannot give us real self-worth, self-esteem, or long-term positive body image.

- ▶ Partnered sex cannot substitute for our own exploration or understanding of our own bodies.
- ▶ Engaging in sex, by itself, cannot give us reliable information about sex or sexual health.
- ▶ Sex in and of itself cannot provide love or emotional affection, friendship, or support, nor relationship commitment or security.
- ▶ Sex cannot substitute for good communication.
- ▶ Sex cannot magically turn anyone into an adult or a mature person.

You might find it helpful to make a list about your expectations. Jot down the things you expect: sexually, physically, emotionally, in terms of your relationship, in terms of your whole life. Let yourself write the whole range of your expectations: the stuff you feel is pretty realistic as well as your ultimate ideals and worst nightmares, even the stuff you think or know is just silly. Just get it all out there so you can have a good look at it and be self-aware. A list like that can also help you bring those expectations to the table when you and your partner talk about being sexually active. No need to show up on a date with the whole thing printed out with a dotted line for them to sign on—having the general gist in your head will do just fine.

A good deal of what we expect includes some of our basic wants and needs. For instance, if you expect to spend time together after sex, snuggling and talking, you can figure out how important that it to you: Is it essential, or would it be okay if that didn't happen? Is it something you need to tell a potential partner that you need? If you expect a certain pace or certain activities, are

s.e.x.

those wants or needs? Once you've got that list, you can go through it and get a pretty good handle on your basic own wants and needs even if when it all happens you find you don't need all the things you thought you would or that you want things you didn't expect to.

want. need. huh?

THE difference between a want and a need is that a need is nonnegotiable. Going without what we *want* can suck and be disappointing, but it's not likely to be terribly traumatic. Going without what we *need* can be traumatic, especially in situations like partnered sex, where we're very vulnerable and the risks can run high.

Divide and conquer. Figure out which is which. Don't make exceptions with your needs: it just isn't worth it. Talk about those needs with your partner, listen to theirs, and be sure you both can do your level best to honor and fulfill them. If you can't, figure out if they're needs that, with time, can be fulfilled, or if with a given partner or situation, they're just not going to happen. It sucks, but if your real needs are not going to be met, you may have to change a relationship or say no to sex with someone because of that.

NO HARM, NO FOUL: LIMITS AND BOUNDARIES

Your wants and needs determine much of your limits and boundaries. This can be tricky when you're new to sexual partnership, because it's common to have a better handle on those things when you've been sexually active for some time. Plenty of people don't figure out good limits and boundaries for themselves for decades, and for

obvious reasons, it can be especially difficult for women. So, in terms of having certain areas touched, or engaging in certain activities, you may find that your feelings change as you go. At the start, one of your boundaries may just be that your partner needs to make allowance for you being in a bit of flux, and be supportive as you work it out.

Some limits and boundaries tend to shift and adapt as we grow and change, or to address different issues in different relationships. Since communication is the order of the day in sexual partnership, so long as we keep talking and keep those windows open, it can often be relatively easy for our partners to be kept in the loop, even if all we're saying is, "I'm not sure how I feel about doing this right now for some reason, but I'll keep you posted when I've thought about it more."

Some limits and boundaries can be established and known in advance. You probably already have a good idea of how "far" you want to go in terms of the sexual activities you want to do and the risks you're willing to take in regard to safer sex. Those are limits. There are probably some lines you won't or don't want to cross, like having sex in public, having heterosex without birth control, having a partner engage you in sex while you're asleep, or having certain parts of your anatomy looked at with a magnifying glass during sex. Those are boundaries. Again, as time goes on, you can adapt, erase, or add to those as need be, and you probably will. But keep your starting points in mind when you're making sexual choices.

SEX ETHICS AND PERSONAL VALUES

Your own system of personal beliefs, ethics, and values is a big part of who you are: ignoring or disrespecting it, or allowing others to, is usually a recipe for disaster. For example, if you believe very strongly that sex outside of marriage isn't okay, then having sex before marriage probably isn't going to make you feel very good about yourself. If you believe that sex has to be 50/50, right down to the money spent on condoms, but your partner isn't taking any responsibility, that's not going to be workable for long. If there are certain codes of sexual conduct that show responsibility, care, or just plain good manners that you or your partner aren't following, everything isn't going to be copacetic. If honesty is a big deal for you, then putting yourself in a sexual situation where you feel compelled to, or are asked to, lie is a crappy idea.

You may not discover what some of your sex ethics, limits, or boundaries are until after you cross those lines; that happens to nearly everyone at some point. But even when you're just starting out with part-nered sex, you likely have plenty you *are* aware of, so be mindful. If you're not sure about them, deal with them the same way you'd cross a busy street: be cautious and slow, rather than running out into heavy traffic. And talk to your partner to see how your ethics, values, limits, and boundaries mesh with theirs, to be sure you can be mindful of one another.

WHAT'S THE RIGHT AGE?

Age in years is a factor when it comes to the legal aspects of sexual partnership, and sometimes when it comes to certain sexual health services. But in many ways, age in years isn't a very helpful way of determin-ing sexual readiness. Most partnered sexual activities require basic physical sexual devel-opment and a good measure of emotional maturity, but those vary a great deal among people of every age.

But nothing magical happens to every single person on their fourteenth, sixteenth, eighteenth or twenty-first birthday. Not physically, not emotionally, not sexually. The right age for you to have sex is when you can deal with the things on the Sexual Readiness Checklist, and when it feels like it's right for you and yours—feels right to *both* of you.

 MANY young adults assume that the majority of their peers are sex-ually active or having intercourse, even when statistical data actually shows us that's not so. Many studies have shown that a scary percentage of people in the world—of all ages—lie to friends and partners about their sexual experi-ence, especially young people. It's a vicious cycle: if everyone assumes everyone else is already sex-ually active, a whole lot of people start exagger-ating or lying about their level of sexual activity. In the United States, the average age at which teens who have heterosexual intercourse report they do is between sixteen and seventeen, but just **over half** of all American teens have had intercourse by the end of high school.

TO PLAN OR NOT TO PLAN, THAT'S THE QUESTION

Being prepared is smart: talking about becoming sexually active with the intent of getting there, having safer sex tools and birth control in advance, getting STI screenings done, finding spaces and times that are safe and private.

Planning special times for sex—especially when you've got something pretty unique cooking—is also fine and fun. But spontaneity

s.e.x.

is often an important part of sex, too. Being spontaneous, or flexible, is important because, especially once people are out of the honeymoon phase of a relationship, one partner may want to have sex, or engage in a certain sexual activity, while the other partner may not be interested. So, we all need to be able to make allowances for that, and have those allowances made for us.

LIGHTS, CAMERA, ACTION!

A lot of people are concerned with looking and acting "the part" during partnered sex. Worries about shaving or not shaving, about the size and shape or taste and smell of body parts, are common. Wondering when one should be moaning and when one shouldn't, if laughing or being silly is okay, if there are "right" things to say during sex, when eye contact should or shouldn't be made, and even what one's face should look like when they reach orgasm aren't atypical concerns. A lot of folks stress out about doing something the "wrong" way.

It may sound tired and clichéd, but the only person you should be when you're having sex with someone is yourself. If you usually shave or wax, fine. If you don't, that's fine, too. If you taste and smell like a person, good: you *are* one. If sex with you and yours isn't like sex in the movies, that's as it's supposed to be: this is real life, not the movies. Sex in the movies is no more accurately depicted than say, cartoons depict accurately what happens when someone has a piano dropped on their head. If you don't look like a supermodel or an action figure, congrats! Welcome to at least 95 percent of the population. Sex with a partner shouldn't be a performance or a beauty contest; it should be a place and an experience where you're able to enjoy being

yourself, intimately, with someone you know wants to be with exactly that person.

WORST-CASE SCENARIOS

Many young couples (though not the majority) who first become sexually active together never have sex together again, and for plenty of people, sex may change a relationship in negative and unexpected ways. Commonly, one partner won't reach orgasm easily or will feel sexually dissatisfied, physically or emotionally. Sometimes, things happen during sex we're embarrassed about or ashamed of: vaginal bleeding, loss of erection, farting. With the high rates of STIs and unplanned pregnancy in youth, it's pretty obvious that plenty of people get unwelcome surprises from partnered sex. Some people discover during sex with a partner that they may be an entirely different sexual orientation than they thought. For some, becoming sexually active creates big problems with friends or family.

When something that can feel so wonderful, that's supposed to be so wonderful, nets bad results, it can be hard to handle. Being ready for some bad stuff is smart. Remember that sex DOES carry risks, physical and emotional, and keep in mind what those risks are. Be sure in advance that you think you can at least handle them— even if it won't be easy.

UNTIL MARRIAGE

If you're a proponent of marriage and want that for yourself, that's absolutely A-OK. If you feel you want to wait to become sexually active until marriage (though if you're gay, that may be a far longer wait), that's also a totally valid choice to make.

s.e.x.

If you'd like to wait for marriage, but think that may be unrealistic for you—or you know it already is—there's no reason not to do some *preparation,* in case you *do* choose to become sexually active sooner. You can get started with sexual healthcare, gather safer sex items (remember, marriage isn't safer sex, so the same guidelines apply to newly married couples as apply to any other couples), and think and talk about your expectations, wants, and needs.

One of the cardinal rules of sex is that you *always* can change your mind, whether we're talking about liking an activity one day and not wanting to do it the next, or being sexually active and later opting out, or being sexually inactive and opting in. It's completely okay to get your mind set on a given sexual choice for a while, and stick to it, then find that it doesn't fit you or serve you well, and adapt as need be. That's what you're supposed to do.

BEING A PRUDE (and Other Really Crappy Names for Choosing Not to Be Sexually Active)

If you choose to let partnered sex and/or dating sit on the shelf, you may have to deal with heavy stigmas and negative messages from your peers, culture, and even your parents, which isn't surprising, considering all the pressures we get—at every age—to pair up and "settle down." People may label you a prude, a loser, a baby, a Mary, or assume that you're unattractive, a social outcast, "behind," or immature in sexual or social development.

"Waiting" for sex isn't always about waiting at all: it's often about pursuing all sorts of others things that interest you. What's sometimes pictured when someone says they're "waiting" is some lonely, sniffling, woebegone guy or girl staring at the unringing phone, or continually pushing a partner away who is avidly pursuing them. Plenty of people—teen and adult—who don't currently have sexual partners are busy with a million things, and doing no real waiting at all. They're just trying to fit more into their lives, and they're not going to rework things to make room for a partner or sex until they feel it's really worth their while, and they feel ready and strongly compelled to do so.

▪ INTIMACY: ▪
Bonding Basics

Therapists generally define intimacy as an emotional space in which two people can be free to be themselves without reservation, both accepting and supporting one another. Sometimes, emotional intimacy (becoming close via feelings or emotions) and physical intimacy (becoming close through touch, be it sexually or platonically) are differentiated. When people talk about intimacy in a sexual context, they're either talking solely about physical intimacy ("intimacy" and phrases like "we were intimate," are sometimes used as delicate ways to refer to sex) or about emotional intimacy, which can occur during sex as well.

Studies like *Greater Expectations: Adolescents' Positive Motivations for Sex* show that a desire for intimacy is often one of the biggest motivations young adults have in choosing to become sexually active. It's important to bear in mind that partnered sex cannot, all by itself, cement or deepen a relationship, or create emotional intimacy that isn't there already, but many aspects of partnered sex *can* enable *greater* intimacy.

s.e.x.

When we share our sexual selves with another person, we are potentially taking physical risks, and risking rejection, disappointment, or deeper feelings and attachment. So, much of the time, we're engaging in sexual activities or relations with people we already feel some degree of intimacy with, or want more intimacy with (even if it's only for an evening).

ARE YOU *MENTAL?* YES!

Often, sex with someone we already have an emotional bond and intimacy with can elevate our feelings, both during and after sex. While saying that one sort of sexual relationship or another is "better" or "worse" for everyone is biased and usually inaccurate, we *can* say that sex with greater levels of intimacy is experienced differently, physically and emotionally, than sex with less intimacy.

No sex is *just* physical. **None.** Because sex is a whole-body process, which utilizes the brain more than any other body part, and because it involves all of our senses, including our sense memory, there are always emotional aspects to partnered sex. That doesn't mean sex must be or always is *romantic,* or that love is required for enjoyable, healthy sex. It doesn't mean that one can't have sexual partners outside romantic relationships, primarily or purely for sex alone. But it does mean that even very casual sexual partnerships, like hookups or FWB scenarios, do have some emotional aspects—such as seeking out companionship or company, wanting to explore various feelings through sex—and do involve varying levels of intimacy, just like romantic or longer-term relationships.

No one relationship model or type of sex automatically equals more or less physical or emotional intimacy than any other. Physically, some people may feel most connected to another person during vaginal or anal intercourse, while others may feel most intimate kissing deeply. Someone in a romantic, close relationship may sometimes feel distanced or unable to communicate freely during sex, while someone else having casual sex may have an emotional epiphany and feel incredibly close to the other person, able to be sexually freer because of the anonymity or a sudden connection. Or vice-versa.

Our levels of intimacy within relationships and during various kinds of sexual activities are all going to vary based on who we are, whom we're with, what we both want and need, what the relationships are like, where we're at in life, what social conditioning and life experiences we've had, how we're feeling on a given day, and how we nurture and protect that intimacy.

INCREASING INTIMACY

If you're looking to increase the intimacy in your sexual relationship(s), and want sex to support and benefit that, here's some good news: the way to do it is the same way you increase your physical satisfaction in sex physically enriching and satisfying—communication.

Touch, all by itself, is a form of communication. When and how you touch others speaks about your feelings for them. It's also about more subtle things, such as whether your partner is touching you with attentiveness to what you enjoy or not, or whether you're both comfortable making eye contact or touching each other after sex. So, spending time with partners involved in caring, loving touch does increase intimacy, because you're using yet one more way to communicate deeply.

When you pair that with open *verbal* communication, about yourself, your relationship, and the sex you're having, you add an awful lot to the mix besides just figuring out how to get off. Sharing feelings about your body, your sexual wants and needs, what you'd like to do with a partner and why, asking about ways to make them feel good, and really working through sexual conflicts builds closeness and intimacy. When you are tackling tougher issues with sex, it's often a good idea not to do so while you are HAVING sex, but instead, when you're just hanging out casually on the couch or taking a walk together.

How and what you communicate to outsiders about your sexual relationship is also a part of intimacy. Most people like at least some of their sex lives to remain private. So, a partner talking up a van full of friends about every detail of the sex they just had with their partner, or going online and announcing a partner's personal worries, insecurities, or the entirety of last night's argument, can be a real roadblock to intimacy. Because intimacy involves trust, betraying that trust in any way is a real problem. Be mindful of your partner's boundaries, and ask your partner to respect yours: talk together about your feelings about privacy, about what you're comfortable sharing, and with whom.

Caring for yourself and your partner is also part of intimacy. That means nurturing ALL the aspects of your relationship and your partner, not just what happens in bed or on a good day. It may mean supporting a partner through a tough life choice or a death in the family, it may mean having to work out compromises with their parents,

it may even mean agreeing to back off from sex for a while, for any number of reasons, or switching your sexual relationship to a platonic friendship.

Limits and boundaries don't inhibit intimacy: **they increase it.** Being open doesn't mean being open all night like a mini-mart. Being open is being honest about your feelings, wants, and needs, even when they don't align with your partner's. Part of getting close to someone else means increasing your compassion and empathy with them, and theirs with you. Some limits and boundaries may be temporary (like say, waiting to have intercourse until you've been together a certain amount of time) and some not so temporary (like not engaging in anal sex, ever). But we've all got them, and they're part of who we are.

Limits and boundaries aren't just a big NO. They are the support systems that give us the trust, safety, and freedom to be able to say a big **YES** to the things we do want, need, and feel ready for.

▪ VIRGINITY: ▪
Past and Present

When people talk about a "virgin," they're usually talking about someone who has not had heterosexual intercourse.

The concept of a virgin as someone who hasn't had penis-in-vagina intercourse leaves a lot of people out in the cold. Defining sexual partnership as male-to-female intercourse would make a lesbian who has had over one hundred female partners, but no male partners, a virgin. The standard definition of virginity also suggests that a woman is not a fully sexual being until she

S.e.x.

has had intercourse with a man, and that heterosexual couples who engage in sexual activities other than intercourse, or who don't even want to have intercourse, are somehow not having "real" sex. On a similar note, the emphasis put on intercourse can cause people to engage in sexual activities they don't really like, because they want physical intimacy, but are ashamed or afraid of having intercourse. People who have been sexually assaulted—who in no way have participated in consensual sex, or really even sex at all—are often thought to have "lost their virginity."

that mysterious hymen

ONCE upon a time, staying a virgin until marriage guaranteed that a woman would uphold family honor and establish a good marriage by passing from father to husband as an object that was owned. Her body was an object of value that would be guarded by her father, until such time as ownership was transferred to her husband. Some of the reason for this were to establish a higher "bridewealth," to ensure the most materially beneficial marriage. Given the lack of reliable birth control before modern times, having strict controls on virginity also helped to reduce illegitimate childbirths, and to verify paternity.

Folks in the third century cared little about technicalities: if a woman was found rolling around naked with a man, she was no virgin, even if penetration had not occurred. In the Middle Ages, you wouldn't have been able to get around virginity standards by saying "But, I only had oral sex, not intercourse!" Rumor traveled fast, and neighbors (and potential in-laws) would have found out about liaisons. What a woman did and didn't do

had little relevance if she had been with a man sexually, she was unchaste.

In the past, "tests" of virginity were often performed on women, few of which had any validity, and many of which were painful and cruel. A urine test may have been done, for instance, because it was believed that a virgin's urine should always be clear and never cloudy. Some looked at which way a woman's breasts pointed: a virgin's breasts were supposed to point up. Women were sometimes given a magic cup to drink from, and those who spilled the wine were thought to have proved that they were not faithful to their husbands. Of course, all of these beliefs were fallacies.

For centuries, many people have believed that the most obvious proof of a woman's virginity is found at her vaginal opening–the presence of a hymen. The lack of a hymen , or a hymen that is not fully intact, has long been considered indisputable evidence that a woman has been sexually active. Although this belief is still widespread, it is normal, as you know, for the hymen to become less visible over time due to any number of things that aren't intercourse or sexual. There are some women who aren't even born with easily visible hymens, and some with hymenal openings so large that their fully "intact" hymen doesn't look any different from one that isn't there at all. It's stretchy, too, and even after it has worn away–from hormonal changes, menses and vaginal fluids, general activity, and solo or partnered sexual activity–small folds of it remain around the vaginal opening for the rest of a woman's life. A "broken" or unbroken hymen is no reliable test of virginity. For more on the hymen, see page 20.

Neither is bleeding during first intercourse, another typical piece of "evidence" often used to "prove" virginity. While some women do experience bleeding, plenty of others do not. Another typical myth is the idea that the difference between someone who is and isn't a virgin can be felt, physically, by their male partner. A virgin is "sup-

s.e.x.

posed" to be "tight." A woman having first intercourse very well may be tight, but that is likely due more to nervousness, fear, and anxiety than it is to whether or not she has had partnered sex before. It's also typical to think that first intercourse MUST be painful, and if it's not, then clearly a given women has had intercourse before. But for plenty of first-timers, intercourse isn't painful—often those who are relaxed and aroused, who are as lubricated as they need to be, who have gentle partners, or whose hymens may have already worn away a good deal or are very flexible.

It's worth a look at the root of a lot of these beliefs and their cultural contexts, when you decide whether or not to sign on to them. Idealizing things like women's pain and bleeding, putting a monetary or moral value on the appearance of the vulva or a woman's sexual history, and putting women through embarrassing and shaming virginity "tests" at all is serious woman-hating. Even defining "real" sex as only the one act that gives a majority of women the least physical satisfaction is pretty warped, when you think about it.

SO WHO'S A VIRGIN AND WHO ISN'T?

What it means to be a virgin really can only be defined by you, and it has to do with how *you* define sex. Someone else can't do it for you, and you shouldn't allow anyone else to do so. (If abstinence or virginity is being asked of you by your church or parents, ask them to define it, explicitly, because what they think it means and what you do may be very different things. Ask questions: If you're going to agree to something, you should be sure you understand, and can live with, all of it.) Virginity shouldn't be a standard by which you judge others, or by which you should be judged. It shouldn't be a symbol of status or a lack thereof. Sex—

or abstaining from it—isn't something that should be used as a bargaining chip for anything, or used to manipulate anyone.

Out-there as it may seem, you might give some thought to abandoning the concept of virginity altogether. However nicely, or in different contexts, it is presented by some now, it is an idea that, throughout history, has been sexist, heterosexist, classist, and oppressive, and virginity as an ideal has actually done the opposite of what many would think it aspires to do: it has *de*valued sexuality and intimacy—and women—rather than making them more valuable.

You can't "give" someone your genitals, and someone else can't "give" your sexuality to you. You both can share them, and sharing (duh!) is the name of the game when it comes to partnered sex. Your value as a person and as a partner is not and should not be merely or primarily sexual. It's about the whole person you are, no matter your previous sexual experience or your lack of previous sexual experience. What makes something special isn't not having done it before: it's bringing your whole self to the table whenever it is that you *do* do it.

▪ BE A BLABBERMOUTH! ▪
Communicating with Partners about Sex

You can read everything from the *Kama Sutra* to *The Joy of Sex,* have a ton of sexual experience, or psychically channel Mata Hari, but if you don't know how to communicate with your partner, chances are good neither of you is going to have truly healthy, beneficial, and satisfying sexual experiences, especially long-term.

Communicating clearly and well about sex and relationship issues, before you

s.e.x.

become sexually active with someone—the whole works, not just when whispering sweet or saucy nothings into a lover's ear—not only puts you in a place where you can have satisfying sexual relationships, short- and long-term, it also helps keeps everyone safe and sound both physically and emotionally.

If you have a car, you know that you've got to keep a pretty good eye on the oil in the engine; if you run out, your car's not going to keep working, even if it's in great shape—and it may well explode in your face. Communication is the oil that keeps the engine of your sexual relationships running smoothly.

HOW TO TALK ABOUT SEX

Talking with your partner about sex isn't just about asking what one person has or hasn't done before, wants to do, or gets hot just thinking about. Talking about sex with a partner also involves discussing the pace you're comfortable with; your sexual health and your partner's; what you want or need, to be comfortable engaging in a given sexual activity; how you masturbate; how you feel about your body; what feels good and what really doesn't; safer sex and birth control; your sexual ethics and beliefs; the relationship model that works for you both; the works. Good sexual communication means you are creating and maintaining an environment in which you and your partner(s) can really talk openly about sex, in and out of bed, even when what you have to say isn't very sexy or isn't what the other person might want to hear. It means being able to say no and having no be accepted and easily respected, without pressure to say yes; it means being able to say yes knowing that it doesn't mean you, or they, have to say yes every time.

It's no big shocker that talking about sex openly and intimately isn't very easy. Many adults in long-term sexual partnerships don't have the hang of it, and plenty prefer to avoid sexual discussions rather than practice them. A rare few of us grew up in households where sex was discussed healthily and openly. Good sexual communication generally requires more than a single-word response. For a lot of people of all ages, honest and open sexual communication is brand-new terrain.

Before you become sexually active with a partner, take a look about how you communicate with them about other things. Are you able to talk openly and freely about your feelings for each other, relationship models, time management, previous romantic/sexual relationships, peer and family relationships, and dealing with crises? If not, it's wise to take a pause and evaluate if that partner is a smart sex partner for you yet: after all, if you don't feel comfortable talking about needing a little more time together or what's going on with your family, it's going to be a serious challenge to talk about wanting to be touched more here or there, or about having a yeast infection. If daily communication, especially about things that are very close to your heart, doesn't feel pretty easy just yet, work on that first, or consider that this person may not be an ideal partner for you. Look at your own existing sexual communication in other parts of your life. Are you able to discuss sexual issues with your friends or your physician with a decent level of comfort and honesty (even if things sometimes feel a bit awkward)?

If you're already at that point, then you've got a good foundation for sexual communication. You can lay it down from the outset just by saying something as simple as (but likely less formal than), "Before we get sexually involved, I want us to be able to talk about sex together honestly and freely." Just making your intentions clear like that opens the door, allowing both you and your partner permission to talk, and to be honest when you do.

If it feels to you as if sexual issues cannot be discussed by you and your partner—either because you don't feel ready, or because you think talking about them will bring on anger, upset, jealousy, or massive insecurity—then you might want to wait for partnered sex with that person until you both do feel able to talk more comfortably You can get more practice talking outside of bed, since any conversation tends to be a lot more loaded between the sheets.

Once you have some basic solid communication dynamics down, it's pretty much just a matter of basic care and feeding: if and when you do start having partnered sex, you'll keep talking to one another, all the time, and it should become second nature to always be communicating, sharing ideas, feelings, and experiences without trying too hard. It's not unusual, when you first start having partnered sex, to go without heavy verbal communication for a while, because it's new, because you're both caught up in all the things that feel good, and because things that aren't as you like them, yet, will just take time. Communication is important, but the sex you're having also doesn't need to feel like a lecture series to be healthy.

It usually takes a few tries—and often more than that—before we meet someone whose needs and wants are compatible with ours, or can work with a partner to find middle ground that works for both of us. Because of that, it's tempting to let things go unsaid, when we really need to be talking about them—things like limits and boundaries that aren't being respected or communicated, wants or needs that aren't being met, relationship models we know we can't deal with, or sexual velocity that is just going too fast. Resist that temptation if it happens: you don't want to set patterns or precedents for things that aren't okay with you or aren't working for you, because that makes it even harder to work them out in the long run. Put your limits and boundaries onto the table as soon as they come up. Even if that feels difficult, awkward, or risky to do, it'll be a lot easier to set limits earlier rather than later.

SEXUAL LINGO

Part of sexually communicating well involves using terms that both of you know the meaning of and are comfortable with. So, you and yours may hit roadblocks to productive sexual communication if, say, you're talking about "tea bagging" or "fingering," and your partner has no idea what you're referring to, or if your partner calls your genitals a "pussy" or a "prick," and those terms are offensive to you.

Be sure that when you are talking about sex, you do so without making too many assumptions, and think about the language you are using to express yourself. Be open to making changes or clarifying in order to better that communication. Ask what words work for your partner; tell them what words and language feel best to you.

On a related note, everyone has different levels of comfort when it comes to "pillow

s.e.x.

the top ten really crappy reasons to have (any sort of) sex with someone else

1. To try to keep them from leaving or having sex with someone else

Sex to keep someone around is manipulative and is emotional blackmail for both people (and also rarely works).

2. To prove your maturity or independence

If you really need it, the best "proof" of maturity and independence is making choices based on what's best for you and what you really want and need—choices that aren't harmful or hurtful to you or others—no matter what anyone else may think of them.

3. As a substitute for exploring your body yourself

Nobody can know your body as intimately as you can. Some people report that they "just can't get into" or enjoy masturbation, and that's fine. Or they complain that it just doesn't feel the same as sex with a partner—and that's not surprising, because they're different things, and they generally don't feel the same. So, masturbation doesn't have to be your favorite thing. But find your own clitoris or prostate by yourself first, rather than asking a partner to seek it out for you. Get to know your favorite places or your ick-zones by yourself, as well as with a partner. Learn about the names for your own anatomy and where everything is, rather than going out for a road trip without a map.

4. To make your parents mad or get their attention

The trouble with this one is that most people don't even realize that's what they've done it until ten years later, and then they get to suck it up and feel pretty stupid when it's clear that's exactly what they did. It's not fun, and it rarely produces the desired result. You may be putting yourself at risks for no good reason, using others or hurting their feelings, and ripping yourself off of the experience of having sex in an environment where it can actually be pleasurable and make you feel good about yourself.

5. Because someone else did it

I know you know what your mother would say, so I don't need to talk about cliff-jumping here. To sum up: Someone else isn't you. The best choices for you are the ones you make FOR you, based on your own needs, wants, and abilities, not someone else's.

6. To fit in with friends or gain status with people

Sex for this reason is often a double-edged sword. While it might net you status with some, it'll decrease your status or reputation with others. People who are your friends accept you as you are, and like you for who you are, including your own sets of values and choices, even if they aren't the same as theirs.

7. Because your partner wants it, even if you're sure you really don't

Having any sort of sex based on feelings of obligation or pressure tends to leave a really nasty taste in your mouth for quite some time, and doesn't do a lot for your self-image. If your partner wants to do something you don't, you can communicate that with a simple, "I'm sorry, but I'm not interested in/ready for/willing to do that. If and when I am, I'll let you know. How about we do this instead?" And any partner worth having isn't going to argue that point. If what's being suggested is a really big deal to them and just not workable for you, now or ever, you may have to deal with sexual compatibility issues at some point (see page 178), but even the least desired outcome of that is going to be easier to live with than participating in activities you really don't want to.

8. To just get it over with

That's an understandable thing to want to do with a job interview, taking out the trash, or getting your cheeks ritually squished by an overzealous aunt. But partnered sex is supposed to be enjoyable and satisfying, and, like most good things in life, it often requires the right set of circumstances, the right time, and being in a good place, all around. Partnered sex doesn't have an expiration date like a carton of milk, nor is it a requirement at any given age or time.

9. Because you're bored or restless

Get a hobby. Get a job! Go hang out with friends. Read a book, see a movie, go biking or skating. Write a novel. Clean your room, surf the Internet, give your dog a bath. Heck, masturbate. Sex with a partner is rife with emotional and physical risks, on both sides. If someone who told you that they decided to climb Mount Everest or learn to swallow knives because they were kinda bored, you'd think they were a little whack, and the same goes with sex because of boredom.

10. To spite someone, even just yourself

Maybe you want to make an ex jealous. Maybe you want to prove to someone who questioned your readiness, attractiveness, or orientation that they're wrong. Maybe you want to sting your best friend for dating someone you also liked by sleeping with him or her. Maybe you cheated on a current partner, and are so mad at yourself, you feel that sleeping with four more people at a party is a justifiable self-punishment.

You don't want your sex or love life to resemble trash TV. You have to live with yourself and the effects of your actions for your whole life—you can't just change the channel. Make sexual choices you feel pretty confident you can live with, and will want to.

talk"—talking about sex during sex, for the effect of heightening arousal. Some people may like a partner to "talk dirty" during sex, but their partner may not be comfortable with that, or not yet. Again, these tend to be matters of compatibility, and by discussing them, even partners with some divergence of opinion can often find middle ground that works for both of them.

▪ BODY OF EVIDENCE: ▪
Legal Issues in Your Sex Life

When we're making sexual choices, we often need to concern ourselves with the people immediate to us: ourselves, our partners, our friends and family. We also have to concern ourselves with our larger community, including the laws of our counties, states, and/or countries. Knowing what risks you and your partner are taking when it comes to the law is important in considering your choices. For instance, taking a chance by sleeping with a legal adult when you're a minor often just isn't worth the risk of landing the adult in jail with permanent sex offender status, something which can and does happen, and ruins lives. Sending someone a racy photo over the Net or asking for one may be something you think twice about when you're aware that it could be a crime, not just a safety risk. You may even be a victim of, or accessory to, certain crimes and not know it.

Laws vary widely internationally, so a list of all the specific sex laws pertinent to every area in the globe would not only be beyond the scope of this book, it's generally beyond the scope of your average law library. To discover which laws apply to you, and if you are a minor, how they apply to juveniles, you have to do a little simple legwork yourself, either visiting your library or the Net. It's helpful, though, to know what sort of thing you're looking for, what the terms mean, and how specific laws may apply to you.

Age of consent: The age established by a state, county, or nation at which a person can legally give consent to sex with another person. Age of consent laws—which were actually initially designed to deal with prostitution of children by their parents—differ between states and countries. The youngest age of consent worldwide is currently twelve (in several countries, including Chile, Panama, and the Netherlands), and the oldest, eighteen, is found in several states in the United States, including California. On average, the age of consent is around sixteen, but what's relevant to you is what it is in *your* area. Some places have AOC laws that differ for men and women. Some AOC laws allow for those who are underage to legally engage in sex together; others do not. Several areas have a different age of consent for same-sex partners than for opposite-sex partners. What "sex" is in terms of AOC laws often differs: in some areas, it is limited to intercourse; in others, petting may be included. If you're a minor or dating a minor, do look up the AOC in your state, and research what *exactly* it covers and doesn't.

While you may have questions about the fairness or "legitimacy" of AOC laws, the intent behind them is to protect minors, however flawed aspects or applications of those laws may be. When used as they were designed to be, they can protect youth who truly couldn't give full, informed consent, who were coerced

S.E.X.

into sex by someone with far greater power than they have, mainly by virtue of being older. They also may make adults who are predatory regarding sex with minors less likely to seek minors out. The partner under the age of consent in any age of consent case is not criminalized; it is the partner over the AOC who is considered to have committed a crime.

Statutory rape: The crime of a legal adult, or person over the legal age of consent, engaging in sexual activity with a minor, or person under the legal age of consent. Depending on the age of the minor, this may instead be treated as child molestation, but generally, when a teen is involved and he or she consented to the sexual activity, it falls under statutory rape. Sometimes, statutory rape or similar charges can occur if a person is over the age of consent, but is still a legal minor and has had sex with a legal adult.

Statutory rape used to be something of an empty charge, but in the United States it's possible for a statutory rape charge to translate into sex offender status for a person's whole life. That's no small deal. A state law known as Megan's Law requires communities to be informed when someone charged as a sex offender moves into their neighborhood. The person convicted may even be required to go door to door to tell neighbors who they are and what they have done. Being a registered sex offender can have a heavy impact on availability of jobs, places to live, custody agreements and parenting—the works.

To put it bluntly, this can mean that a sixteen-year-old boy, over the age of consent, who has had consensual sex with his girlfriend, only six months younger but under the AOC, could wind up charged with statutory rape and registered as a sex offender. Sadly, while rare (most states have "Romeo and Juliet" exceptions to statutory rape laws, for cases where two partners are very close in age), such things have happened. Even when sex offender status is not applied, having a statutory rape charge on your record can mean not getting into college, not being considered for a job, or being turned down for leases because you've got a criminal record.

How could someone get charged? By a parent, teacher, friend, doctor, or neighbor reporting the known or suspected sexual activity. By someone under the AOC who originally said yes, but has decided in retrospect, sincerely or maliciously, that they really were not able to give full consent. For the record, parents cannot override these laws. So, even if a given person's parents approve and are okay with a minor teen having sex with a legal adult, if someone else reports the activity, charges can still be filed.

The younger party in cases like this is rarely charged with anything, but needless to say, that doesn't mean they don't suffer. As well, parents may find themselves charged with negligence if they knew what was going on and didn't report it themselves. Gender is a nonissue here: both men and women can be and have been charged with statutory rape.

Indecent exposure: This is the term for public acts of nudity, masturbation, or partnered sex. A lot of people participate in indecent exposure without even knowing it, because what they consider public and what is LEGALLY public are

s.e.x.

two different things. For instance, having any kind of sex in a car in a public garage, or parked out on public property, like the street or a park, is public rather than private sex, and thus, indecent exposure. "Public nudity" generally applies to exposure of body parts deemed sexual, such as genitals and breasts.

Solicitation: In the most basic sense, sexual solicitation occurs when some form of sex is offered, accepted, or suggested in exchange for something else, such as money, higher job status, or a place to stay. Prostitution is a form of solicitation.

This can include Internet activity. For instance, if you ask someone in a chat room to send you explicit photographs, offer to do the same, or ask for certain sex acts, you're soliciting (and then some—especially since, if you're a minor, you'd also technically be distributing "child pornography").

On a related note, it's important to know that sex work is not legal for minors in the United States. And unlike the way some other sex laws are enforced, a minor can be charged, punished, and/or incarcerated for solicitation.

Sodomy: Sodomy laws are those that criminalize any act of oral or anal sex, even between consenting adults. These laws have almost exclusively been applied to homosexuals and bisexuals.

Starting in the sixties, states have been repealing these laws, usually with the help of the American Civil Liberties Union. At this point, fewer than twenty states in the United States still have sodomy laws on the

books, and most sodomy cases at this point are tossed out of court or repealed. *Lawrence v. Texas,* a 2003 U.S. Supreme Court case in which two gay men sued—and won—over state sodomy laws, has essentially made even sodomy statutes that still exist basically unenforceable.

Rape: Rape occurs when a person is forced into a sexual act against their will, with physical force or some form of strong coercion. If a person consents to sex under duress, such as threats to harm friends or family, or if the victim has been given drugs or alcohol to produce consent, that is also rape.

Rape often has subcategories. "Forcible rape" generally implies physical force or full-body violence. "Date rape" or "acquaintance rape" applies to a rape committed by someone known to the rape victim. "Spousal rape" refers to a rape that has occurred between married people. "Gang rape" is the term for a rape in which more than one rapist is involved. "Attempted rape" and "assault with intent to rape" are terms used to describe an instance in which rape did not take place, but was intended or attempted. Rape may also be classed as sexual assault, abuse, or molestation.

While very few people are confused about what forcible rape is, many people are in denial about other types of rape. Coercion—pushing and pressuring a partner to have sex until they finally give in—can be rape. Pursuing sex with someone who is clearly inebriated, under the influence of drugs, or distressed is also rape, if sex does ensue. Organizations such as the Guttmacher Institute and SIECUS have stated that nearly 60 percent of women under fifteen who are sexually active have reported some sort of involuntary or coerced sex.

The vast majority of people raped are female—as many as one out of every six women have been a victim of rape or attempted rape—and the vast majority of rapists of women and men alike are male. However, men are also raped: about one out of every eight rape victims is male, according to the National Crime Victimization Survey in the United States. For more on rape and sexual assault, see chapter 10.

Sexual harassment: Unwelcome and uninvited sexual advances, requests for sexual favors—even in the form of jokes—or other sexually-loaded verbal or physical conduct are sexual harassment, when accepting or rejecting that behavior or those advances could affect a person's employment, interfere with a person's performance, or create an intimidating, hostile, or offensive environment. While it's most often applied in job environments, sexual harassment can also occur in schools, community centers, and other areas.

Sexual harassment has the power and impact it has for the same reason it's so rarely reported: because in a culture where sex is often seen as shameful, it's very easy to shame someone into silence where sex is concerned, and our culture also has a tendency to blame the victim of a sexual crime, especially when that victim belongs to a sexual or general minority. The girl who gets called a whore again and again may not say anything because that makes her feel like

one; the person getting unwanted sexual attention may stay silent for fear that reporting the harassment will cause even more of that attention—or they may feel that the situation is their own fault. Sexual harassment isn't rape, so a lot of people being harassed figure they'll just suck it up and it'll go away. A lot of people also think it's funny or harmless, when it very often is neither.

Loitering: Loitering—being "in a place at a time or in a manner not usual for law-abiding individuals" and arousing "suspicion" among others or from the property-owner—isn't a sex crime, per se, but it can be treated like one. Again, loitering laws are most often used against groups (like gays and lesbians or teens) whose sexual activity isn't socially acceptable in a given area. Loitering laws can also be used to discriminate against transgender persons by being applied, for instance, when a TG person uses the "wrong" bathroom. Trying to evade or argue with security or law officers in any situation where you're on private property that isn't yours (which includes malls, stores, schools), even if you are in the right, is a bad idea and likely to result in a charge. So, if loitering is being suggested and clearly used as discrimination that you want to counteract, your best bet is to leave the situation, complying with the officer, then later report it to another officer or talk to a lawyer or legal aid group.

Be careful and aware when it comes to the law. Certainly, some laws, and the ways they're applied aren't fair, and certainly, it's a bit strange to have to consider the courts

_s.e.x._

when making sexual choices for yourself. But legal issues exist all the same, and unless you're willing to go to jail to protest them, it's a really good idea to obey the law as best you can. And if you're going to take a risk, seriously consider not just the emotional or physical consequences, but also the possible legal ramifications.

However, take comfort in the fact that if you're making sound sexual choices based on criteria like the factors in the Sexual Readiness Checklist, sex laws are not likely to be a big issue for you, so there's no need to freak out or obsess.

popular mechanics:
the ins and outs of partnered sex

NOBODY NEEDS COMPLETE step-by-step instruction manual for sexual activities, which is why this section isn't one.

It's often assumed that there is one "right" way to perform any sexual activity and/or that there is one "right" order in which to engage in sexual activities. Sure, most people kiss before oral sex or intercourse. But sexual activities aren't simply a matter of a progression that builds up to penis-vagina intercourse or anal sex for everyone, and the order that feels right for a given person, or with a given partner, can vary a lot. While any one sexual activity can be performed by itself, for most people a combination of activities, with full body contact, is what's most satisfying.

What is essential is feeling able to communicate on the same page, to do what comes naturally, to be creative and spontaneous, and to learn what each of you enjoys by experimenting and communicating together. If you don't worry too much or overthink it; if you're talking, listening, and attentive to your partner's nonverbal cues (when they smile, moan, turn a body part toward you more closely, or pull away slightly), and when you are giving cues yourself and respond truthfully and authentically, it's pretty impossible to do any sort of sex "wrong." It's common to get all hung up on touching "right" and forget that it usually does come naturally if you let it. **There aren't rights and wrongs** when you're paying attention to and respecting your partner, and they you.

Much of sexual pleasure is psychological and emotional. That doesn't mean what goes on physically is irrelevant or unimportant—

it's very important—but if you're feeling good about what you're doing; if you're emotionally and practically prepared; if you feel safe, trusting, and relaxed with your partner and are simply enjoying being close to them, and they with you, then most things feel good without trying too hard. The only person who could make a sex manual for how to please your specific partner IS that partner; the only person who could make one for you is *you*.

The sexual activities listed below aren't in a progressive order you should feel the need to follow, nor is the list meant to imply that each activity needs to or should be a be-all and end-all. It's ordered in terms of increased intimate contact, STI and pregnancy risks, and prevalence of practice. The list here also isn't divided by gender or orientation. There are heterosexual men who engage in receptive anal sex with their girlfriends, there are lesbian women who participate in blow jobs or vaginal intercourse with dildos or hands. Obviously, some form of phallus is required for fellatio, some sort of vulva for vaginal intercourse, but those bare basics aside, there isn't any form of nearly any sexual activity that any combination of partners can't do.

About the Pregnancy and STI Risk Assessments

You'll see that after each activity, the level of risk for pregnancy and STIs is noted. These assessments are for the level of risk incurred when birth control and safer sex are NOT used. So, for example, vaginal intercourse is listed as high risk for pregnancy and STIs, but those risks can be substantially reduced with a reliable birth control method and safer sex practices. (For specific information on birth control methods and effectiveness rates, see chapter 11, and for specific information on reducing STI risks, see chapter 9.)

low risk

medium risk

high risk

▪ KISSING ▪

AKA: Making out, macking down, sucking face, smooching, snogging, pecking, French kissing.

What is it, and how do you do it?
You know this one. Kissing is when two people press their lips together, and enjoy exploring one another's mouths or any other part of the body with their lips, teeth, and/or tongues.

Most folks know how to deliver a closed-mouthed kiss, but with a sexual partner, you shouldn't want to grimace or hold your lips super-tight for fear of too much slobber from Uncle Joe or Aunt Gladys: you are opening yourself up to your partner through your mouth.

Some partners test the waters by kissing a partner on the cheek first. For a lip-lock, you just lean forward and press your lips gently to theirs, tilting your head a bit to get noses out of the way. You can have a session of closed-mouth kissing for quite some time, just by repeating the kisses for as long as you'd like, and kissing whatever parts you and your partner choose.

Openmouthed, or "French," kissing means just what it says: your mouths are open. That may mean using your tongue to explore your partner's tongue or lips, slight nibbles on the lips or tongue with the teeth. Kissing is a whole lot like dancing: both partners are taking steps and following the other's lead and rhythm. So, it's good to pay attention to the subtleties of what your partner is doing, and go slowly until you get in the groove together.

Kissing isn't just reserved for mouths only: you or your partners can kiss any part of the body! Many people find kissing and outercourse (like petting, cuddling, and "dry sex") to be some of the most enjoyable and intimate sexual activity there is.

You might also want to be aware that, because kissing (especially deep or extended kissing) does feel so intimate, it may be something you and/or your partner are hesitant about, or that you or a partner may be comfortable with other sexual activities before kissing, and that's okay. In that regard, it's also probably safe to say that if you really, really don't feel comfortable kissing someone, or if they're continuously hesitant to kiss you, that can be a sound cue that either you or they aren't feeling ready for sexual intimacy yet, or that you may not be a good fit as sexual partners altogether, for any number of reasons.

STD/STI risk: No risk to low risk. (No risk for dry or closed-mouth kissing; low risk for wet or openmouthed kissing, although if there is a mouth sore or injury present in either partner, there is a greater risk.)
Pregnancy risk: No risk.

▪ PETTING/MASSAGE ▪

AKA: Feeling up, rubbing, necking, petting, touching up, outercourse.

What is it, and how do you do it?
It's exploring and pleasuring one another's whole bodies with the hands. For some people, the major draw is parts of a partner's body they think of as sexual, or those that aren't touched in common, platonic

S.e.x.

contact: the neck or back, breasts or chest, stomachs, hips, thighs, buttocks, genitals.

Petting and massage can be anything from heated to really mellow and relaxed. You may even just be giving your partner a backrub because they're tense or sore, or because it feels nice, and it may or may not become sexual.

How someone likes to be touched differs from person to person and area to area. For example, one woman may like some squeezing on her breast or intense nipple play, another may just like light, feathery stroking. Sometimes partners limit touch to one area, as a way of working with it or as an extended "tease." As with all intimate contact, communication is a good thing, and many people figure it out as they go by just asking, "Does this feel good?" or "Should I rub more gently?" Feedback like "I love it when you touch me like that there," or "You can do that harder," keeps communication open.

During petting, massage, or cuddling, you can rub, stroke, knead, or pull your partner's skin with your hands and fingers, varying in intensity from very light, almost tickly touching to very deep kneading or massage. Sometimes you might add your mouth to the mix, licking, sucking, or kissing parts of the body.

People tend to forget that our genitals aren't the only sensitive or sexual parts of our bodies. Touching the whole body can increase intimacy with partners, and increases overall sexual sensation and arousal. Plus, it feels good! Some people can even reach orgasm due to intense petting or massage, or from touch to parts that aren't genitals: the breasts, neck, thighs.

When you're with a new partner, you might want to start by setting limits and checking with your partner about their limits. You or your partner may have certain body parts you don't want, or don't feel ready, to touch or have touched. There may be parts of your body you still feel awkward with, and you can let a partner know about that. If you want to stay fully or partially clothed, communicate that, and encourage your partner to communicate their preferences.

STD/STI risk: No risk, so long as no body fluids are shared.
Pregnancy risk: No risk.

▪ MUTUAL MASTURBATION ▪

AKA: Circle jerking/jilling, flop-whacking, wankwatching (okay, so I made that one up).

What is it, and how do you do it? When partners masturbate in each others' presence, it's called mutual masturbation. (Sometimes, mutual masturbation is also the term used to describe partners giving each other manual sex at the same time, but that's not what we're talking about here.) During mutual masturbation, there is not genital contact between partners: it is *self-contact* with your partner present. Both partners may be masturbating at the same time, one after the other, or only one person may be masturbating with a partner looking on.

It's not unusual to have mutually masturbated with friends during childhood, puberty, or adolescence; plenty of people do or have done that, no matter their gender or sexual orientation. It's also not unusual to feel a little weird about mutual masturbation, especially at first or with a new partner. Usually when we masturbate, we're alone, and often feel freer with our bodies without the self-consciousness we may experience in the company of even a partner. You or a partner may feel that if either of you "needs" to masturbate during partnered sex, it's because you aren't good enough at pleasing each other. Not so! Try to remember that none of partnered sex is a "need" scenario—any of us may just *want* to do different things at different times. And masturbating with a partner isn't a replacement for partnered sex, it IS a form of partnered sex, one that can be a pretty great way to learn about things you and your partner like, such as the kinds of genital touch and sensation you enjoy.

STD/STI risk level: No risk.
Pregnancy risk level: No risk.

▪ FROTTAGE OR "DRY SEX" ▪

AKA: Dry sex, humping, grinding, freaking, body rubbing, tribadism—or tribbing—outercourse.

What is it, and how do you do it?
It's when two people grind their genitals together (or their genitals against a

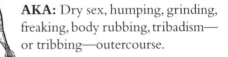

Premature Ejaculation

Young men tend to reach orgasm and ejaculate fairly soon after any given sexual activity begins. In fact, the average length of time for a man to reach orgasm after he gets an erection, according to Kinsey, is around twelve minutes in the early teens (and as few as two minutes for nearly 20 percent of all men) The interval can climb to forty minutes in the late teens and early twenties (shooting up about ten minutes more over the next decade, then declining again in the thirties). Overall, according to Kinsey studies, men on average, of all ages, ejaculate within less than five minutes of intercourse.

The term "premature ejaculation" is a bit bogus. It assumes that there is one "right" length of time or minimum time that is acceptable for erection, and that's just not true. It's not "premature" for a young man to orgasm or ejaculate within a few minutes: it's completely normal. Should the male partner ejaculate when his female partner still wants more intercourse, that's very easily achieved. Take a tip from women who sleep with women: hands can be used to create the same sort of sensations, and you can even find different positions and angles with the fingers that provide variations.

If, as a man, you feel like you're reaching orgasm or ejaculation in such a short time that you just don't feel satisfied, or if you want to try to extend the length of time of erection for other reasons, you can also try masturbating before a partnered sex date; taking pauses of a few minutes from sexual activity when you feel close to orgasm; or making sure that the sex you're having is more full-body than just genital. An added bonus of condom use is that the ring of the condom applies pressure to the base of the penis, often aiding in maintaining erection.

S.e.x.

partner), but usually while dressed (thus the "dry" part), and without direct genital intercourse.

In any position where there is (covered) genital-to-body or genital-to-genital contact, both partners simply move their hips back and forth to stimulate the genitals via pressure and friction. Some male-female or male-male couples also enjoy dry sex by pressing the penis from behind into the buttocks; some female-female couples position themselves to use each other's thighs or genitals for simultaneous genital frottage. Because genitals are sensitive, you can get quite a bit of sensation from the warmth and motion of another's body, and since partners are often face to face, and are usually engaged in full-body contact, it can be very emotionally intimate.

If you are nude or wearing very thin garments, a latex barrier (a condom or dental dam) is a good idea, to prevent accidental fluid contact (for more on barriers and how to use them, see chapter 9). For frottage between women who are nude or wearing thin clothing, a dental dam won't work as a barrier without a harness (see page 212), but there are dam latex "hot pants" on the market that can be used this way, or you can fashion a pair out of a roll of cling film.

STD/STI risk: Low risk.
Pregnancy risk: Low risk.

▪ MANUAL SEX ▪

AKA: Hand job, fingering, finger-fucking, whacking off, wanking, jacking off, jilling off.

What is it, and how do you do it?
Manual sex is when one partner is engaging a partner's genitals with their hands.

For men, receiving manual sex can mean stimulation of the penis, testicles, perineum, anus, and surrounding areas; for women, the vulva, including the mons, inner and outer labia, clitoris and vagina, and/or the perineum, anus, or surrounding areas.

"Fingering" is often assumed to mean vaginal entry only, when, in fact, more women enjoy either clitoral stimulation or a combination of clitoral stimulation and vaginal stimulation.

Bear in mind that the vaginal canal is curved, not straight. So if you are going to engage in manual vaginal sex, putting a rigid finger or three in there as if pushing an elevator button isn't likely to feel so hot. Instead, try to keep your fingers curved inward a little, as if you were holding a ball, and work one finger at a time, gradually, as feels good for your partner.

If you are going to enter the vagina or anus with fingers, gloves and lubricant are advised, primarily for comfort and pleasure, not just for safety. Handwashing can cut some STI risks, but not only do latex gloves do a much better job, they also make manual sex feel better, protecting the genitals from scrapes and abrasions from calluses on the hands, hangnails, or fingernails. Lubrication (what's lube? See page 210) is really important, as is starting slowly and gradually.

For clitoral play, if you're not in a position to look at your partner's genitals and need help finding the clitoris, just ask: so long as she knows her own body well, it's pretty easy for her to place your fingers where it is. Experiment with different

Deeper Manual Sex: Fisting

Deep manual sex, or manual sex with more than a finger or two, is NOT called fisting because you make a fist and try to put it into a vagina or anus, which is unlikely to be anything but painful, if not impossible. Rather, fisting involves starting manual sex with one or two gloved fingers (and lube, added as you go) and slowly working up to more, as is pleasurable for the receptive partner. If a whole hand is wanted by both partners, and four fingers feel good, the performing partner can then tuck his or her thumb into their palm or inside the fingers to make the whole hand as slim as possible, and then slide upward. Once it's all inside, that partner can then turn the hand back and forth, slowly open the fingers up gently and rhythmically, or go up and down, as is comfortable for their partner.

Fisting isn't all that common. Fewer people will likely be interested in full-on fisting, especially at the beginning of their sex lives, and more people are generally interested in vaginal fisting than anal fisting. While both canals really CAN make room for that much inside, and it can feel good, this can be hard to imagine if we're still getting used to the idea of single fingers, a penis, or a dildo inside the vagina or anus. As with any sort of entry to the vagina or anus, if the idea of deep manual sex makes you very nervous, it's smarter to opt out, because being scared or nervous not only inhibits arousal, but keeps the muscles of both canals from relaxing enough for deeper entry to be comfortable and pleasurable.

Very deep manual sex carries a much higher STI risk than less intrusive manual sex does.

levels of pressure and speed, and with what part of the clitoris you're touching. For some women whose clitorises are very sensitive, indirect clitoral stimulus might be better; for others, very intense, direct pressure may be ideal.

With men, it's not unusual to assume that the head of the penis is where all the good stuff happens, but that isn't necessarily so: the whole penis—head, shaft, and base, and for uncircumcised men, the foreskin—is sensitive to touch, pressure, and sensation. It's common for many men to find they're most sensitive along the coronal ridge under the head, around the frenulum (especially for uncircumcised men), and on the underside of the shaft,

but as with anything else, people vary. Experiment with varying pressure to different areas, and with different speeds and ways of touching. You might curl your whole hand around the shaft and stroke up and down, slowly or briskly, but you can also pat or tap more lightly with fingertips, use a thumb or fingers to apply more focused pressure to certain areas, or roll the shaft between your fingers. An erect penis isn't required for manual sex, so you don't need to wait for an erection, if your partner likes manual sex when he's flaccid or only partially erect.

Since genitals are *sensitive,* using lubricant—and saliva is a substandard lubricant, as well as an infection risk—for

s.e.x.

a handjob is a good idea, though some men may prefer manual sex without. If you have an uncircumcised partner, take your time finding out how far is comfortable for him in terms of pulling the foreskin back on your "downstrokes." Per usual, taking your time and starting off slow is usually a good habit.

If you're engaging in anal manual sex, make sure to switch gloves or wash hands between anal and other genital contact. For people of any gender, before partnered anal play, experimenting alone and gently with the anus first is wise, both to understand how delicate the area can be, and to be prepared for how intense the sensations can be from anal play.

STD/STI risk level: Low risk.
Pregnancy risk level: No risk.

• ORAL SEX: •
Cunnilingus

AKA: Eating out, licking out, going down on, going south, giving head, tipping the velvet.

What is it, and how do I do it? Stimulating a woman's vulva externally (inner labia, clitoris, vaginal opening, perineum) and/or internally (the vagina) with lips, tongue, and/or teeth.

While for many women, the clitoris is the preferred center of activity for oral sex, remember that the inner labia and the clitoral hood are also connected to the clitoris and full of nerve endings, too, so stimulation there often also feels good.

Some women like external licking or sucking of the vulva. You can circle the clitoris and vaginal opening with your tongue, lap at it top to bottom or side to side, flick at it with your tongue, suck on it and the labia, even give your partner's vulva loads of soft kisses. Some women enjoy having their vaginal openings explored with the tongue. Even teeth, with *gentle* nibbling or grazing, can feel good. You may wish to hold your partner's outer labia open (and she can also do it with her own hands), to be able to see where you're going or provide more intense sensation to the whole area. Sensitivity differs among women, so you will need to adapt for your own partner.

Many women also enjoy vaginal or anal stimulus during oral sex, either with fingers or a sex toy, and some also enjoy oral stimulus to the perineum or anus (see rimming, below). If you're using a latex barrier for oral sex and are going to incorporate anal play, just be sure to use a new dam for that area, rather than sliding the same one back and forth.

STD/STI risk: Moderate risk.
Pregnancy risk: No risk.

• ORAL SEX: •
Fellatio

AKA: Blow job, blowing, giving head, sucking off, hummer, teabagging (for oral sex on testicles).

What is it, and how do I do it? When a man's penis is stimulated with mouth, tongue, lips, and often, also hands. There isn't usually any actual blowing involved; in the fifties and sixties, "blow" was slang for ejaculate, which is probably the source of *blow job* as slang for fellatio.

Generally, fellatio involves licking, lapping, and sucking the head of the penis, the ridge beneath it, and the shaft. It can also include oral contact with the testicles, perineum, and/or anus.

There's all sorts of crude commentary on what NOT to do when giving head, but we can sum it up, far more respectfully, by merely saying this: A penis is part of a person, not an object, and a pretty sensitive part.

choked up

IF you're the receiver of fellatio, a quick etiquette tip: Imagine, if you will, someone roughly shoving an unpeeled banana fully into your mouth and throat. Not a pretty picture. Holding a partner's head gently or guiding their mouth with your hands during fellatio is completely fine, if they're down with it (not everyone is—some people find that it feels threatening). Pressing your pelvis very intensely or quickly into a mouth isn't anything but a good way to choke somebody, so just be sure to be attentive, if holding a partner's head, to what your hands are doing and to what their limits are.

Guard your teeth behind your lips. Don't suck on a penis too roughly: start slowly and softly. Even when you use a little more intensity, remember that the skin is delicate there. If you're giving fellatio, know this: You do NOT have to try to fit the entire penis in your mouth. You can use your hands as an extension of your mouth, instead, to stimulate the parts of the penis not covered by the mouth.

While the penis may look simpler than female genitalia, it really isn't, and just like the vulva and clitoris, it is a sum of several different parts. Don't be in a hurry: like women, many men enjoy more delicate or subtle sensations at first, too.

There's a pervasive myth out there that every single man not only loves blow jobs, but loves receiving oral sex most of all. The truth is that most people of *all* genders enjoy oral sex, male and female alike. And there are plenty of people, of all genders, who either just don't like it, or who prefer other things at other times.

STD/STI risk: High risk.
Pregnancy risk: No risk.

▪ ORAL SEX: ▪
Analingus

AKA: Rimming, rim job, tossing the salad, hitting it.

What is it, and how do I do it?
One partner orally stimulates another partner's anus or rectum with their lips or tongue. Rimming is one of those activities often assumed to be practiced only by gay men, but people of all genders and orientations may enjoy rimming, as well as stimulus to the perineum.

It's strongly advised to use a latex barrier during analingus, because traces of fecal matter often carry bacteria that can cause infection, especially if you're also using your mouth on other portions of your partner's genitals. While it's unusual to have direct contact with substantial amounts of fecal matter during anal play,

s.e.x.

oral sex freakouts

A LOT of people are concerned about tastes and smells during oral sex, especially with new partners. But if you're with someone you haven't been with monogamously for at least six months, practicing safer sex, you should use a barrier method to avoid STI transmission, so taste is really a nonissue. When that time has passed, you'll likely feel more comfortable with your partner and less worried about that. Healthy body fluids tend to taste like . . . well, body fluids. Like sweat, they're a little salty, sometimes a bit bitter or sweet. Same goes for smells: nobody's vulva or penis smells like roses. Genitals often smell a little musky and intense. Ultimately, no one in sound sexual health is going to taste or smell "bad." If you know or suspect you do, check in with your sexual health-care provider: a seriously foul, fishy, or overly strong taste or scent often signals an infection.

If you're curious, it is safe and okay to taste and smell your own genital fluids. If you feel funny about them, that's a good reason to hold off on partnered sex that involves your genitals; until you can enjoy and feel comfortable with all the aspects of your own body, it's awfully hard to do so with someone else.

Lastly, if you feel fearful, intimidated, or in some way freaked out by getting up close and personal with your partner's genitals—or by having someone get up close and personal with yours—by seeing, tasting, or smelling more of them during oral sex than you might with other activities, or if you feel that some form of oral sex is required of you, have a think. Let's come out with it: there's no need to tiptoe around issues many of us know can be common problems. Some prevalent attitudes about oral sex are pretty unhealthy, especially between men and women. Plenty of men who sleep with women don't want to engage in cunnilingus. They may feel that they don't understand female anatomy, or they may be intimidated by it. Many are influenced by cultural attitudes that say that giving a woman oral sex is somehow subordinate, dirty (despite the fact that the vulva is no more or less clean than the penis) or unmasculine. Plenty of women who sleep with men find that some male partners don't really make fellatio optional. Women may give blow jobs as a way to say no to something else—for instance, to get men to cease pressures to have intercourse—or they may come up against cultural attitudes about serving "male needs," being dominated, or women being responsible for getting male partners off.

If you've gotten this far into this book, none of these people should be you. You understand the anatomy, you understand crappy cultural and gender mandates and roles, you understand that part of sexual readiness is feeling ready to get very intimate with all of your partner's body. You already know that it's not such a swift idea to do one activity with a partner as a means to try to "earn" the same for yourself. You should always be doing only things you want to do, but it's also smart to evaluate why you do or don't want to do them, and make sure your reasons for either are sound and healthy.

bacteria and infections are often present because feces have passed through the rectum and anus.

Culturally and/or personally, some people may find the idea of anal play repulsive because they have such negative associations with excrement, and because of strong cultural stigmas, especially for male receivers, straight, gay, or otherwise. For some who only associate anal stimulation with gay men, homophobia may make anal play unappealing. As with anything else, it's perfectly okay *not* to want to engage in anal play. But it might be a good idea, even if you pass on it, to reevaluate how you think, even just about your own anus. No parts of the body are dirty or bad, and learning to love ALL of our parts is pretty essential to loving our bodies and feeling good about them.

STD/STI risk: High risk.
Pregnancy risk: No risk.

▪ VAGINAL INTERCOURSE ▪

AKA: Sexual intercourse, heterosexual intercourse, having sex, screwing, fucking, making love, shagging, hitting it, nookie, getting laid, the horizontal mambo.

What is it, and how do I do it? Vaginal intercourse is often the assumed "default" sex, as in, that's what many people mean, and assume others mean, when they say they're "having sex." Vaginal intercourse is when the vagina is entered, generally by a male partner's penis, and those parts remain interlocked, generally moving in an in-and-out motion, for sexual satisfaction. Lesbian couples, though, can also engage in vaginal intercourse by using dildos with harnesses (AKA strap-on sex), or can experience a similar sensation with manual sex. Obviously, there are no pregnancy risks

between women, but a shared dildo that hasn't been or cannot be boiled, and is not covered by a condom, poses moderate to high STI risks, and a hand not washed or gloved also poses those risks. For the most part, the same tips that apply to heterosexual vaginal intercourse also go for strap-on vaginal intercourse.

For many women, intercourse, all by itself, is not entirely satisfying, nor is orgasm likely to occur from intercourse alone. If I had a nickel for every young woman who thought there was something wrong with her, or that she was doing something wrong, because she didn't reach orgasm from intercourse— or even like it all that much—I'd be writing this from spacious oceanfront resort property. The reason for this is simple: the design of the vagina is such that most of the vaginal canal is not rich with nerve endings, unlike other parts of the vulva.

That doesn't mean intercourse isn't enjoyable for women, or that all enjoyment from it is only emotional or intellectual. It's just to say that pairing intercourse with OTHER sexual activities—before, after, and/or during intercourse—is what's optimal for most women.

Men, as well, may not find that vaginal intercourse is the very best sexual activity for them. Some men find that not being able to feel where they end and a partner begins, which is common during intercourse, is too vague for their enjoyment; that more friction is desired for more sexual sensation on their part. Like women, plenty of men may also need or like a varied combination of sexual activities, rather than intercourse alone.

That isn't to say that all cheers for intercourse are hype and bluster. LOTS of

s.e.x.

people enjoy intercourse. For many people, intercourse feels more intimate than other sexual activities, perhaps because the experience of interlocked genitals and the positions assumed for intercourse can give the feeling of an incredibly full and complete whole-body embrace.

As with any form of vaginal entry, it's key to take things step by step. For men, erection is required for intercourse; for women, arousal and lubrication beforehand and during are needed for pleasurable, "successful" intercourse.

Take your time working up to intercourse, with other sexual activities beforehand (sometimes called "foreplay"), even to the extent of both partners reaching orgasm or feeling fully satisfied with those other activities *first*.

The vaginal symptoms of arousal aren't all that difficult to figure out: if a woman is aroused, she feels good with a few fingers inside her vagina, and a penis or dildo entering the vaginal opening feels good and isn't a struggle. If a partner feels very "tight," or if that initial entry is painful for the woman, then chances are good she's not yet fully aroused (unless her inner labia are being tugged on painfully, or because of a hymenal issue or vaginismus—in which case, you can just gently move them aside with fingers).

How deeply to have intercourse is up to both partners, but the receiving partner is the one most likely to experience discomfort if a penis or dildo is inside too deep for her, especially if she's not fully aroused, so be mindful and stay in com-

Vaginismus is a persistent condition in which vaginal contact, entry, or intercourse causes the vagina to essentially clamp up or close, which can make intercourse or manual sex with vaginal entry very painful. It's relatively rare, affecting less than around 5 percent of women, and may be caused by previous sexual trauma or abuse, by repeated incidences of painful or uncomfortable sexual intercourse, or by intense fear or nervousness about intercourse or other vaginal entry. Because women with vaginismus expect pain, repeated attempts or pressure to engage in intercourse can create anxiety, which only exacerbates the condition. If you and your partner are only having intercourse once full arousal and relaxation are present, with plenty of lubrication, but vaginal entry, manual vaginal sex, or intercourse is still painful, check in with your doctor. There are various therapies available that are effective for the majority of vaginismus patients. Be sure in the meantime, though, to just engage in other, external activities, as continuing to try over and over again when it hurts can make vaginismus more persistent and intense.

Remember that if a woman is not fully aroused, is scared or nervous (which is often compounded when birth control or safer sex practices aren't used), doesn't really want to be having intercourse, and/or isn't properly lubricated, intercourse is likely to be uncomfortable or painful, and that isn't vaginismus or any special medical condition.

s.e.x.

munication throughout. (And if discomfort from depth is an issue for the female partner, choosing a position where she has control over that, like on top, can be helpful.) Men and women alike may find the most sensitive stimulation they feel from intercourse is from shallower depth. Having intercourse at a shallow depth—only entering a couple of inches—can stimulate the textured G-spot in women with the sensitive coronal ridge of the penis: in other words two of the most sensitive parts of both the male and female genitals are engaged at the same time.

Since different people are different shapes, including their genitals, a position that was great with one partner may not be so great with another. There are a gazillion books out there with huge lists of sexual positions, but most can be summed up simply: bodies can fit together a whole lot of different ways, and which ways are best generally depends on what feels best for the specific bodies involved.

There are some schools of sexual thought that concern different ways to engage in intercourse to meet certain ends. Tantra, for instance, focuses on slowing down movements during intercourse and delaying or withholding orgasm or ejaculation (mainly for men). But overall, most people generally find that what they like has some constants (depth or angle, certain favorite positions) and some variances (how fast or slow, or additional sexual activities) from day to day and partner to partner.

STD/STI risk: Very high risk.
Pregnancy risk: Very high risk.

HIP TO THE HYPE: COMMON INTERCOURSE PROBLEMS AND EXPECTATIONS

A lot of people are raised with the idea that not only are all sexual activities only a lead-up to heterosexual vaginal intercourse, but that intercourse is THE sexual big deal, THE one thing we'll all like best (or the ginormous thing we'll be missing out on, if we have same-sex partners only), feel most intensely, and have the most emotional connection during. Many heterosexual people, when they talk about "sex," are only talking about intercourse, and heterosexual intercourse is in a tie with masturbation as the most common sexual activity people engage in. The media often depict intercourse as falsely as it depicts most anything else. We're told, all over the place, that intercourse is the most special, the most intimate sexual thing we can do with another person. That's some pretty intense advance billing and some heavy hype.

So, it's not too surprising that when many people do have intercourse they're scratching their heads wondering what they did wrong, or trying to figure out what all the fuss was about. For some people, it really is everything they expect the first time round. But for many, it isn't, and for most, there are going to be at least a few times—if not a lot of them—when heterosexual intercourse just isn't all it's cracked up to be.

Design Flaws

One of the major issues is that intercourse—or manual vaginal stimulus—all by itself usually doesn't stimulate some of our most sensitive parts. The vaginal canal and opening actually aren't rich with many nerve

s.e.x.

endings. That's a serious bonus for women in labor—after all, if having an infant pass through the vaginal canal and opening produced any more sensation than it already does, most folks'd pass out as they gave birth. But it's not so great for women who want intercourse to satisfy their every sexual need or to be sent physically out of this world. For men, intercourse also offers very little stimulation of the prostate, which for many—of any orientation—is an area that provides vast enjoyment and sensation, and for some may be even more enjoyable, or likely to bring about a deeper orgasm, than stimulation to the penis only.

The other thing is that heterosexual intercourse requires an erect penis. Penises don't always want to get or stay erect, even when a guy is aroused and feeling amorous. So, if a couple attempting intercourse hits a snag and erection doesn't occur or stay present, that may be viewed as failure, which can put a lot of pressure on a guy, making enjoyment of the act more difficult than it really should be.

Statistically speaking, it takes women at *least* a couple minutes longer to reach orgasm, from any activity, than it does men. So, since erection is required for intercourse, and it's most common for men to lose erection right after orgasm, chances are good that the male partner will "cross the finish line" first. Thus, a single act of intercourse, all by itself, doesn't commonly equal orgasm or full satisfaction for both partners, even for those who can reach orgasm from intercourse alone.

When Intercourse Just Won't "Work"

It's not abnormal to discover that the first couple of times you attempt intercourse, it just won't "work." With everybody nervous and keyed up, in an activity that's unfamiliar to you, it's so easy to space out the simple stuff, or get stressed, that the easy fixes aren't obvious. This can happen with any number of other genital sexual activities, too. Here's what to do:

▶ **Where to go:** Having trouble finding the vaginal opening at all? A woman at the point where she's really ready for intercourse knows where it is (and to be honest, either of you doesn't know, you might want to slow down and wait until the anatomy is more familiar to you both). So, if you're a partner and you're having trouble, just ask, or slide your fingers to the vulva and feel for it with your hands; when your finger slides into the vaginal opening, it should be pretty obvious. If you're female, and your partner is having some trouble, step up and show them yourself with your own hands. It's also possible that the female partner may have a partial, or even fully intact, hymen blocking the way. Hopefully, if you're at the point of intercourse with a partner, you're familiar enough with their or your anatomy already to know the state of their vaginal opening, and whether or not a full or partial hymen is present. If an intact or resilient hymen seems that it may be an issue, that's something to talk to a gynecologist about.

▶ **How to get in**: If vaginal entry is problematic, chances are good it's one of two things: lack of adequate lubrication, relaxation, and arousal (for one or both partners) or an angle that just isn't working out. If the vaginal opening feels very "tight," it's a strong signal she isn't aroused enough. Full arousal is what causes the vaginal opening and canal to loosen and self-lubricate so that intercourse is possible, comfortable, and pleasurable. So, be sure you've taken the time—step back from intercourse and take more time, if need be—to engage in other enjoyable activities first, and create an environment where the both of you can be relaxed, not overly nervous or anxious. Even when a woman is fully aroused, you may also need to use some extra latex-safe lubricant. Lube really can never hurt, it can only help and make intercourse feel better, no matter what (as well as keeping condoms from breaking).

If both of those things are under control, you may need to adjust your angle. The intercourse position where the woman is on top is often the best in terms of an easy angle of entry. Other positions feel more comfortable for different people, physically and emotionally; just bear in mind that the vaginal canal isn't a straight line: it curves slightly upward, from the opening, in the direction of a woman's belly.

► **When to take a break:** If intercourse is uncomfortable or painful (or just a big yawner) for either party, at any point, just stop. Some people try a different position, add more lubricant, slow down, or add other sexual activity to the mix, like clitoral stimulation with manual sex, masturbation, or a vibrator. If the male partner is having a hard time maintaining erection, give it a rest. Engage in other sexual activities that don't require an erection, and are enjoyable for both of you, or just talk, make out, or cuddle for a while. If you've been going at intercourse for a while and one or both partners isn't reaching orgasm, or is starting to feel less aroused, stop for now. You can engage in other sexual activities, or just halt sex altogether until another day; sometimes, we just hit peak capacity for sex and feel finished, even if orgasm hasn't taken place, and that's perfectly okay.

Intercourse Underwhelm

Lots of people can't reach orgasm from vaginal intercourse, either on a given day, or at all. Most women cannot achieve orgasm from intercourse alone, for the anatomical reasons described earlier, as well as for other reasons. The idea that all men can reach orgasm from intercourse is also false: plenty will not always be able to. Even men or women who CAN achieve orgasm from intercourse may not always want to: orgasm that arises from a different sexual activity may feel better to you or your partner. Intercourse, for both partners, is often most enjoyable when it isn't isolated, when other activities or stimulation are involved. Orgasm is also completely reliant on arousal, and arousal is reliant upon relaxation. Nerves, worries about performance, appearance, relationship, secrecy, pregnancy, disease, or infection, or just not feeling fully ready—all can undermine the ability to achieve orgasm.

You may even discover that intercourse just isn't your thing. Rest assured that not liking it doesn't automatically mean you aren't heterosexual, aren't sexually mature, or don't

s.e.x.

like your partner. It doesn't mean that something's wrong with you or yours. It just means you don't like it or don't like it best, the same way you may not like certain foods, and some foods just aren't your favorite.

Intimacy That Isn't

Emotional intimacy is something that can increase—or not—during ANY sexual activity. You might feel increased intimacy or closeness during intercourse because there is something unique and special about having both sets of genitals engaged at the same time, or because someone is literally inside your body, or you are inside someone else's body, but that can also happen with other sexual activities, like manual or oral sex. Or you might feel that at a given time, with a given partner, or even overall, deep kissing feels more intimate than intercourse. Ultimately, there's no right or wrong answer here: Whatever you find feels most intimate or close with a given partner, or at a different time, is valid and right for you.

Some people find that the expectation that intercourse will or must be the most intimate act, must make both partners feel the most close to each other, creates disappointment for them when one or both partners *don't* experience that fully, or even at all. Some people push for intercourse to try to force a romantic relationship to happen, or to hold onto a lapsing relationship, and sadly discover that it doesn't produce the results they desired.

If your disappointment or discomfort was due to things that are solely up to you to manage (if, for instance, you discover you're only comfortable having intercourse with a committed, long-term partner, or if you just need to learn what turns you on more, by yourself), you've got all the time in

the world to take care of, or wait for, those things before engaging in intercourse again. As with any other sexual activity, both intimacy and enjoyment with a partner tend to deepen and increase over time, as both of you get to know one another and yourselves better, sexually and personally. As your bond deepens, the unfamiliarity of intercourse passes, and your comfort level and confidence increase, it's very likely things will only get and feel better.

is sex better when both partners reach orgasm at the same time?

NOT necessarily, and most sex therapists advise couples against aiming for simultaneous orgasm. Trying to have sex like synchronized swimming isn't such a great idea because it makes it harder for both people to simply enjoy themselves, thereby making any orgasm more difficult, let alone doing it at the same time. When it happens on its own, it's a very happy accident but it's more likely to happen naturally than to be forced, and it's pretty rare. More times than not, when people try to force it, one or both partners will end up faking an orgasm, which sets a bad sexual pattern, and isn't any fun for anyone.

▪ ANAL SEX/INTERCOURSE ▪

AKA: Buttfucking, asslove, backdoor action.

What is it, and how do I do it? Anal sex is entering the anus and rectum for sexual satisfaction of both partners.

It's not uncommon for young hetero-sexual couples of late to engage in anal sex, either to try to avoid the pregnancy, or because it's seen as "adventurous" by one partner. Sadly, it's also not uncommon for the receiving partner to either not be all that interested in it, or not enjoy it at all, because their partner isn't aware that anal intercourse involves MORE patience, preparation, and precaution than vaginal intercourse, not less.

butt b.s.

- Sometimes, with activities that all genders can engage in, the best way for a partner to learn how to make it pleasurable for everyone is to be both giver and receiver. In other words, when a couple wants to explore something like anal sex, since all partners have an anus, taking turns giving and receiving—even though preferences may vary—can give both partners some direct experience and information, as well as increasing intimacy by sharing both roles equally. Men, gay, straight, or otherwise, don't just have to be the "givers" during anal sex. Many men also enjoy receptive (getting) anal sex—especially since it provides stimulation to the prostate gland—as do plenty of lesbian women. For men sleeping with women, and women sleeping with women, this is usually accomplished with fingers, toys, or with a dildo and harness.
- If you're using toys or dildos for anal sex, be sure the object has a flared base that is a good deal larger than the anus. While things can't get "lost" inside the vagina, they can inside the rectum.
- Anal sex is not "safe sex"; it's not a less risky alternative to vaginal intercourse. It is just as

important to have protected anal sex as it is to have protected vaginal sex, and not just because of high STI risks. For opposite-sex partners, pregnancy can't occur *through* the anus: it isn't connected to the uterus internally. But what CAN happen is that during unprotected anal sex, if the receptive partner is female, ejaculate can run down the perineum and into the vulva, and pregnancy can occur that way. So, if you're thinking unprotected anal sex is a good birth control method, rethink it.

- Let's be frank: With rectal tissue as delicate as it is, using anal sex as some kind of powerplay is really uncool. Plenty of people set up anal sex as a form of control or domination over a partner—or, conversely, as a "gift" to a partner, even when it's not pleasurable or even comfortable to receive. If those are roles you want to play with, it's vital both that the receiving partner is feeling pleasure and that the "giving" partner is especially sensitive.

Anal sex shouldn't hurt. But if it isn't done right, or happens too quickly, it can be painful for the receiving partner. Doing it right means a few things. First, BOTH partners need to be interested in it and relaxed. Second, anal intercourse should be **very** slow and gradual.

Unlike the vagina, the rectum doesn't produce any of its own lubrication. The anus is also a tighter, smaller orifice. So, latex-safe lubricant is an *essential* with any anal sex. Because of the risks of infection AND small tears or fissures due to rough hands during manual anal play, gloves or finger cots are also essentials.

If one or two gloved, lubed fingers feel good to the receiving partner, and he or she wants to move up to a fuller sensation,

s.e.x.

then you can do that—again, slowly and gradually, and with a condom on the penis or other object. The person doing the anal entry shouldn't be pushing or forcing their way in: if they/you go slow, the anus will slowly "accept" and pull in more of what's introduced to it. After that, how deep, fast, or slow one should go is up to the person on the receiving end, so communication is as important here as ever. Like other sexual activities, anal play or intercourse can be combined with oral sex, manual sex, or even vaginal intercourse by using fingers or sex toys such as butt plugs.

STD/STI risk:Very high risk.
Pregnancy risk: Moderate risk.

▪ CYBERSEX OR PHONE SEX ▪

Talking "dirty."

What is it, and how do I do it?
Talking "dirty"—even though there's nothing dirty about sex or talking about it—in person, on the phone, or over a computer, to a partner for the purpose of sexual arousal or satisfaction. Some partners use this to tease or incite a partner before an upcoming date; for others, it's an end unto itself, whereby both partners may masturbate to orgasm. Some couples may also talk explicitly about sex during other sexual activities. For partners in long-distance relationships, it's a great way of enjoying sexual intimacy between visits.

What language is used is up to the both of you: some people are turned on by explicit or directive lingo, while others find they're more excited by a more subtle approach.

STD/STI Risk: No risk.
Pregnancy risk: No risk.

▪ SENSATION PLAY ▪

What is it, and how do I do it?
Experimenting with different sensations, throughout the body, not just genitally (in fact, it need not be genital at all).

Some people do this by applying hot and/or cold items to the body, by stroking the body with different items, such as feathers or silky or rough fabrics, by adding food or liquid items to sexual play. Others might use clothespins for a pinching sensation, snakebite kits for "cupping" certain areas of the body for a feeling of suction, safe forms of electrical play with static electricity machines configured for sexual use, or hands, whips, or paddles to strike the skin.

Some use sensation play as part of SM or BDSM activity (see page 168). But those roles structure aren't at all required for sensation play; many people engage in sensation play without incorporating them at all.

So long as skin isn't broken in any way, or direct oral or genital contact isn't being made, sensation play is 100 percent safe sex.

STD/STI risk: No risk.
Pregnancy risk: No risk.

▪ "KINKY" SEX ▪

Just about everybody's heard it, but no one really knows what it means. That's because *kinky* (like *deviant* or *perverse* or *obscene*) is a pretty arbitrary term: everyone defines it a bit differently. But what most people mean when they refer to "kinky" sex is either an uncommon practice or one typically thought of as unconventional. Typically, bondage and restraint, fluid or blood play, the use of sex toys, "edge" play, powerplay or role-play, and some sensation play are filed under "kinky." Whether you feel that any or all of these are "kinky" or not is completely your call.

ROLE-PLAY

What is it, and how do I do it? Just like "make-believe" or "playing doctor" as a kid, some people do the same in a sexual context with partners. That may mean a couple pretends that they're in a different place, that someone is watching, or that they're different genders—what have you. Some bring costumes and props into the scene; for others the fantasy is solely in the imagination. Role-play can be a way for couples to play out sexual fantasies together.

Some people may incorporate hierarchal roles into their fantasy scenario; some may be about "powerplay," in which partners explore different power relationships between them, or sexual fantasies in which power or hierarchical elements are in place, such as student/teacher or employee/boss. Some people explore scenarios that would either be harmful, dangerous or taboo in actuality, such as incest, rape, or sex with strangers. Others may use role-play to explore existing gender roles or stereotypes, or enjoy sillier fare, like playing doctor, cops 'n' robbers, Amazon and captured guy, Bert and Ernie—whatever floats your boat.

Role-play that plays with risk, consent, taboo, or hierarchy power can be very charged and loaded, and also more easily coercive. After all, many of those things are problematic in our culture, and/or based on violence or abuse, and it's really easy to have unacknowledged, internalized ideas about sexual roles that can limit one's awareness of real problems.

Be mindful. Talk about limits and boundaries in advance, and be open to adaptations over time. For instance, you or your partner may find that, while certain activities within a given role-play session are just fine, certain language may be unpleasant, scary, or unwanted. As well, one person's idea of what a given role entails or involves can be pretty different from another's. So, not only is it important to discuss expectations, limits, and boundaries, but it's also a good idea to put fail-safes in place that allow either partner to make clear, pretty immediately, when and if something isn't okay and the action needs to stop. It's also worth talking about where the role-play stays. For instance, if one partner agrees to being submissive during a given "scene," make sure both parties understand that there's no obligation or agreement to always be that way, or bring those roles into other aspects of the relationship.

s.e.x.

BDSM: top to bottom

D/S is a term usually used to describe sexual dominance and submission play, in which one partner "tops" and another "bottoms," and/or one partner is dominating and another submitting. The top or bottom may be of any gender, and the action may involve extending pleasure past a point of physical or emotional comfort; "punishing" a partner via humiliation, sexual play, or withholding sexual activities; and utilizing bondage, sensation play, or verbal enactments. *SM* or *S/M* is an abbreviation for sadism and masochism, or sadomasochism, which means that one partner is giving pain (sado-), and the other is receiving it (-masochism). The "B" in BDSM usually refers to bondage.

BDSM educators recommend what's often known as the *SSC rule:* safe, sane, and consensual. In other words, whatever is being done is agreed upon by both partners, and is performed in ways that are both physically *and* emotionally safe and sane–the same sort of guidelines advised for any kind of sex. Safe and sane includes partners truly being able to consent (including legally) and fully understand what they're agreeing to, both in the short term and the long term (that is, how these sexual choices may affect the individuals, their relationship, and the other areas of their lives). Any sort of sex or role that is forced, sexual coercion, or a malicious use of power roles or sex is NOT safe, sane, or consensual.

D/S play may involve sex acts most people are familiar with, such as oral sex or intercourse. D/S may also incorporate sensation play, bondage, or other "kinky" sexual activities. Many people engaging in D/S play incorporate *safewords* into their play: phrases or gestures understood by both to express thresholds, limits, and boundaries. Saying a safeword stops the role-play or sexual activity at any time, immediately and without question. Like polyamory, D/S or BDSM play often requires more discussion and negotiation than other sexual activities might. D/S roles shouldn't be dictated by sex or gender: both men and women can be tops, bottoms, or "switches," people who enjoy both roles.

Stay self-aware if you're considering or involved with D/S play. It's not atypical for some people to use D/S as a way to make an abusive relationship seem acceptable or sexy, or to employ it as a means to extend self-injury or controlling behavior, even unconsciously. If your partner is in any way physically abusive in the whole of your relationship, or you're not having deep discussions negotiating sexual roles; if your partner verbally abuses or humiliates you outside a "scene," or as a general practice; if you feel that there's a required, implied, or given–rather than agreed upon and optional–power dynamic or imbalance, then it's entirely possible that D/S or S/M play is merely an extension of abuse. With relationship abuse as prevalent as it is for everyone, it's not sensible to entertain the delusion that somehow BDSM relationships or communities are immune.

This is also a particular risk for anyone who has previously been sexually or otherwise traumatized or abused, or has a history of self-injury. As shown in such studies as Stephen Southern's "The Tie That Binds: Sadomasochism in Female Addicted Trauma Survivors," Darren Langdridge and Trevor Butt's "The Erotic Construction of Power Exchange," and Moira Carmody's

"Ethical Erotics" (see the Resources section), attraction to or participation in a D/S or S/M relationship or play, for some abuse survivors, may be reenactment of abuse or simply the only familiar dynamic, rather than one expressly chosen. Some people do choose to process—or find they are processing—abuse issues through BDSM, but again, self-awareness is key, to be sure that it is really beneficial, that it is choice, rather than habit/pattern, and that you are prepared for all the things BDSM can trigger for survivors. (If you're recovering from abuse, checking in with your counselor or therapist is a good plan, before stepping into BDSM.)

Since the sexual activities involved in any BDSM play will vary, pregnancy and STI risks are dependent on those specific activities.

Sometimes, people may find that role-play isn't so good for them, especially if the roles they're playing aren't completely wanted or consensual, if they're sexualizing or reinforcing negative or destructive patterns. For example, a rape survivor wanting to reenact a rape again and again may be trying to process issues via sex that would be more productively and healthily processed in nonsexual situations.

Lastly, it's not unusual for a lot of role-play to be hierarchal, or based on roles of dominance and submission. One reason that is so common is that this power structure is so old and pervasive in our society and culture: those are the roles a lot of us learn. But you can also explore sexual role-play that's outside those structures; nobody has to be tied to any given roles if they don't want to be. If your sexual role isn't 100 percent optional, it isn't healthy (and that goes for our sexual roles even when we aren't outrightly role-playing).

STD/STI risk: Risk levels are dependent on what sexual activities are engaged in during BDSM.
Pregnancy risk: Risk levels are dependent on what sexual activities are engaged in during BDSM.

Bondage/Restraint

What is it, and how do I do it?
Bondage or restraint is the practice of having one partner (or less often, both partners) restrained in some way during sexual activity, for the purpose of increasing pleasure, usually with ropes, cords, other types of fabric or cuffs, and other restraints designed for that purpose. Some people self-restrain during masturbation. Others use rope or cord to create intricate and creative patterns of knot-tying on the body. The Japanese tradition based on that practice is called *shibari*.

It's really important to understand that tying up or restraining a partner against their will is an absolute Big No. **That is assault or kidnapping, and it is criminal and abusive.** As with any other sexual activity, for this sort of play to be at all emotionally safe, it's vital that *everyone* feels *good* about it and consents to it, that everyone is clear on their limits, and that the intent isn't malicious or punitive, but about pleasure and intimacy.

"Edge" Play

Edge play generally refers to sexual activity that crosses the line of what is physically or emotionally safe, sane, or consensual, by taking serious risks with one's life or health. Some examples are breath restriction or bloodplay, engaging in "planned" abduction, some forms of humiliation, and exploring fantasies that may trigger fears or particularly strong adverse reactions, like incest. Many aspects of and approaches to BDSM can be edge play, but so can things like having intercourse without birth control, neglecting safer sex practices, and engaging in any kind of sex you know you don't really want or feel ready for. Given how much we talk in this book about safety, health, and consent, as well as about interpersonal equality and self-esteem, it shouldn't be a surprise that "edge play" is something I'd suggest you steer away from. Not only can sex easily be fun and fulfilling without being physically or emotionally dangerous, but I feel strongly that, in the long term, you'll have better sex, enjoy better sexual relationships, and feel better about yourself, when the sex you're having is safe and responsible.

Like sensation play, sometimes bondage and restraint are incorporated into BDSM or role-play, but just as often, they aren't. Bondage can be used to allow a partner to be selfish in terms of being given all the pleasure, being unable to reciprocate during a given sexual activity, because they can't use their hands or mouths. Some people enjoy being bound or restrained in certain ways that keep them from engaging in behaviors that may be habitual for them, as a way to seek out other avenues of pleasure; for instance, a person who typically masturbates during intercourse may enjoy having their hands bound and then having to seek out other forms of extra stimulus.

Discussing bondage in advance of the activity is important, as is establishing some code or means of communication so that if the bound partner begin to feel uncomfortable or unsafe, it's easy for them to clearly express that and halt the action.

If you're going to be tying or restraining a partner, remember that circulation is a good thing, and cutting it off isn't. To assess healthy circulation, especially in limbs, doctors and nurses use the code CSM: color, sensation, and movement. Color should be normal, a person should be able to feel the same sensations on that limb as anywhere else, and they should be able to move extremities easily. Make sure whatever restraints you're using are comfortable for your partner, and that he or she still has at least some mobility. If he or she is tied to something, make sure that it's stable and safe, and that they are not left alone. While some people like the feeling of some restraint on their necks during sexual activities, restricting the airway, for a partner or yourself, is incredibly dangerous.

Not everybody will want to engage in activities like bondage. For plenty, it may ring of servitude, slavery, or imprisonment, conditions that many people don't find erotic or pleasant at all. For others, consent and care being present erase those negative associations. As with anything else, if you're interested in an activity and your partner just really isn't, don't push.

STD/STI risk: No risk (as long as skin is not broken).
Pregnancy risk: No risk.

BODY FLUID OR BLOOD PLAY

What is it, and how do I do it?

Some people enjoy any number of body fluids sexually: ejaculate, vaginal fluids, menses, urine, or blood. They may simply enjoy tasting, feeling, or smelling them during other sexual activities, or they may engage in activities specific to enjoying those fluids, such as "golden showers" (being urinated on) or having a partner ejaculate on them. Some enjoy this because it feels taboo, or naughty, to have intimate contact with body fluids. For others, fluid play may be enjoyable because a certain intimacy or sacredness is experienced in fluid-bonding.

But from an infection and disease perspective, this can be very dangerous, especially when body fluids have contact with incredibly sensitive sites like the eyes. While urine itself is sterile, it does pass through the urethra, where an infection may be present. Ejaculate can carry several different infections. Contact with blood, or cutting or piercing partners in any way, opens the door to some of the deadlier diseases and infections out there, like Hepatitis B and HIV.

So, for the most part, this sort of play is quite risky, especially for younger couples, the majority of whom will not have sound or regular sexual healthcare. Most younger people have not had safer sex practices with a monogamous partner long enough to be safely "fluid-bonded."

STD/STI risk:Very high risk.
Pregnancy risk: No risk, unless male ejaculate has contact with the vulva.

SEX TOYS

What is it, and how do I do it?

Sex toys come in many varieties. From vibrators—electric and battery-operated, big and small, swanky and silly—to silicone dildos, anal plugs to masturbation sleeves, cock rings to clitoral suction devices, toys and tools run the gamut. People use them not just for masturbation, but also for partnered sex, by themselves or in conjunction with other activities.

Generally, sex toys aren't available for purchase by minors, and are sold in sex toy shops, through catalogs, or at Internet sites. Some people will also make their own sex toys, or use household objects as sexual toys or aids: foodstuffs, plastic bottles, socks, pillows, and all sorts of other objects.

So long as simple directions are followed for those items sold as sex toys, they're usually safe for use. For instance, using something electrical in a bathtub isn't safe or smart, and using an item not designed for anal use—and without a flared base—in the anus is a bad idea. Anything with sharp edges should generally not be used on or in the genitals. Anything that is being used as a sex toy, especially if it is shared, needs to be able to be covered with a latex barrier or boiled; otherwise, you could brew and

S.E.X.

pass around infections and bacteria. Shared (and uncovered) toys are often a very common route for infections to be spread between female partners, something lesbian women often aren't even aware of. Using household items—such as electric toothbrushes, the zucchini for dinner, or shampoo bottles—as sex toys, when they ARE shared by household members, who are unaware of what they're being used for by you, is decidedly on the Not Okay list.

Phthalates

Some sex toys may contain toxic substances, such phthalates—a family of chemicals which has been linked to reproductive problems for men and women and potential cancer risks in some studies. Some toys will say that they are phthalate-free on their packaging, and sex toy sellers can usually direct customers to phthalate-free goods, but many manufacturers do not list these ingredients, and because many sex toys are sold as being "for novelty-use only" they can dodge health regulations. Toys which are made of "cyberskin" or "jelly toys" are most likely to contain these substances: silicone, hard plastic or acrylic, glass or metal sex toys usually do not.

There are so many different kinds of toys, and so many different ways to use them, a whole separate book would be required to cover all the bases. But men and women alike can and do enjoy a multitude of toys, and many women who have trouble first reaching orgasm find that a vibrator can help get them there. Women may like vibrators or suction toys used on their clitorises or labia, men on the penis or testes, men and women both on the perineum or anus or the nipples. Dildos, plugs, and insertable vibes can be used in and around the vagina and for anal sex (if, again, they have a flared base). Women can use dildos paired with harnesses, worn on the hips, for vaginal intercourse with female partners, or for anal intercourse with male or female partners.

It's often asked if vibrators can "desensitize" areas they're used on, and the simple answer is that they can do so only as much as any other sexual activity. Very fast or intense friction or sensation can, temporarily, cause less sensation to be experienced in the genitals, because heavy friction can tend to numb things slightly. Clap your hands together very intensely for a while, for instance, and you can get an idea of how that can happen, and also how quickly sensation comes right back. Right after the clapping, the tingling in your palms will be intense, and touching your palm with fingers may not feel like much, but shortly, the tingling subsides and your touch will feel more sensitive again. No big. Too, any one form of stimulus can, after a while, feel old or become a mere habit. But vibrators and other sex toys don't have the ability to permanently make any area of the body less sensitive.

Some partners may feel threatened by the suggestion of adding toys to partnered sex, feeling that if a toy is "needed," they or their genitals or other body parts are inadequate in some way. Explaining the difference between "need" and "want," in these situations, is often helpful, as is making clear that wanting to add toys to play is really no different from wanting to try any new sexual activity. Toys that can be enjoyed by both partners, in whatever ways, are also often helpful for dealing with feelings of insecurity about toys. Some partners may feel that sex toys are "unnatural," but nowadays, so much of our environment, from our sex lives to the foods we eat, is man-made or inorganic, that while the desire to stay close to nature is understandable and important, sex toys aren't a major inhibitor to that.

 A WORD of warning: If you are of age to go into sex shops and shop for toys, be particular about where you go, especially if you're female and/or by yourself. Adult shops situated off highways, in rural areas, or those clearly catering primarily to men for sexual entertainment, are often not safe spaces to be in. While it may be relatively safe—albeit possibly unpleasant, on several levels—for you inside, you may not be safe after you leave the store. If you're shopping for toys, seek out independently owned, clean, friendly shops or reputable online vendors. There are even plenty around the country that are women-owned and/or intended to be female- and couple-friendly. There are a lot of good sex toys on the market, but there's also a whole lot of junk out there. A reputable, all-gender-friendly and independent vendor also usually weeds out a lot of the garbage and can help you find the best of what you're looking for. See the Resources list at the end of the book for some suggestions.

If you're a minor without access to manufactured sex toys, life WILL go on without them for the time being. Sex toys can be completely great, but as with most things made for sale, the marketing hype (especially since they're seen as very adult or adventurous) can often be far greater than the actual value. Anyone can have a healthy, enjoyable sex life—solo or with partners—without sex toys as well as with them.

STD/STI risk: No risk to moderate risk.
Pregnancy risk: No risk.

▪ THE OL' GIVE AND TAKE: ▪
Sexual Symmetry, Reciprocity, and Equality

Inequities, imbalances, and mismatches in love and in partnered sex can manifest in many ways. Perhaps there was something you did with a previous partner that sent them straight to heaven, but that leaves your present partner completely unaffected. Maybe you performed oral sex on a partner, and so feel they "owe" you the same, even if they aren't as interested in it as you are—or maybe you only performed that oral sex to try to earn some for yourself. Perhaps you always initiate sex in your partnership, and would really like the shoe to be on the other foot for a change. One partner might feel that the other always gets what he or she likes, but that they never get what's good for them. And sometimes, one partner may have a satisfactory experience, while the other just doesn't, and that might feel unfair.

RECIPROCITY, RELOADED

I'm going to suggest you look at reciprocity in sex—the idea that one person gives something, so the other should get something of equal value back—in a different way than you might be used to.

With activities like sexual intercourse, dry sex, or kissing, where the same or similar parts are getting used and stimulated at the same time, we assume reciprocity: that both parties are giving and getting the same thing. That in and of itself is often a false assumption, because no activity guarantees that both partners are having the same experience, or that their enjoyment in that activity is identical.

With activities like oral or manual sex, people usually assume that one partner is giving and the other getting, and that the giver and the getter can't be both giving and receiving unless they're "performing" the same activity on each other simultaneously. Assuming that assumes a lot. For starters, the assumption that only one partner is sexually engaged or pleased is based on the flawed idea that our genitals are our only pleasure center, that if one person's genitals aren't involved in a sexual activity and someone else's are, that only the person whose genitals are getting some action is "getting" sex.

If during any partnered sex activity, either partner feels they aren't getting *anything* out of a given sexual activity, or getting pretty equal satisfaction, then something really isn't okay.

Partnered sex involves more than just you, and there can be many things going on for each person—both giving AND receiving pleasure. If we're with someone who is a good partner for us, we're not just getting off on being pleased, we're getting off on our partner experiencing pleasure with us.

If both the giving and the receiving aren't pretty fantastic, no matter what role you're in during a given activity, then that's something to evaluate. Check to make sure you're sleeping with someone you really like, for instance, and who you know likes you—inside *and* outside the bedroom. Be mindful for hidden trouble spots in the relationship, like feeling constantly taken advantage of, feeling that your needs are ignored, or that you always have to be the leader. Double-check with yourself to be sure that partnered sex, rather than masturbation, is really what you want at the moment, and that you're not engaging in any sexual activity out of obligation, rather than desire.

It's also worth making sure that neither of you is just being a selfish creep. It happens, even to the best of us, sometimes. Even otherwise good, sharing partners can get so caught up in having sex that's all about them, that they space out their partner's wants, needs, or limits.

▪ SEX AND OBLIGATION ▪

Nobody "owes" anyone sex. We don't lend and borrow sex the way we lend and borrow money or our favorite sweaters. Yet, plenty of people engage in sex or certain sexual activities out of feelings of obligation. Obligatory sex usually feels crappy and boring at best, and horrible—emotionally and physically—at worst, especially over time if it becomes habit. When you're really not interested in partnered sex at all and agree to it, it may even feel like rape. When your partner is doing their homework in their heads during sex, rather than being fully present with you, or just saying yes to avoid an argument, it can feel pretty weird, and create some unhealthy patterns.

Maybe your partner performed oral sex for you, so you feel that you're obliged to perform a similar or understood-to-be-equal activity, whether you like it or not. You may feel that your boyfriend or girlfriend is someone you don't deserve, or is somehow above you, and sex seems like a good way to even the scales. Friends may push you to become sexually active for their own agendas. Perhaps your partner has had a level of previous sexual experience you feel you've got to live up to. Maybe you've been together for some time, and it seems sex should happen, by some arbitrary and invisible timeline, or it's been a few weeks since you had sex, and even though you're not in the mood, you feel you owe it to your partner to have sex with them.

 ONCE you or your partner engage in any given sexual activity, you're not then forever obligated to keep doing it. If you find there's something you just don't like or have no interest in; if at any given time, something you usually like just doesn't have appeal; if at any point you feel you want or need to take a break from sexual activity or partnership altogether, it is ALWAYS okay. If we go swimming once, we don't feel obligated to do it every day, or always at the same lake or with the same stroke, and the same goes for any sort of sex.

If your partner performed oral sex for you, and they're expecting something in return that you aren't interested in, let them know you aren't interested in whatever that is, and fill them in on the things you ARE interested in instead. If you feel that your boyfriend or girlfriend is too good for you and you've got to compensate by engaging in sexual activity they want, then deal with the self-esteem issues or relationship imbalances that are causing you to feel that way. If you've been together a while, and some arbitrary timeline seems to require that sex should happen, start talking to your partner about feeling that way, and discuss, between you, what your own individual timelines are, and what you feel ready for and want. If it's been a few weeks since you had sex, and you're still not in the mood, start talking: look into why that might be, like relationship or sexual problems, stress, depression, low libido, or just not feeling up to sex. You owe your partner communication and honesty, not sexual favors, and they owe you patience and understanding.

If you find yourself in a situation, or you're putting a partner in a situation, where sex is NOT 100 percent optional, where anyone feels owed or obligated, regardless of *any* actual shared desire, you two need to be talking, not schtupping.

• FAKING IT •

Plenty of women—and even some men—fake orgasm, for a variety of reasons: They may feel that if they don't "come," they are ruining something for their partner; they may be worried that they'll look sexually immature or inexperienced if they don't have an orgasm, or that they'll hurt a partner's feelings. Whatever the reason, while you'd be hard-pressed to find a person who has never once in their life faked it, it's a *seriously* bad habit to get into. Faking orgasm is not only dishonesty that can break down the trust and intimacy in your relationship, it

s.e.x.

gives your partner false cues about what is turning you on. You fake it a few times, you may find you've closed the door on building the sexual communication you need to make a real orgasm happen with a partner. Eventually, to get back on track, you may have to 'fess up that you've faked it, setting both of you up for hurt feelings and a loss of trust, both in and out of bed.

If you've never faked it, great. Do yourself a favor, and don't start. If you feel that you have to fake it, or are stuck in a pattern of doing so, talk to your partner. It's not the easiest conversation to have, but it can be done sensitively. Make it clear that your faking isn't about your partner being "bad in bed," but about your failure to explain or explore what does work for you, or maybe it's about trying to live up to unrealistic expectations one of you has. Make clear that you don't *want* to fake it, you want to work on communicating and exploring what you both DO enjoy, with or without orgasm. Be sure to express that it's okay if either you or your partner doesn't have an orgasm; your self-esteem isn't (or sure shouldn't be) dependent upon their orgasm.

VIAGRA (sildenafil), a medication intended for older men having trouble achieving or maintaining erection, has gained some popularity as an illegal recreational drug among younger men. Viagra and other similar medications aren't generally intended for young men and shouldn't be used recreationally. Viagra aids in relaxing the muscles and arteries leading to the penis and increasing blood flow to the penis, and is intended for men with decreased circulation due to age or certain disabilities. In young, healthy men, this isn't usually an issue unless they just aren't feeling aroused, in which case there's no sense in having any sort of sex anyway. Viagra is neither a hormone nor an aphrodisiac: it can't make you feel aroused when you aren't.

It's typical for both men and women to have trouble achieving full arousal when they're under the influence of alcohol, so some people use Viagra recreationally then. If you're having trouble with erection, arousal, or orgasm when you've imbibed, the answer is pretty simple: stop getting smashed. Sex is usually a lot more enjoyable for everyone when you aren't wasted, anyway.

Beyond the illegality of using Viagra without a prescription, Viagra can have some serious and uncomfortable side effects, including headaches, stomach upset, dizziness, blurred vision, uncomfortable erections that persist for hours, dangerous interactions with other drugs (including other recreational drugs, like amyl nitrate), stroke, or heart attack.

If you are having persistent problems achieving or maintaining an erection, talk to your doctor. In young men, this is most often a psychological, rather than a physical, issue, but some medical conditions may be contributors.

People don't always reach orgasm, even with satisfying sex. They may be tired, stressed out, emotionally overwhelmed, or physically exhausted. If you're expecting yourself or your partners to achieve orgasm with every sexual experience, you're being unrealistic in your expectations.

• HAVING TROUBLE REACHING • ORGASM OR FEELING AROUSED WITH A PARTNER?

Take a look at these common culprits (even just one may be your roadblock):

s.e.x.

- Are you moving too fast—not just in terms of getting sexual with someone, but in the way you are sexual? Are you giving yourself time to savor EVERY nuance, or are you in a big hurry because one or both of you are nervous, in an unsafe place, or afraid of being caught?
- Can you have a good sense of humor during sex, or are you afraid to laugh with your partner?
- Are there aspects of your sexuality or sexual choices that feel forbidden or taboo? If so, are they enhancing your experience, or keeping you from satisfaction? Do you feel ashamed or guilty before, during, or after sex?
- Are you comfortable with the power roles or (lack thereof) between you and your partner? Do you feel that you're pretty equal, for instance, in initiating sex, setting limits and boundaries, and sexual reciprocity? Do you feel that either of you is passive in any aspect of your sex life?
- Do you feel safe, physically and emotionally? Can you say no and have it respected, without argument? Do you have protection from pregnancy and STIs?
- Are you comfortable communicating with your partner, and do you feel they're communicating wit you, in terms of what you both want and need, like and don't like? Can you discuss what could be better, what you'd like done differently, what you need included in your sex but aren't getting?
- Do you feel under any pressure to reach orgasm, to be or feel "sexy," or to please your partner?

- Do you have any current conflicts, doubts, or worries about your relationship?
- Are you comfortable with your sexual fantasies, wants, and needs? How about your partner's?
- Are you really recognizing and communicating that you are or are not aroused? Do you feel 100 percent comfortable saying no when you're not aroused, or do you feel obligated to go ahead anyway?
- Are you dealing with depression, anxiety, recent illness, surgery, a major health complication? Are you sleep-deprived, or have you not been resting well recently? How about recent stress or trauma, like college acceptance issues; tests or grades; arts or sports competitions; a death, illness, or separation in the family; sexual or other assault?
- Do you feel that your partner has to supply all of your sexual satisfaction, or are you down with providing it on your own, via masturbation, both when you don't have a partner and when you do? Are you comfortable with having or trying masturbation as part of your partnered activities?
- Do you feel comfortable reaching orgasm or being aroused, or do you feel self-conscious about aspects of arousal or normal body functions (like erection or ejaculation, clitoral enlargement, vaginal lubrication, menstruation, farting, body scents, or the effects of orgasm)? If you have a disability, do you feel comfortable making any needed modifications with your partner? Does sexual response make you feel uncomfortably

out of control; do you trust yourself when aroused or sexually engaged? Do you feel overexposed physically with a partner, nervous about nudity? Do you experience body-image problems with a partner?

▶ Are you getting hung up on things that appear to be problematic, rather than seeing ways in which your obstacles can enhance your erotic experience? Are you overthinking sex, and finding yourself unable to relax enough to turn off your analytical brain for a bit so you can actually enjoy yourself?

WHO'S IN CHARGE?

The structure of our society often gives us the impression that relations between people have to be hierarchical: leader/follower, top/bottom, boss/employee. But they don't. In a healthy sexual relationship, BOTH of you should be active partners, in initiation, in decision making, and in performing actual sexual activities.

Are you worried about asserting yourself, about stepping up and talking about what you really want and need, about taking charge just as much as your partner is? Do you feel that you'd be threatening your relationship by doing so? If you feel threatened or usurped by a partner doing those things, step back and evaluate the situation. Are you and your partner both really ready to be in an intimate relationship with someone else, or not? Are you involved with someone who's really not right or appropriate for you? Are you ready to truly make full allowances for someone else's needs and wants, and learn to work out yours with theirs, even when it's hard or disappointing?

Do you feel confident enough in yourself to both assert your own needs and desires AND make some compromises sometimes? Do you feel secure and safe enough with your partner to screw up sometimes and deal with that? All of those things are worth looking at to be sure that you're both able to share the wheel.

▪ SEXUAL DIFFERENCES ▪ VS. SEXUAL INCOMPATIBILITY

It's very rare to encounter a sexual partner with whom your sexual wants and needs are an effortless, perfect match. More times than not, you will find yourself and your partner making allowances and compromises. That might mean skipping an activity you've liked with other partners, avoiding a position you like that is uncomfortable for your partner, trying something new, or accepting that your favorite fantasy has just got to renew the lease in your head for another year, rather than moving out into the real world.

Those things shouldn't be that big a deal. Engaging in a sexual activity with someone who isn't into it takes the fun out of that activity, and you usually find that fun and satisfaction in activities both partners *do* enjoy.

If a partner is being honest with you about what they like and dislike, what they do and don't want to do, you've just got to accept those things. You can talk it over and work to find middle ground, but pushing, guilt-tripping, or otherwise pressuring a partner into any sexual activity isn't part of healthy, consensual sex.

It **IS** okay to opt out of or terminate a relationship when there is big sexual incompatibility. Some people have the idea that doing so is shallow or insensitive, but strong sexual

s.e.x.

wants and needs aren't different from any other sort of wants and needs, such as wanting to be married or not, wanting a given amount of time alone, wanting or not wanting monogamy. We wouldn't think it was shallow if a person terminated or didn't pursue a relationship with someone who didn't want the level of commitment they did, or didn't share their emotional feelings, after all.

It might be hard to fathom that you will meet people who meet most, if not *all,* of your needs—sexual, emotional, practical—without either of you trying too hard. That can seem especially improbable when you're young, when you've been single for a long time, or had a long run of relationships that didn't even come close to meeting your needs and wants.

But they are out there. And part of finding them is becoming and staying aware of your wants and needs, of reciprocity and equality, of what's genuine and what is forced.

▪ AFTERCARE ▪

Part of what makes partnered sex so intimate and so intense is the openness and vulnerability we experience with each other, no matter what sex act we've engaged in.

When we've finished with sexual activities for the night (or day), it's pretty common to want a little comfort, to want to reaffirm and extend that intimacy together. Snuggling, gentle stroking and kissing, lying around and talking, taking a bath or a walk, going to sleep curled up together, or even good-natured roughhousing and laughing (pillowfight!) are all kinds of aftercare plenty of people appreciate and savor.

It's just as common for some people to want a little personal space, or even to feel a little *over*exposed, a little *too* vulnerable, and to want a *lot* of space. Sometimes, that's due to not-so-great sexual choices being made, but it can also be due simply to differences in personality, chemistry, emotional nature and style.

Just as people differ in what they want and need during sex, what one partner wants and needs after sex may not be what the other does. We've all heard the complaints about those with a partner who "just rolls over and falls asleep," as well as about partners who are too "clingy" after sex. But aftercare is just another aspect of sexual compatibility—your partner may naturally fall into the exact sort of aftercare you need . . . or they may not. Communicate your aftercare wants and needs, limits and boundaries, and seek a middle ground when need be, just as with anything else.

▪ "GAY" SEX AND "STRAIGHT" SEX: ▪ What's the Diff?

Queer sex involves the exact same sort of things that sex with partners of the opposite sex does: kissing, hugging, snuggling, petting, touching, frottage, mutual masturbation, manual sex, oral sex, and vaginal or anal intercourse and stimulation—the works. Any and all of those activities are just as fulfilling, satisfying, and orgasm-inducing for same-sex couples as they are for opposite-sex ones.

The biggest general difference is how the people involved feel about their partners in terms of gender. If you're heterosexual, opposite-sex-partner sex of any kind is likely to feel better, or seem better, to you, because that's how you're wired. If you're homosexual, sex with someone of the same

s.e.x.

sex or gender, and all that may entail, will tend to have more appeal and feel more natural. If you're bisexual or pansexual, you may find that you have a slight to strong preference for one gender or another, or you may be completely impartial, and varying activities with varying genders will feel more or less "right" or fulfilling for you based on those preferences. Same-sex partners may often find their sex has a different "flavor" than sex with opposite-sex partners, because certain common gender roles between men and women aren't present. The limited, pervasive gender roles that men and women are reared with can really louse up sex and sexual relationships sometimes, so it is common enough to find that queer sex *can* be a bit more diverse, as that conditioning can be easier to escape or unlearn with a same-sex partner. But that's nothing hard-wired: straight folks can diversify their sexual activities and gender roles, too. As is probably obvious, it's also typical for people to feel differently about, or safer with, sex when there's no risk of pregnancy.

But ultimately, what feels good or doesn't, what one person likes or dislikes in sexual activities, is less about orientation than it is about life experience, individual sensation, and individual attraction and chemistry.

▪ SEX AND DISABILITY ▪

"Disability" is a word that can cover a wide range of things. A person may be physically, neurologically, psychologically, developmentally, or learning disabled in ways that are obvious: they might be deaf, blind, or wheelchair-bound; have a missing limb or a speech impediment; or suffer from a condition like narcolepsy or an obsessive-compulsive disorder (OCD). Some disabilities, such as epilepsy, fibromyalgia, eating disorders, depression, attention deficit disorder, or Asperger's syndrome, may be fairly invisible or harder to notice.

When it comes to sex and disability, it's pretty simple: most disabled or differently-abled folks are like most people who aren't disabled. Most disabilities do not remove the desire for sex, sexual partners, and romantic and/or sexual relationships. Partners of a disabled person may or may not also be disabled, just as persons of one race may or may not have partners of that same race. The same sexual risks that apply to those who aren't disabled usually apply to those who are: disabled people can contract STIs like anyone else, and can often become pregnant like anyone else. Being disabled doesn't take away humanity, nor does it elevate a disabled person to a level "above" being human.

Like most other people, those of us who are disabled are going to have individual wants and needs, and sometimes some special adaptations need to occur to make sex work for us, while some things just don't work. With certain physical disabilities, some sexual positions or activities may be uncomfortable or just not doable. Some medications for psychological disabilities may decrease libido or have other sexual side effects. Some disabilities may require special modifications during sex to make communication possible: for someone blind, verbal communication is going to be important; for someone hearing-impaired, having the lights off may not always work. If you're disabled, you may find you've got to work a bit harder at communicating with your partner than those without a disability. That may have its rough spots and get frustrating sometimes, but it's actually a blessing in disguise: the better any set of partners gets at communicating with one another, the better their relationship and their sex life tend to be.

Ask for help managing your sex life when you need it—not just from your partner, but also from friends, parents, doctors, or therapists. It's hard enough for many young people to talk to their doctors or counselors about sex, and it may be an even larger challenge for those who are disabled—especially if a doctor or counselor thinks that a disability makes someone less of a sexual being. If you are disabled and need to know about issues pertinent to your sexuality (like if your disability impacts your fertility, how to engage in a certain sexual activity with limited mobility, what type of birth control you can use, how to talk to partners about sexual specifics pertaining to a disability), ask questions of your healthcare providers, and insist on getting the answers you need. If you have a healthcare provider who insists on treating you like a nun or a eunuch because of your disability, find a new one.

If you're disabled, you may also find you have social challenges when it comes to dating, relationships, and sexual partnership. Whether or not you date, or want to date, someone who is also disabled, you may find you have to fight for your right to live, date, and love like anyone else. You may face discrimination or a lot of silly questions about your capabilities, even when they aren't asked with the intent to be insensitive or malicious. You may find that some people just will not even consider dating a disabled person, for any number of reasons, both fair and completely stupid. That's a disability of *theirs,* not yours.

If you're dating a nondisabled partner (or are a nondisabled person dating a disabled person), you may both have to deal with tricky and difficult social adjustments. Talk it out among yourselves, your friends, and your families. Ask all the questions you need to, even if they seem stupid. If your partner is disabled, inform yourself about their specific disability. Seek out support groups or help intended specifically for those with disabilities and their partners. Try to be patient, and have a relationship that's full and fun, not tense. No one should feel as if they're walking on eggshells all the time. If a disabled person tells you something won't break them, hurt them, or make them ill, trust them. If you're disabled and your nondisabled partner tells you they're cool with adaptations you need or things you can't do, believe them.

▪ THE POPULAR MECHANICS ▪ ROUNDUP:
The 5 Most Important Things to Remember During Partnered Sex

1. **Communicate!** Talk openly and plainly. Let your partner know when something feels good, and let them know—kindly—when something doesn't. Ask them to tell and show you what they enjoy. It's okay to feel shy, but when you're naked in bed with someone, being physically intimate, you've pretty much tossed shy right out the window. So, if you don't yet feel comfortable about communicating clearly and openly during sex, then wait for partnered sex until you DO. If you feel unable to do so with a given partner, that can be a strong

signal that either you're not with the right partner, or not at a good point yet to be sexually active with that partner.

2. **Start slow.** Something doesn't have to be fast from the onset to be intense and charged. Genitals, mouths, hands, and other body parts are sensitive, but too much fast action and friction, especially from the get-go, can actually make things feel LESS intense rather than more. When you're communicating with your partner during sex, if he or she wants to go faster, all they've got to do is say so.

3. **Forget about the "right" way.** It's fine to feel clueless: in fact, it's better to feel clueless when you really are than to think you know what to do when you really don't. Experimenting is good, asking questions is good, finding out as you go . . . it's all not only good, it's the only way to truly find out what you and your partner enjoy most.

4. **Partnered sex is for mutual pleasure, care, and intimacy.** That means that the following are Really Bad Reasons to have sex with someone: to fulfill perceived obligations or expectations, to impress someone or yourself, to try to gain status or a given reputation, to prove your worth or sexual value, to avoid problems in a relationship or try to keep a partner from leaving, to replace masturbation or self-only pleasure, to "just get it over with," to boost your self-esteem, to comfort someone you feel sorry for, or to get back at somebody else— or any other number of other reasons that are NOT about mutual pleasure,

care, and intimacy. That doesn't mean, for instance, that casual sex, sex with multiple partners, or with a friend, if that's what you want, has to be a no-go. It just means those scenarios, too, should be about mutual pleasure, care, and intimacy, above all else.

5. **Feeling good in terms of sexual activities isn't just about getting off, nor just about feeling good DURING those activities.** It's also about being intellectually, ethically, and emotionally okay with whatever you're engaging in; about taking care of everyone's hearts, minds, and bodies as best you can. A great many of us have woken up with feelings of regret for something we did the night before, when something that seemed or felt great at the time felt really lousy, physically or emotionally, afterward. It happens. But it's less likely to happen when you're mindful and aware of how the choices you're making and the things you're doing might impact you, as well as your partner; when taking care of your sexual health is done before the fact, and routinely, not just in crisis situations; when you're protecting yourself from physical and emotional risks smartly; when you're with partners who will be attentive and caring, not just before and during sex, but afterward; when you choose partners who will hear and respect "no" at any time, and when you can do the same; when you're seeking out sex for good reasons, rather than destructive or self-destructive ones; and when you treat yourself and your sex partners with the respect you all deserve.

safe and sound:
safer sex for your body,
heart, and mind

SEXUAL SAFETY ISN'T just about avoiding pregnancy, abuse, or the most deadly infections and diseases. It's about doing what you can to safeguard yourself and your partners in body and in mind, via smart, preventative sexual and general healthcare, awareness of your physical and emotional risks, and smart sexual practices. Safer sex, a group of practices proven to greatly reduce your risks of sexually transmitted infections, will help keep you and yours as safe as possible, allowing you to enjoy yourself and your sexuality, not only now, but in the long run.

Whether you're having any sort of sex or not, the best place to get started in protecting your sexual health is with regular, preventative sexual healthcare.

▪ TAKING CARE DOWN THERE: ▪
Sexual Healthcare

Sexual healthcare doesn't need to be different from any other sort of healthcare. If you take care of your sexual health vigilantly and in cooperation with your healthcare professional, both preventatively and in response to worries or concerns—even if you aren't sexually active—it's very likely you'll stay healthy, avoid infections and serious conditions, and enjoy your sexuality even more than you would otherwise. So, read up! Find out what you need from healthcare pros, when, how, and where to get that care, how to keep yourself well *by* yourself, and what steps to take to get started on a life of great sexual health and well-being.

STI or STD?

In this book, the term *STI* is used to discuss sexually transmitted infections. Some people use the term *STD* (sexually transmitted disease) instead, which is not inaccurate, as *disease* can mean any sort of illness, but STI is the preferred medical term at this time, and it's also a lot less loaded. In this chapter, we discuss sexual healthcare, safer sex, some general infections, and issues pertaining to all the STIs out there. For specific information on each of them—what they are, how widespread they are, what symptoms they may have, how they're tested for and treated—refer to Appendix A.

YOUR BUSINESS, THEIR BUSINESS: HEALTHCARE CONFIDENTIALITY AND PRIVACY

The American Academy of Pediatrics has reported that the main reason teens and young adults are hesitant to seek out healthcare is worry about confidentiality. They say that it is important for doctors who serve young people to develop office policies that ensure confidentiality, and that those policies—available to patients and staff—should include information about when confidentiality must be waived, guidelines for reimbursement for services, medical record access, appointment scheduling, and information disclosure to public (such as to public health agencies) and/or private parties.

At the current time, no U.S. state's policies require parental notification for STI testing or treatment (and only one state,

Iowa, requires parents to be notified about a positive HIV test), birth control services, prenatal care or delivery, or other basic sexual healthcare. The same is true of mental health and substance abuse services. In the case of abortion, laws regarding young adult autonomy and parental notification/permission vary wildly. When in doubt about any of your state's policies, you can ask your doctor or the office staff via phone in advance of visits.

Whatever the politics (which are ultimately about politicians, not doctors), know that all of the major medical associations advise healthcare professionals to respect and ensure the privacy and confidentiality of young adult patients, and most medical professionals are in strong agreement, taking their patients confidentiality, and their legal rights to it, very seriously. Ultimately, the golden rule most doctors hold—echoed in the mature minor doctrine—is that what is best when it comes to young adult healthcare is what is best for the young adult patient; most doctors take advocating for their patients, no matter their age, very seriously. So long as you are clear that your privacy is important, and are able to advocate for yourself and demonstrate a clear understanding and ownership of your health, there is no reason to let worries about privacy stand in the way of getting the healthcare you need. Only if your doctor determines that you do not understand the situation, and/or that your privacy is endangering your health, should he or she discuss notifying parents with you.

If you are using a parent or guardian's insurance plan, understand that your exam and any other fees will likely appear on their bills, so for 100 percent privacy, you will need to pay for your healthcare yourself. If the issue is just keeping test results private, you can ask to have them sent only to you (such as at a college address), or see if you can call in to the office for your results rather than having them sent.

BEFORE YOUR FIRST APPOINTMENT

▶ When you call to make your appointment, be sure you express to the receptionist or doctor that it is your first visit, and feel free to let them know if you feel nervous or have any special concerns. During that call, as well as when you have your appointment, you can ask that the doctor explain what she or he is doing, and why, though most doctors with a patient new to sexual health exams will do that, anyway.

▶ If you feel more comfortable with a doctor of a certain sex, you can seek one out, and/or ask for a nurse of a given sex to be in the room during the exam. If you are able to choose your doctor yourself, you can ask friends or family for a recommendation of someone they have liked. If you have any special needs the nurses, doctors, or staff should be aware of, such as any mobility disabilities, or issues from sexual trauma, let them know these things in advance of your appointment, as well.

▶ If you will want a parent or guardian in the room with you, let them know. If you want privacy from a parent coming in with you, but feel that you'll have a hard time asking for it in the office, discuss this over the phone in advance, and request a note be left for your doctor or nurse to please ask your parent to stay in the waiting room. If you have any specific billing requests—such as whether or not to bill a parent's insurance plan, or if you need a payment plan—state them up front.

▶ Prepare a list of all your questions in advance (such as if your genitals look normal, if you can do anything about your menstrual cramps, if a lump or bump on your genitals is okay, why you're experiencing pain during sexual activities, etc.). Sometimes, the doctor's office can feel a little intimidating, and having a list in your hands is helpful in being sure to have all your needs addressed.

▶ Do what you can to relax about your upcoming exam. Tension and anxiety, no matter the situation or your sex, always increase physical discomfort during exams.

GYNECOLOGY FOR BEGINNERS

After a woman begins menstruating, she should begin having a yearly pelvic exam with an OB/GYN (an obstetrician/gynecologist), with a family doctor who also handles sexual health, or via a sexual health clinic. Some people say that a woman should begin having annual exams at eighteen, others when she becomes sexually active. But nothing special happens to your body when you turn eighteen, and your reproductive system functions on its own, with or without sexual partnership. Many complications that can occur—such as infections, hormonal imbalances, vaginal itching or discomfort, labial cysts, painful menstruation, or delayed menarche—have nothing to do with partnered sex or age of majority.

s.e.x.

There's really no need to be scared about your first gynecological visit. It's normal to feel a bit awkward about it, since in our culture, the genitals are often presented as "special" or private anatomy, but to a doctor, your genitals or breasts are really no different from any other part of your body. Doctors who work with sexual and reproductive health are in a specialized practice, just like someone who chooses to specialize in heart surgery, and sexual healthcare professionals are those who simply have a strong interest in ensuring good sexual and reproductive health. There is no reason to feel it is dirty—you aren't and it isn't. You're taking care of yourself, and your healthcare professional is there to help you do that.

General sexual healthcare and annual pelvic exams are available through private OB/GYNs (some of whom specialize in adolescent OB/GYN), through general practitioners and family doctors, sexual health clinics like Planned Parenthood, and some school health services. Which is best for you is going to depend on what you can afford, how much distance or privacy you'd like from your general or family doctor, if any, what is within easy reach of you in terms of transportation, and what setting you feel most comfortable in.

What to Expect during Your Exam

After you have changed into an examination gown (and sometimes you'll also be given a sheet to drape over yourself before you sit on the table), your doctor will:

▶ Ask some questions about your medical history that you—and your parent, if present—can answer. Your doctor should ask if you are sexually active. It is vital that you be honest about this (and volunteer that information if your doctor does *not* ask), so that your doctor can do their job and give you screenings and tests you may need. Being "sexually active" generally includes participation in any of the following: manual, oral, vaginal, or anal sex with a partner of any gender, and when you answer, you can specify this.

▶ Give you a basic physical exam, just like at a "regular" doctor's visit, including checking your blood pressure, height, and weight.

▶ Give you a breast exam, during which the doctor will feel your breasts and chest area in pressing movements, to check for any lumps or irregularities. She or he may also ask if you do regular self-exams and show you how to do so.

▶ Take some blood samples to check your hormone levels, if necessary (in the case of abnormal periods, for instance, hormones may be out of whack). You may also get blood and urine screens for STIs, if you've requested them, or your doctor includes them as policy.

A gynecological table—which you'll likely be sitting on for some of your basic exam, like your breast exam—has metal stirrups at the end of it, and the doctor will pull them out and ask you to move your torso down the table so that your bottom is on the edge of the table, and slide your heels into the stirrups. The doctor will then sit between your legs. Plenty of women find that a gynecologist's table is intimidating, as it does look pretty funky. The stirrups are there to help

S.E.X.

make your exam physically comfortable for you, and to give your doctor a good position in which to perform your exam properly. However, some gynecologists feel that stirrups and the doctor's position between them make the exam more psychologically uncomfortable for women, and may give pelvic exams standing to the side of the patient, while she lies on the table with her knees up and her feet flat on its surface.

can you have a pelvic exam during your period?

 IT'S often suggested that you do not have annual pelvic exams when you are menstruating, because menses tend to make examining vaginal discharges and cervical cells more difficult. However, if your OB/GYN is difficult to get an appointment with, or if you have a serious crisis or emergency, give their office a ring and ask; in some situations, it may be just fine for you to go in with your period.

Your doctor will first just look at the appearance of your vulva, looking for any signs of irritation or infection, such as chafing, redness, swelling, unusual discharge, cysts, lesions, genital warts, or other problems. She or he may put a finger on your vaginal opening to see if your glands produce any pus or mucus when touched.

You may or may not get a speculum exam and Pap smear (a sample taken of your cervical cells to make sure your cervix is healthy) at your first pelvic; women who have not yet become sexually active do not usually need a speculum exam. A speculum (Latin for *mirror*) is a sanitary plastic or smooth metal device that is used to hold the vaginal canal open so that the doctor can examine your vaginal walls and cervix. If you are not used to the feeling of your own vaginal walls being stretched a bit, this may hurt a little, but the doctor will choose a speculum size that is right for you, so that it is not too uncomfortable. You may feel some pressure in your bladder when the speculum is in, and if you do, let your doctor know, and they will make adjustments so that you are more comfortable. Sometimes the speculum might feel a little chilly. To do the Pap smear, your doctor will use a long cotton swab or curette to collect cells from the cervix for tests. This doesn't hurt, it just feels a little weird, especially if you're not used to feeling something on your cervix.

(If you're curious, you can ask your doctor to get a mirror and show you what your cervix looks like when the speculum is in: it's really pretty cool.)

At this point, the doctor will remove the speculum, and will insert gloved fingers into your vagina while they put their other hand on your abdomen and torso. They'll press different spots on your abdomen and hips, and ask if anything feels painful or tender. It can be a little strange to have someone you don't really know with their hand in your genitals asking you questions, but it's really no different to a doctor than looking down your throat or in your ears.

The next thing your doctor may do is a rectal exam, which involves putting one finger in your anus, and another in your vagina. This is so your doctor can see how your uterus is aligned with the other parts of your reproductive organs. In general, this is the part of the exam most people find the most uncomfortable. If the doctor knows it is your first exam, you can feel confident she

s.e.x.

or he will be gentle and careful, and try to cause you the least discomfort possible.

 SOME doctors do NOT give full STI screenings during annual GYN exams without a patient asking for them, and that's even more common with young adult patients. If you're sexually active, or thinking of becoming sexually active, it's very important to get those screenings every year. Condom and barrier use are only a part of practicing safer sex. Behaviors and annual screenings are the other portions. So, don't just assume your annual exam includes those screenings; ask your OB/GYN for those screenings, for ALL sexually transmitted infections, not just HIV. For more information on STIs and screenings, read on.

And that's it! If you have any questions or concerns you haven't addressed before or during the exam, now is the time to ask them. Remember: part of the service a doctor should provide is *information,* so take advantage of your time there to ask pertinent questions. Results from a pelvic exam, Pap smear, and STI screenings are usually ready in a week or so; if you don't hear anything back in a couple weeks, call in. If all your results come back normal, you won't likely need to have an exam for another year, unless a new issue crops up in the interim.

Special Concerns

▶ **Virginity:** A doctor (or other person, for that matter) cannot accurately tell whether or not you've had vaginal intercourse by the width or tightness of your vagina, or by the state of your hymen: that's an old wives' tale. A gynecologist also cannot "devirginize" you via a GYN exam.

▶ **Pubic hair:** OB/GYNs have seen every type of vulva under the sun, and about any configuration of pubic hair you can imagine. Before you go to see the GYN, practice basic hygiene by showering or bathing that day, and by avoiding use of any vaginal creams or douching, as well as any vaginal intercourse, for at least forty-eight hours before your visit.

▶ **Judgment for being sexually active:** When discussing whether you are or are not sexually active, your OB/GYN should not be doling out lectures or heavy-duty value judgments. If yours does, or you feel you can't be honest with your doctor about your sexual activity, find a new doctor. For more on this and other types of healthcare discrimination, see page 199.

▶ **Birth control:** If you would like to discuss birth control options with your OB/GYN, let them or your nurse know that in advance of the exam; there's no need to have extended conversations about all your options while you're freezing your buns off in an examination gown. If there are specific methods you're interested in, your doctor can be on the lookout for health issues during the exam that may make a given method a bad fit for you. When you're finished with the exam itself, you and your doctor can decide on a method that is best for you. If you are seeking out birth control that requires a prescription, such as oral contraceptives, or a method that requires measurement, such as a cervical cap, your doctor can tend to that during this time. For specific information on contraceptive options, see chapter 11.

A visit to the gynecologist isn't a punishment, nor does it need to be something you dread; it is a necessary part of keeping yourself healthy. Your gynecologist can turn out to be a great source of honest, accurate sexual health information and support for you, for years to come. Keeping your sexual health in tune regularly is one of the steps that you take to be a responsible adult with smart sexual behavior.

MALE SEXUAL HEALTHCARE

Many men go without annual sexual healthcare, because there isn't really the equivalent of a gynecologist for men. As well, male sexual health is often taken for granted. There are a few reasons for that: for one, men usu-

ally have lesser risks from STIs or other sexually related conditions than women do, and young men are not at a substantial risk for reproductive cancers or infertility due to sexually transmitted diseases and infections. It is also more difficult to test for some STIs in men, because many of them are asymptomatic in men or we do not currently have accurate means of testing.

But men need sexual healthcare, too. Not only do existing STIs in men require treatment, but just like women, men may develop certain conditions unrelated to STIs, and men also may have questions or concerns about their sexual and reproductive health, birth control and/or sexual partnership issues, genital appearance, and other related matters. And because men are more often the carriers of STIs, it's really important to be extra-responsible when it comes to sexual health to keep your partners safe, too. So, once a year, men should get a general sexual health exam if they are or have been sexually active, or are soon to be sexually active;

did you know . . . ?

There are not currently many available STI vaccines, though more are in development. For now, your family doctor likely already takes care of your hepatitis vaccinations, but there is a new vaccine, Gardasil, available to help protect you against many strains of HPV, a virus that commonly causes cervical cancer—a cancer that, according to the FDA, results in the deaths of over 230,000 women worldwide every year. At this time, the vaccine is only available to women, and is ideally given to girls between the ages of eleven and twelve, or to young women up to the age of twenty-six who have not yet been in any way sexually active (and thus, have not been exposed to the virus). However, even if you have been sexually active, you will likely benefit from the vaccine, since it provides protection from four different strains of HPV: few young women will have been explosed to all four, even if they have been sexually active. Be sure to ask your doctor or gynecologist about it. For more on HPV and hepatitis vaccinations, see Appendix A.

are experiencing any unusual sexual symptoms such as genital sores, redness or chafing, discharges from the penis or anus, or any pain or irritation with urination or erection; or have general concerns about their reproductive health or appearance, such as intense penile curvature or general groin, testicular, or pelvic pain or discomfort.

Men may receive annual sexual healthcare via their general practitioner or family doctor, from a urologist or proctologist, or through a sexual or general health clinic. Whom to see boils down to individual preference: some patients may be most comfortable with their usual family doctor, and others may feel their privacy is better protected by a sexual health clinic.

What to Expect during Your Exam

The exam will begin with a written and verbal review of individual and family health history, as well as any current symptoms or concerns the patient may have. It's important to be as specific and honest as possible so that the doctor or clinician can do their job as best they can.

Overall, a male sexual health exam is a lot less complicated and shorter than those for women. During your exam, the doctor or clinician will:

▶ Do a general physical (taking blood pressure, measuring height and weight, etc.)

▶ Do an external examination of the penis, testicles, and anus, feeling the penis and testicles, in search of any unusual lumps or bumps, and testing for any pain or discomfort from gentle pressure. The doctor may also perform a rectal exam by putting one gloved finger gently into your rectum, feeling for any swelling or tenderness.

▶ Perform swab, blood, and/or urine tests as needed and as available, if you are or have been sexually active, or have requested STI screenings. You will likely not be able to simply be "tested for everything." For STIs like herpes or HPV, without visible sores or warts to sample, reliable tests may not be possible, though better means of testing are currently in development.

On the Down Low

Honesty with your doctor or clinician includes honesty about the gender or orientation of your partners, and specific activities with them. Some men who have had or currently have male partners may find it difficult or uncomfortable to be fully honest. Just remember that a doctor isn't a priest or a parent: it's not their job to sit in any sort of judgment about your sexual behavior or your sexual identity, and it is their responsibility to respect your privacy. Their job is to safeguard and assess your health, and to help them do that, you need to be forthright.

Urethral Swabbing

If you're having any STI testing done, or have had any sort of urinary problems or concerns, your doctor may want to do a swab test. A urethral swab involves a *very* slim, tipped swab inserted a few millimeters into the urethral opening of the penis, turned briefly, then taken right out. Like Pap smears for women, urethral swabbing really shouldn't be painful—it just feels unusual—but the idea of swabbing does freak a lot of guys out. Just as with women's exams, wigging out about it can create a situation healthcare pros refer to as a *perceived body injury* (or *insult*): if we expect pain, we're much more likely to trick our bodies into feeling it, even when it isn't really there. Your best bet is just to relax: ask any questions you need to beforehand, or have the doctor show you the swab and explain how it works so that you can feel less stressed out about it.

That's really all there is to it! But that needn't be all that happens in your exam. If you have questions about your sexual health, about birth control or reproduction, about genital appearance or sexual function, this is your golden opportunity to ask. You may feel awkward or embarrassed, but pretty much any question you can think to ask is one your doctor has heard and answered before, and that's part of what your doctor is there for.

DIY SEXUAL HEALTHCARE

A big part of keeping yourself sexually healthy is maintaining your sexual and reproductive wellness in the first place, and paying attention to your sexual health as a habit so that you can get the jump on any problems. While having GYN exams and sexual and general health checkups every year, as well as using safer sex practices, is important preventative care, so are these ways to care for yourself every day, for your whole body, not just your genitals:

▶ **Do you really WANT to be what you eat?** Poor eating habits and nutri-tion can take a real toll on your sexual health. Sodas, refined sugars, fried foods or junk foods, alcohol, choco-late, caffeine, and foods that have been treated with chemical pesticides can all contribute to yeast infections or jock itch; bacterial, UTI, or bladder infec-tions; menstrual problems (such as severe cramps and PMS); and issues with arousal and libido, as well as interfering with your overall sexual health and enjoyment and your over-all physical and mental health. A poor diet can compound issues like depres-sion and anxiety, or contribute to poor functioning of neurotransmitters that send sexual messages to the body. A poor diet also keeps your immune sys-tem from working at its best, which can put you at a great risk of STIs. The same goes double for smoking, drug and alcohol abuse.

▶ **Rest and motion:** Plenty of rest and plenty of exercise are a big part of staying healthy. Good circulatory, car-diovascular, respiratory, and hormonal health, and reduction of stress are key to having a good sex life. When any of those things aren't doing so well, you may find yourself having problems with libido, arousal, and orgasm.

▶ **Cleanup: daily genital hygiene:** When washing your genitals, no mat-ter your sex, use only a gentle, unfra-granced soap. Fragranced or deodorant soaps, vaginal "cleansers," and douches should be avoided. It may be that a doctor or naturopath will pre-scribe a woman a vinegar or other type of douche for a given condi-tion, but that's the only time douch-ing should be done. Women only need

s.e.x.

to concern themselves with cleaning the external genitals: the mons, around the clitoris, the inner and outer labia, and the rectal area.

For circumcised men, a simple, gentle wash of the penis, testicles, and rectal area is all that's needed. For uncut men, with foreskins, when cleaning, just gently pull back the foreskin and clean lightly beneath or around it—and water alone will do—to get rid of the normal dead skin cells and secretions from the sebaceous glands (otherwise known as *smegma,* which also may sometimes be found in women, inside the hood of the clitoris), which help keep the foreskin lubricated for comfort and often accumulate beneath the head of the penis and foreskin.

If at any point, whether you're male or female, your genitals have the appearance of not being clean, despite normal hygiene—either from a profoundly funky smell, or with profuse or discolored discharge, itching, or the like—then talk to your doctor and make sure you aren't dealing with an infection.

What's good for your general health is what's good for your sexual health. Healthy, fresh foods that are both enjoyable AND good for you, an active lifestyle, plenty of sleep as well as plenty of relaxation and rest, and daily hygiene are great big deals if you want to be healthy and feel healthy sexually.

Check Yourself Out!

Men: Check Out Those Testicles

Testicular cancer is the most common cancer in men aged twenty to twenty-five,

so a testicular self-exam each month is a must. It's best to perform self-exams after a bath or shower, when the heat has relaxed the scrotum. Standing in front of a mirror, first look for any unusual swelling. Then, using both hands, check out each testicle, one at a time. With your index and middle fingers under a testicle and the thumbs on top, roll the testicle gently between your thumbs and fingers, comfortably. Feel around for any unfamiliar lumps; it's normal for the testicles to already feel a little lumpy, and the epididymis, which is behind the testicle, normally feels a little lumpy. Lumps that can be cancerous are usually on the sides or front of the testicles, not the back. Remember, too, that a difference in size between testicles is also normal.

If you discover any small, pea like lumps that are unfamiliar to you, seem unusual, or are painful to the touch, then talk to your doctor or clinician. Same goes for any general discomfort, soreness, swelling, or feeling of heaviness of the scrotum or testes that lasts for more than a couple of days.

Women: Check Out Those Breasts

Every month, do a breast self-exam. These are best done lying down and then standing, with the arm raised on the side of the breast you're checking, or in the shower.

With your three middle fingers of the hand from the opposite side (if you're checking your left breast, raise your left arm, and use your right hand to check that breast), you want to feel for lumps in the breast. Use enough pressure that you can feel the different texture of the breast tissue, starting with light pressure, just to move the skin, then a bit more to feel more of the tissue, and finally the most pressure, to be able to feel your ribs beneath the breast.

mouth matters

ORAL herpes is incredibly common, found in one out of four people, even in those who have not been sexually active (the majority of herpes cases begin in childhood), and it can be sexually transmitted, both orally and genitally. So, be on the lookout for cold sores.

There's a lot of confusion as to what cold sores are, and where they appear.

Cold sores are **not**:

- Mouth ulcers, which are caused by biting into the mouth or cheek accidentally, by burns or other mouth injuries, or by hormonal changes
- Canker sores

Cold sores **are**:

- "Fever blisters" that appear on the lips or on the skin just around the mouth
- Caused by the oral herpes virus

If you have cold sores, you have herpes and can transmit it to others, orally or genitally, even when sores are not present.

If you think you have found a cold sore and you have not seen a doctor about them before, make an appointment as soon as you can: it's best for the doctor to see the sore while its active. While there is not yet a cure for the herpes virus, there are many treatments that can help suppress outbreaks and symptoms substantially. If you have already been diagnosed with oral herpes and find a cold sore or see one cropping up, just slow down a little bit and take care of yourself: cold sores are a sign that your immune system is stressed out. If you're sexually active, wait for oral partnered activity until the sore is gone, or use latex barriers that can **fully** cover your mouth (dams can, but condoms often do not). For more information on herpes, see page 303.

Feel around the whole breast in circles, from the outside in, or by going up and down from one side to the other. It's best to pick one way to do your exams, because that way, you'll become familiar with how the breast is supposed to feel in that pattern, which will make it easier for you to recognize anything abnormal. You'll need to do this for both breasts. If you did the exam lying down, you'll want to stand or sit up when you've done the exam and go through it once more: some parts of the breast feel different when standing.

Do a visual exam as well, keeping an eye out for any changes in your nipples, skin dimpling, puckering, unusual redness, or swelling.

Should you find an unusual lump, see your doctor. Most breast lumps in young women are not cancerous, so if you do find something, don't panic, just get it checked out.

Men and Women:
Check Out Those Genitals

Genital ingrown hairs and pimples are pretty easy to identify. They either have a small white head, or they are just tiny bumps,

s.e.x.

slightly red, that may smart a little bit, but should not itch or develop a raw, open, or very crusty top. As with pimples or ingrown hairs anywhere else, it's best not to pick them. If a hair is sticking out of a pustule, you can use a tweezers to pull it out, which can alleviate soreness and help it to heal. Hot compresses can also help heal pimples and ingrown hairs. Generally, just keep the area clean and let it heal on its own.

You should see your gynecologist or sexual healthcare provider—and take a break from any partnered sex until you do—if you notice any of the following symptoms:

▶ Any open, raw, raised, or reddish sores
▶ Hard lumps that can be seen or felt inside the outer labia or on the mons, testes, scrotum, foreskin, or penis
▶ Small white cauliflower-like growths or warts
▶ Persistent itching or scratching
▶ Unusual lumps or bumps that can be felt but not seen
▶ Any unusual discomfort with no visible cause

Men and Women:
Check Out Your Discharges

Vaginal discharge that is NOT normal, but a likely signal of infection or illness may:

▶ Be chunky or very heavy, with small curds like cottage cheese
▶ Be very watery
▶ Have a strong foul, metallic, or fishy odor
▶ Be grayish, yellow-greenish, yellow, pinkish, or tinged with bloody spots or streaks
▶ Cause excessive discomfort, burning, or itching

Penile discharge that is NOT normal, but likely a signal of infection or illness may:

▶ Be ANYTHING that is not ejaculate, pre-ejaculate, or urine
▶ Be any color from clear to yellow or greenish
▶ Contain blood or appear pinkish
▶ Appear with pain or burning during urination, a frequent need to urinate, any sort of genital rash, or swollen glands in the groin area

As well, any sort of discharge from the anus—in men or women—that is not clearly fecal matter should always be investigated.

The above sorts of discharges can be due to an infection like those listed below, or to an STI like gonorrhea or trichomoniasis. If you have any of the above sorts of abnormal discharge, or related symptoms, please see your gynecologist or doctor.

URINARY TRACT, BACTERIAL, AND YEAST INFECTIONS

Sexually transmitted infections are called that because they are most often transmitted through sexual contact. But there are also common genital infections that straddle the boundaries: they are genital, and sometimes sexually transmitted or exacerbated by sexual activity, but they often can, and do, occur without a person having had any sex at all.

Bacterial Vaginosis (BV)

What is it? A bacterial imbalance in the vagina, when the normal healthy bacteria of the vagina are essentially outnumbered by other not-so-nice bacteria.

Who gets it? Women—lots of them; BV is very common. It's estimated that as many as two million American women have it at any given time, and it is the most common cause of vaginitis—any irritation of the vagina characterized by discharge, odor, swelling, and/or itching—though many women with BV have no obvious symptoms.

How do you get it? The why and how of BV are not clearly understood, but your chances of developing it are increased by: douching, sexual activity (especially with new partners), switching between vaginal and anal sex (either unprotected or by using the same condom for both), sharing sex toys that can't be or weren't boiled or covered with a latex barrier, improper wiping after bowel movements, or antibiotic use.

What are its symptoms? Those with BV may discover a fishy, bad-smelling (especially after sexual activity) vaginal discharge that is creamy and grayish-white.

What do you do to treat it? BV needs to be diagnosed by a gynecologist or other doctor or sexual health clinician, and is usually easily treated with antibiotics or naturopathic or nutritional remedies. It is important to get treatment, as untreated BV can lead to serious conditions like pelvic inflammatory disease. BV isn't often passed on to male partners, though among women who sleep with women, it's common for both partners, especially when they are new to one another, to wind up with BV if one partner has it.

Urinary Tract or Bladder Infections

What are they? Just as BV occurs when "bad" bacteria are introduced to the vagina, a UTI (sometimes called cystitis) or bladder infection occurs when bacteria—from the anus, the external genitals, clothing, hands, toys, or partners—get into the lower urinary tract or the bladder.

Who gets them? Men and women. Urinary tract or bladder infections are most common in women, due simply to the design of the female genitals, but men can wind up with them as well.

How do you get them? UTIs or bladder infections can develop from improper toilet wiping, which can bring bacteria from the rectum into the urethra, and from sexual activity (namely, manual, oral, or vaginal sex, though "dry" sex can cause a UTI) in both men and women. Other culprits can include "holding" urine in too often, rather than urinating when you have to, wearing garments or undergarments made of synthetic fibers that don't allow the area to "breathe," spermicide use, kidney stones, or diabetes.

What are its symptoms? Most people with a UTI experience pain or burning with urination, difficulty urinating at all (often coupled with a persistent feeling of having to go), blood in the urine, or very strong-smelling urine. Fever and lower abdominal pain may also occur.

What do you do to treat them? At the VERY first *mild* sign of a UTI—like some minor discomfort urinating, or mild feelings of urinary urgency—you can sometimes fend UTIs off at the pass by drinking a whole lot of water and real (unsweetened) cranberry juice, tablets, or extract (the cranberry "cocktails" have very little cranberry juice in them, so cranberry tablets taken with lots of water, or concentrated or partially diluted pure juice is best). If, after a day or two of self-treatment, symptoms persist or get worse, it's time to hit the doc's office and be diagnosed and treated, because UTIs can spread and cause real problems for the bladder and kidneys. UTIs are diagnosed with a simple urine test, and treated with antibiotics. They tend to resolve very shortly after treatment begins, usually just a couple of days, and you'll often feel a lot of relief the very first day of treatment. (However, even if you feel better, never stop taking your antibiotics until you've used up the whole amount prescribed for you!) Sexual partners don't need to be treated.

For most people, UTIs are temporary and easily managed. However, some may get them chronically. Chronic sufferers are often given stronger antibiotics, and sometimes for much longer periods of time. Unfortunately, some people with chronic UTIs find that, after some time, antibiotics don't do the job anymore, either. If you are having UTIs chronically, your doctor should be evaluating your kidneys, and making sure you don't have any abnormalities of the urinary tract that may be causing the condition. If nothing is found, and nothing else seems to help, it's also important to make sure something simple isn't causing the problem, like not drinking enough water reg-ularly, wiping improperly, neglecting proper hygiene, or consuming things known to irritate the bladder, such as alcohol, caffeine, or even citrus.

Yeast Infection (or Thrush)

What is it & who gets it? *Men and women, both.* A healthy, happy vagina normally has some amount of yeast within it, but it exists in a delicate and acidic balance. When something occurs to disrupt that balance, and the vagina becomes more alkaline and less acidic, the yeasts proliferate and cause an infection. Men can also acquire genital yeast or fungal infections—sometimes it's called *jock itch*—though they are less common in men. Yeast infections can also be present orally or anally in men and women.

How do you get them? Yeast infections can be the result of many things, including an unbalanced diet (especially one high in caffeine, simple carbs, sugars, and processed foods), a food allergy, a preexisting sexually transmitted infection, antibiotics, birth control pills, spermicides, pregnancy, diabetes, or immunosupression as the result of disease. Douching, feminine "hygiene" sprays or lotions, pantyhose, and synthetic or wet undergarments without breathability are also common accomplices. If you're taking antibiotics for something, be sure to eat plenty of organic, plain yogurt, or take acidophilus tablets, while you're taking them, as that helps prevent the yeast imbalances that can cause yeast infections. Genital sensitivities can also be a factor: if you're allergic or sensitive to latex, or certain detergents, lubricants, or

s.e.x.

other substances, use alternatives. It's also possible for yeast infections to be passed from partner to partner.

What are its symptoms? Common symptoms of a yeast infection are itching, burning, chafing, swelling, and/or generalized irritation of the vagina and vulva, or the penis, testes, or anus. The anus, vagina, or vulva may feel uncomfortably dry. It may be painful to urinate or engage in manual sex or vaginal intercourse. Unusual discharge isn't always present, but when it is, it tends to be thick, white, and chunky, sometimes with small cottage-cheese-like curds. A smell may or may not be present (a discharge that smells like baking bread is a sure sign of a yeast infection). Oral yeast infection symptoms generally include a mouth ulcer, usually on the tongue or inside the cheeks, with a creamy, white appearance. A pervasive feeling of dry mouth may also be present.

What do you do to treat them? A doctor can usually diagnose a yeast infection with a visual exam or swab. For women, most doctors prescribe either oral medications or over-the-counter treatments. The latter are used with an application tube that inserts a treatment cream or suppository tablet into the vagina. With that treatment, a woman may also use a soothing cream for her labia and vulva, to relieve soreness or swelling. Men are usually given a simple, topical antifungal cream.

As with urinary tract infections, there are some safe at-home treatments you can try, at the first sign of a mild yeast infection or general vaginitis, before hauling out the big guns. Many people find that plain, organic yogurt (if you're vegan, you can use soy yogurt) with active, live cultures is an excellent treatment: acidophilus in the yogurt kills excess yeast by producing hydrogen peroxide. It can be applied on the irritated external genitals and inside the vagina, by simply spreading it on and in with a finger. Some women fill empty tampon applicators with yogurt and freeze them, inserting them for use that way (the coolness is also soothing when the vagina is irritated). Given that this is more than a little messy, it's really only a good remedy for bedtime.

Eating plenty of natural yogurt (especially when on antibiotics) also helps protect and restore the healthy bacteria in your body. Other natural remedies include inserting cloves of garlic as vaginal suppositories (garlic is a natural antifungal) until the infection clears up, and again, drinking pure cranberry juice or using cranberry supplements can be of help here, though only for very mild infections. If these DIY treatments don't seem to be helping within a few days, see your doctor or sexual healthcare provider for more intensive treatment.

Do NOT self-treat a possible yeast infection with over-the-counter treatments if you have never been diagnosed with a yeast infection. If you do, and you do NOT actually have a yeast infection, you could either reduce the effectiveness of the medication, if and when you DO have one later, or you could actually cause one by disrupting the acid balance of your vagina. Plus, if you have a different sort of infection—like BV, trichomoniasis, or chlamydia—it's important you get that diagnosed and treated as soon as possible.

S.e.x.

So, always be sure to see your doctor first, to be sure it's even a yeast infection that you've got.

It's best to abstain from partnered sex until you've been diagnosed and treated, since yeast infections are contagious, and often sexual activity when you have a yeast infection is incredibly uncomfortable anyway. Informing a partner of a yeast infection is also important; they may have one themselves without knowing it. And to be perfectly plain, yeast infections tend not to look very pretty, so a partner unknowingly engaging in sex with a person with an active yeast infection is likely to be pretty grossed out or freaked if they see (or smell) the symptoms on their partner's genitals.

As with UTIs, some people experience recurrent or chronic yeast infections. Chronic or recurrent yeast infections should be reported to a doctor and looked into, because they can be a sign of diabetes, HIV infection, or another immunosuppressive disease or disorder. They may also be due to dietary issues or food allergies, which can be remedied simply with diet changes.

preventing vaginal infections and stopping the cycle of chronic infections

 BECAUSE of the way women's anatomy is "designed," women are particularly inclined to infections like UTIs, yeast infections, and BV. But you can do some things to help yourself avoid them:

- Avoid spreading germs from the anus to the vagina. When urinating and after bowel movements, always wipe from front to back—vulva to anus. Wash your hands before and after you masturbate, and if sexual partners are not using latex gloves, have them wash hands before manual sex.

- Practice safer sex, using latex barriers for manual, oral, vaginal, or anal sexual activity. Avoid flavored lubricants for vaginal use, or those with high glycerine content, as well as spermicides or spermicidally lubricated condoms. Spermicides often irritate genital tissue, which heightens the risks for developing infections.

- Use good basic hygiene, making sure to wash the vulva daily with a gentle, unfragranced soap.

- **_Do NOT douche!_** According to the National Women's Health Information Center (sponsored by the U.S. Department of Health and Human Services), most doctors and the American College of Obstetricians and Gynecologists suggest that women steer clear of douching. Douches disrupt the delicate pH and bacterial balance of the vagina and the self-cleaning cycle. Some studies show that women who douche at least once a month are over 30 percent more likely to have bacterial vaginosis or a mild vaginal infection than women who never douche, that women who douche have more health problems than those who do not, and that douching can spread vaginal infections into the reproductive organs, which can also cause pelvic inflammatory disease, which often leads to infertility. Recent research has also suggested a link between douching and increased risks of HIV, herpes, other STIs, and cervical cancer.

- Avoid too-tight pants, panties without a cotton crotch, pantyhose, and other clothing that can trap moisture and doesn't breathe. Comfortable natural-fiber clothing is always best.

- Do not try to self-medicate with over-the-counter treatments or someone else's medication for a suspected infection . Not only may it not work, while your infection gets worse, but you may end up giving yourself an infection that you didn't even have to begin with. Yikes!

- Eat a healthy, balanced diet, and avoid processed foods and lots of carbonated sodas. Take good care of yourself.

- If you are being treated for an infection, be sure to take all your medication to the end, as directed, and abstain from sexual activities until you are fully well. In addition, avoid using tampons while infected—if you are menstruating or currently have a genital infection, use cotton pads instead.

- *Do not* let suspected infections go untreated, as they can worsen or spread. Sometimes, symptoms of an infection may go away, but that does not mean the infection itself is necessarily gone. If you suspect an infection, see your doctor or gynecologist as soon as possible.

When You Just Can't DIY

Most of the time, you can manage your own health, especially when you're taking smart daily care of yourself, and being vigilant about annual sexual and general health checkups. But some things are best managed by your doctor or healthcare provider. Among the reasons to contact your doctor or clinic are: pain in the abdomen during intercourse or other sexual activity; unusual appearance of genitals or nipples; itching or burning on or in, or unusual discharge from, the genitals or nipples; skipped or missed periods when there is no pregnancy risk; a suspected pregnancy, STI, yeast infection or UTI; blood in the urine, or difficulty or pain when urinating; unusual sores or discharge on/from the genitals or mouth; extended illness (like a cold or flu that lasts more than a week or two); unusual tiredness or lethargy; and recurring illness or infections. If you are on hormonal birth control and have changes in your health or habits that may pose risks to you while using those methods (such as smoking or high blood pressure), consult your doctor. Serious and persistent concerns about nutrition and activity, about body size or shape, about the ability to sleep and rest soundly, about managing stress, or about depression or anxiety should also be directed to your doctor, nurse, or clinician.

SEXUAL HEALTHCARE DISCRIMINATION: ROADBLOCKS TO GOOD HEALTH

Due to the strong feelings in much of our culture about young adult sexuality, you may bump up against some discrimination that makes taking care of your sexual health more difficult.

That discrimination may be minor and fairly easy to counter: perhaps your family doctor doesn't want to give you a pelvic exam or prescribe birth control for you. It's also not unusual to encounter a doctor or healthcare provider who isn't real excited about your sexual choices—or who outright opposes them—even if those you've made have been as responsible and safe as possible. While your healthcare provider doesn't have to agree with your decisions, it is their job to give you information and guidance to be as healthy as possible, not to impose their moral codes on you. In situations like these, you can voice an objection or make a complaint, switch to another doctor, or visit a general

s.e.x.

sexual health clinic instead, such as a Planned Parenthood branch, where sexual health services are provided without judgment.

It's important to learn to be your own advocate. Find out what your rights are, based on your age and what you're seeking out (STI screenings, GYN exams, birth control or emergency contraception, abortion, confidential testing, sliding fees): your rights will differ some from country to country and state to state. For instance, confidentiality requirements and obligations in terms of your services, records, and results, vary in certain situations and areas, based on local laws, your age, and general practice or clinic guidelines and approaches. As detailed in chapter 7, some states require mandatory social service reporting for doctors and nurses if a patient under the legal age of consent (AOC) reports sexual activity with a partner over that AOC. Some states, counties, or countries may have the right to refuse emergency contraception for patients.

know your rights!

 YOU have a right to seek out and receive quality sexual healthcare, no matter your age, location, gender, orientation, or income bracket.

You have a right, when you choose sexual healthcare, to choose that which is in your best physical and emotional interest, from a healthcare provider who will be your sexual health ally. Shop around with clinics and doctors. Before just making an appointment, call a few different offices. Voice concerns—whether that's about having access to the services you need or simply finding a doctor or clinician who'll treat you with respect. Bear in mind that "respect" may not always mean unconditional or quiet acceptance of everything

you do. A good doctor or nurse, for instance, isn't likely to stay mum if you're engaging in risky activities without protection or playing Russian roulette with pregnancy. But it does mean being treated with courtesy and objectivity. A healthcare practitioner should not be bringing their personal agenda to the table.

A good way to find a good gynecologist, doctor, or sexual health clinic is to ask peers or trusted adults for a referral. In a particular group practice, one of the best ways of finding a good doctor is to talk to the nurses who work there, and let them know what exactly you're looking for: nurses are often the best patient advocates out there.

GLBT patients may face additional challenges. GLBT discrimination can manifest in many ways. A given doctor or clinic may go completely overboard in panicking about sexual health risks for gay men, or in dismissing or ignoring lesbian STI risks and concerns completely. GLBT patients who are not out yet may have special concerns about confidentiality. Bisexual patients may experience assumptions that their orientation means they're promiscuous or sexually irresponsible. Transgender patients may find it difficult to have their boundaries or identity honored.

All that said, finding healthcare that is accepting, informed, and appropriate for GLBT patients is not impossible. Look in the phonebook or online for clinics that expressly serve GLBT populations, or call community centers, therapists, or groups that are GLBT-friendly and ask for help finding safe, welcoming healthcare. Some Internet sites, groups, and resources can also be of help (see the Resource section for some organizations).

If you do encounter discrimination, the

best approach is to find a better doctor, practice, or clinic first, and deal with any reporting you want to do about the discrimination later. Your health comes first. What's most important is the quality of your healthcare and your ability to be honest and open with a healthcare provider, so that you can be sure to get what you need.

It's rare, but sometimes, harassment and very real abuse, sexual and otherwise, can occur in the healthcare system. In those instances, do NOT go back to that doctor or clinic; either speak with your parents or another trusted older adult, and/or contact the medical board, police (if that feels necessary, and always in cases of any sexual or physical abuse), a private lawyer, or a legal aid service. For more on how to handle abuse or assault—from anyone—see chapter 10.

▪ SAFER SEX 101 ▪

STIs can happen to anyone—*anyone*—who is or has been sexually active (and not just those having vaginal or anal intercourse), and they do happen to about nineteen million new people, in the United States alone, every single year. *At least one person in every four will contract an STI during their life.* According to the Guttmacher Institute, over 65 million people in the United States currently live with an incurable STI, and although teens and young adults only make up around 25 percent of the sexually active population, people from fifteen to twenty-five years of age account for nearly *half* of all STI diagnoses every year. By the time you're twenty-four, among you and two of your closest friends, one of you probably will have or have had an STI. Teens also have more of the most common STIs than

anyone else: chlamydia, gonorrhea, herpes, and HPV all have higher incidence in young adults than in their elders. And all too many young adults and teens are walking around with an STI that they don't even know they have, because they don't get annual sexual healthcare and STI screenings; because of wrong ideas about STIs and how they are transmitted; and because so many STIs don't present visible or obvious symptoms.

As a young adult, your risks are higher than those of any other age group: Young adults, especially young women, are physically more susceptible to diseases and infections to begin with; they're more likely to have greater numbers of new sexual partners; they often lack regular sexual healthcare; and, on top of that, they often neglect safer sex practices. In addition, most STIs are more prevalent in young women than their male counterparts, and young women risk greater complications from sexually transmitted diseases and infections than men do, such as PID, reproductive cancers, and complications during pregnancy and childbirth.

STIs can happen to you, whether you've had ten partners or are just starting with your first partner; whether you're had vaginal intercourse or "only" oral sex; whether you're conservative or more freewheeling; whether you're male or female, straight or queer, fifteen or fifty. Viruses and bacteria don't care who is "nice" or who isn't, who is a "virgin" and who's not.

The good news is that in most cases, STIs can be prevented—ensuring both you and your partner's health, as well as the health of all of us worldwide—with an easy combination of smart risk assessment and reduction, safer sex practices, and regular sexual and general healthcare.

s.e.x.

Risk Assessment

Very high risk activities:
▶ Unprotected anal intercourse
▶ Unprotected vaginal intercourse
▶ Body fluid or blood play

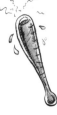

High-risk activities:
▶ Unprotected fellatio
▶ Unprotected vaginal fisting/deep manual sex
▶ Unprotected analingus or anal fisting

Moderate-risk activities:
▶ Shared sex toys without a condom
  or barrier on them (for toys that cannot be boiled)
▶ Unprotected cunnilingus
▶ Unprotected manual sex (all sexes)
▶ Kissing (open-mouth)

Low-risk activities:
▶ Protected oral sex, anal or vaginal intercourse
▶ Unprotected manual sex with handwashing
  before and after
▶ Manual sex (all genders) with gloves
▶ Kissing (closed-mouth, so long as no wounds
  or sores are present)
▶ Oral contact with body parts other than the
  mouth or genitals (hands, feet, ears, necks, backs, etc.)
▶ Dry sex

No-risk activities:
▶ Kissing (closed-mouth, so long as no wounds or sores are present)
▶ Massage and petting (nongenital, and without fluid sharing)
▶ Sensation play
▶ Hugging
▶ Role-play, cybersex, or phone sex
▶ Mutual masturbation

what is safer sex?

 SAFER sex is a combination of **three** basic things, ALL of which need to be done to be practicing safer sex:

1. Have full STI screenings and sexual health exams, at least once a year, more often if you have new or multiple partners.
2. Limit risks during sexual activities through barrier use (condoms, dental dams, latex gloves) and other practices.
3. Make safer lifestyle choices, like limiting the number of your sexual partners, limiting or avoiding high-risk sexual behaviors, limiting or eliminating nonsexual STI risks in general (intravenous drug use, for instance), using clean needles for body modification work, and taking care of your general health.

If you're not doing **all** three of those things—or abstaining from partnered sex until you CAN—you aren't practicing safer sex. Doing any of them certainly helps, but unless you're doing all three, you're not substantially reducing your risks.

Some people are now using safer sex throughout their whole sexual lives, from day one. But for plenty, that isn't the case. Perhaps you started your sexual life without knowing how, or feeling able, to protect yourself from infection or disease. Or maybe in your relationship, you and your partner started taking risks somewhere along the line, and now you're having some trouble breaking those habits. Some people even think that being responsible when it comes to safer sex—or asking a partner to—is insulting or rude. No matter the situation, it can feel awkward, and it might seem difficult to settle into healthy practices without feeling like the Sex Decency Brigade. But it doesn't have to be that way.

It's never too late to start having sex as responsibly and safely as possible, and there's no reason it needs to be a drag: if anything, safer sex often makes sex more, rather than less, enjoyable. Worry and fear about disease, infection, and pregnancy can inhibit our brains from firing off all the pistons that make us aroused and sexually excited. In men, that can mean premature ejaculation, or trouble with erection or orgasm. In women, it can include a lack of vaginal lubrication, vaginal tightness and discomfort, and inhibitors to orgasm. So, aside from the mental anguish, there are also very real and visible physical effects to taking risks we just don't feel good about. And since partnered sex isn't a requirement, but something any of us should only do to feel pleasure, intimacy and joy, if it's riddled with anxiety and fear that keep that good stuff from really happening, there's just no point.

PRACTICING SAFER SEX: A LESSON IN THREE PARTS

Safer sex practices don't make sex 100 percent safe, even if all of them are used to the letter: they make sex safer. A condom may—especially if not used properly—break or slip off. Some STIs, like HPV, herpes, or pubic lice, can be more difficult to protect from, because latex barriers don't cover the entire genital area. And even when we practice safer sex guidelines religiously—including barrier use, testing, and lifestyle modifications—we can still transmit or contract an STI. We need to accept that STI transmission (passing one around) is always possible. Safer sex practices are a lot like seatbelts: even with one, we may still get hurt, but it's a whole lot less likely than if we ditch them altogether.

s.e.x.

why practice safer sex?

IF YOU don't practice safer sex, you are at *high risk* for the following infections and diseases.

Unprotected vaginal or anal intercourse, or vaginal intercourse with a condom that has also been used for anal intercourse, puts partners at risk of contracting (getting) or transmitting (passing on):

- Bacterial vaginosis (page 194)
- Chancroid (page 299)
- Chlamydia (page 300)
- Cytomegalovirus (CMV) (page 301)
- Gonorrhea (page 301)
- Hepatitis (page 302)
- Herpes simplex (page 303)
- Human immunodeficiency virus (HIV) (page 304)
- Human papillomavirus (HPV, warts) (page 305)
- Pelvic inflammatory disease (PID) (page 308)
- Pubic lice (page 309)
- Syphilis (page 310)
- Trichomoniasis (page 311)
- Yeast infections (page 196)

Unprotected oral sex ("blow job," "giving head," "going down," "eating out," "rimming") puts partners at risk of contracting or transmitting:

- Chancroid
- Cytomegalovirus (CMV)
- Gonorrhea
- Hepatitis
- Herpes simplex (oral and/or genital)
- Human immunodeficiency virus (HIV)
- Human papillomavirus (HPV, warts)
- Yeast infections/thrush
- Syphilis

Unprotected manual sex ("hand job" or "fingering") puts partners at risk of contracting or transmitting:

- Bacterial vaginosis
- Cytomegalovirus (CMV)
- Herpes simplex
- Human papillomavirus (HPV, warts)
- Pubic lice

For more information on each of these infections and diseases, see Appendix A, "Sexually Transmitted Infections: From A to Z."

s.e.x.

Most STIs *are* both treatable and curable, so long as you get them diagnosed early. Some are treatable and manageable, but not curable. Some, especially if left undiagnosed and untreated, can cause severe and longstanding health problems, like PID (see page 308), reproductive cancers, or infertility, and a few can actually kill you and/or your partner.

Safer sex doesn't just make things safer for us, it makes sex safer for everyone. STIs, even the curable/manageable ones, aren't just about you and your partner; they affect public health as a whole: the more people practice who sex safely, the fewer STIs there will be floating around out there! What happens in our bedrooms may be private, but our choices can also affect people we'll never even meet, and someone else's choices can have a profound effect on our own lives and health. Whether those effects will be negative or positive depends on the choices we all make.

SAFER SEX, PART ONE: TESTING AND ANNUAL SEXUAL HEALTH EXAMS

Because barriers cannot offer 100 percent protection against disease and infection, especially with common STIs like HPV and herpes, it's important to be tested so that both you and your partners know as accurately as possible what your risks are, and so that if either of you does develop an STI, you can get it treated quickly, and take extra precautions as needed.

Remember that *sexually transmitted* means that these diseases and infections are most often transmitted sexually, not that there is no *other* way they can be transmitted. Oral herpes, for instance, can be contracted by kissing your grandmother. Pubic lice can

did you know . . . ?

Many people feel they don't need annual screenings. Plenty more think they HAVE been screened when they haven't: many women just assume annual pelvic exams involve STI screenings, when they often do not. Some folks who may have been tested for HIV at some point think they also were tested for all STIs at that time, when they likely were not. The majority of young adults have not had full STI screenings, unless they have asked for them explicitly, or exhibited symptoms that made a doctor or GYN suspect they might have an STI. Don't forget that many STIs are asymptomatic, so plenty of folks presently infected with an STI have no idea.

be passed around by sharing towels in a locker room. Hepatitis or HIV can be spread by a tattoo or piercing done with a shared needle. And "sexually transmitted" doesn't just refer to heterosexual intercourse, but to any number of sexual activities. This is why someone who is a "virgin" cannot automatically be assumed to be STI-free. So, screening is even important BEFORE you become sexually active, not just afterward.

What exactly does STI testing involve?

STI testing includes a few simple tests that can be done in your gynecologist's or general practitioner's office, or at a general or

s.e.x.

sexual health clinic. Some may cause slight, brief discomfort. It's important to recognize that when you ask for a full screening, you will get all the tests available to you that will net accurate results. There are some STIs that can't be screened for accurately, under certain conditions. For instance, without an active sore, it's generally not possible to test for herpes. Ask your doctor or clinician to tell you which tests they CAN do, so you're fully informed.

When you go in for a screening—which, as mentioned earlier in the chapter, can be done at your annual sexual health checkup—the clinician or doctor will first ask you some questions regarding your exposure to STIs and your sexual activities and sexual history. It's important that you be honest in answering these questions. Your privacy is protected, and while certain activities, partners, or risks you have taken may be embarrassing or uncomfortable for you to talk about, chances are good they aren't going to ruffle or rattle a health clinician at all—there's very little most of them haven't seen or heard at some point. If you've come in for a screening because you know or suspect that you have been exposed to a specific STI, or you have symptoms that lead you to believe you may have contracted one, give that information to the doctor or clinician during this time.

The doctor or clinician will do a visual examination of your body and genitals, looking for evidence of sores or lesions, abnormal discharges, or unusual skin texture or color. If you are a woman, you will go through the same procedure as you would for a pelvic exam. During the pelvic exam, the doctor will take a small sample of cells

and fluids called a smear or swab. This is similar to a Pap smear test, except that in this case, when the technician or doctor looks at the cells through a microscope, they will be looking for signs of the various microorganisms, antibodies, or cell changes that indicate specific STIs.

For male patients, if you get a swab test (page 190), it will involve the doctor or clinician gently inserting a long cotton-tipped swab into the urethra to get a sample of cells. While most men do find this test unpleasant, it is not particularly painful and it only lasts a moment. The cells gathered on the swab will then be examined under a microscope.

For both men and women, the clinician may also take a sample of cells from your throat (to check for STIs that can be present in the mouth or throat, such as gonorrhea) and/or your rectum, by swabbing the same way your genitals were swabbed.

For a full screening, your doctor or clinician will likely also take saliva, blood, and urine samples, for screenings that require those.

Your healthcare professional may be able to tell you immediately if you do or do not have certain STIs; for most, you may have to wait a few days or weeks for complete results of your tests. Waiting for test results is never fun for anyone—it's normal to feel nervous and anxious. But since you have had your screenings done, so long as you are not taking additional risks while you wait, you should know that you've done all you can currently do. So, try to relax. Take care of yourself. And give yourself mad props for taking steps to take care of your sexual health.

SAFER SEX, PART TWO: BARRIERS AND OTHER GEAR

Condoms (Latex or Nonlatex)

Condoms are used for: vaginal or anal intercourse (with a penis, dildo, or other safe object), for fellatio, and for covering shared sex toys, like dildos or vibrators, especially those that cannot be boiled or sterilized. They can also be used to cover the penis during manual sex, in lieu of latex gloves, or cut lengthwise and opened for use as a barrier for cunnilingus or analingus. For those with latex sensitivity or discomfort, a nonlatex or polyurethane condom should be used; there are a few on the market, and the female condom (see chapter 11) is polyurethane.

How to use a condom

1. Always open a condom package carefully—if you're using your teeth or fingernails, be sure you're only tearing the edge, so you don't rip the condom by accident. **Don't unroll it until you are putting it on.** To increase the wearer's comfort, place a

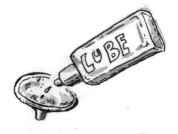

few drops of latex-safe lubricant inside the tip on the unrolled condom. (NEVER use Vaseline, cooking or body oils, lotions, or other lubricants not intended for condom use, as they will corrode the condom.)

2. To put on the condom, pinch the tip of the condom with one hand, leaving about an inch of space. Slowly roll the condom over the shaft of the penis or other object, to the base, pushing out any air inside the condom as you do. To increase the durability of the condom and everyone's pleasure, apply more latex-safe lubricant to the outside of the condom. If you're putting a condom on an uncircumcised penis, pull the foreskin back comfortably and hold it back with one hand while unrolling the condom onto the shaft of the penis. When you have the condom rolled down as far as it will go, release the foreskin and let it roll back up naturally. Adjust the base of the condom if you need to, so it's both secure and comfortable.

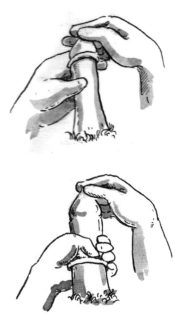

s.e.x.

3. After ejaculation, withdraw while the penis is still erect, while holding onto the base of the condom to make sure it doesn't slip off. Roll it off slowly and throw the condom away.

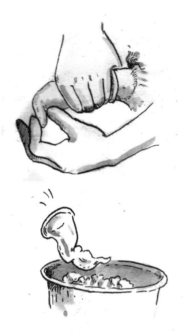

To use a condom as a dental dam for cunnilingus or analingus, simply cut the condom with a clean pair of scissors down the middle, lengthwise, and open it up.

For EVERY new or repeated sexual activity, use a new condom. Do not switch between vaginal, oral, or anal sex without also switching to a new, unused condom. Condoms cannot be reused: once you've used one, it's toast.

The vast majority of condom failure is due to improper use. Condoms and other latex barriers do not have imperceptible holes through which viruses can pass: when a condom is used properly, any bacteria or virus that was within the condom (on the surface of what the condom covered) CANNOT be transmitted. It is when a condom breaks, tears, or slips off that it may be ineffective (as birth control as well as a barrier to disease). Breaks and tears are pretty easy to avoid: be sure you are using a high-quality condom, that it has been stored properly (even before you bought it—gas stations or vending machines are poor places to get condoms for this reason), that you use it with additional latex-safe lubricant, and that you put it on correctly, with enough room left at the tip, and rolled to the base of the penis.

Condoms are very easy to obtain in most areas. You can find them at most pharmacies, megastores, or grocers. You can often obtain them at no cost from sexual health clinics and community centers, though in those cases, you do not often get to choose the type you will get. Condoms can also be ordered by mail online or via catalog, and are generally shipped in plain packages for privacy.

Helpful Hints

▶ **For the most part, most condoms will accommodate nearly all penis sizes, especially lengthwise.** Ring (the condom base) sizes, however, vary more, and are less flexible, so you may need to shop around if the base feels too tight on you or your partner. Condoms termed a "snugger" fit tend to have smaller ring sizes; those with words like "maximum fit" or "larger" tend to have larger ring sizes. There currently are a few custom-fit condoms on the market, and several brands of condoms sized with extra room only at the head of the condom to provide greater comfort. Most men will fit average-size

s.e.x.

condoms, so be sure not to purchase larger ones if you don't need them: if you do buy them, and they're slipping off at the base, go back to an average or snugger size.

▶ **Thin is in.** Choose thinner condoms for greater durability, sensation, and comfort. With thinner condoms, less friction occurs, and as a result, thinner condoms tend to be more durable and less likely to break than thicker ones.

▶ **Avoid condoms with Nonoxynol-9.** Nonoxynol-9, a spermicide used on spermicidally-lubricated condoms, is only added to condoms at this point to make users *feel* more secure. However, not only do spermicides cause irritation for many people, thus inflaming genital tissue and making infection transmission MORE likely, but spermicides (which aren't very effective to begin with) only get a chance to work if a condom breaks. When high-quality condoms are used correctly, with additional latex-safe lubricant as needed, the chances of them breaking are truly minimal. So, it's best to buy either unlubricated condoms or those lubricated without spermicides.

▶ **Don't double up.** Putting one condom over another increases friction, so BOTH are actually more likely to break than one used alone (not to mention that a man wearing two condoms is not likely to feel very much).

▶ **Hold the chocolate.** Do not use flavored condoms for anal or vaginal intercourse. The flavored lubricant contains sugar, which can make yeast infections more likely to occur. Flavored condoms are intended for oral sex use.

▶ **Be aware of latex sensitivities.** Anywhere between around 1 and 6 percent of people are latex-allergic or latex-sensitive. Some people who are latex-allergic experience symptoms with immediate contact, others after a few hours or even days after contact with latex. So, if you experience any genital swelling, burning, redness, blistering, fissures, scaling, any nausea or vomiting, a dizzy or faint feeling, or cramps after using latex condoms or other barriers, you may be allergic to latex. If you suspect you are, try using polyurethane condoms, and see if you have the same symptoms. You can check for a severe latex allergy in advance of condom use by wearing a latex glove on your hand for about twenty minutes.

▶ **Keep cool.** Keep your condoms in a cool, dark place to prevent the latex from degrading. So, vehicle glove compartments, wallets, back pockets, and the like are not good places to keep them, except for very short periods of time.

▶ **Accept no substitutes.** Lambskin condoms do NOT offer protection against STIs. Cling film or Saran wrap, plastic bags, or a latex glove CANNOT be used in place of a condom.

▶ **Sensitive guy?** For some men, condoms may reduce sensitivity to a point where there is great difficulty reaching orgasm or ejaculating. If this is the case, you have some options: You can use the thinnest condom possible, and choose condoms with ribs or dots inside the condom. Place some lubricant inside the tip of the condom before use. Make sure other issues aren't

s.e.x.

involved in the matter, like antidepressants or other medications with sexual side effects, latex allergies, lack of full arousal, lack of lubrication, or the biggie: negative attitudes about barriers.

Lubricant

Lubricants are used for: any sexual activity, especially with latex or polyurethane barriers—condoms, dental dams, latex gloves—or simply for extra pleasure, during vaginal or anal intercourse or manual sex. Women using hormonal birth control methods, such as the pill or patch, may also find they need extra lubricant, because those methods can cause extra vaginal dryness.

How to use lube:

To use with a condom, place a couple of drops inside the tip of the condom before putting it on, then apply lubricant on the outside of the condom when it is fully unrolled, and/or on the vulva or anus, if vaginal or anal intercourse will occur.

To use with a dental dam, apply lube on the genitals before the dental dam is placed on them.

For manual sex, apply lubricant to both the outside of the glove or hands and the other partner's genitals.

How much or how little to use is a matter of preference, but there should be enough lube, at all times, to keep the barrier from becoming dry or tacky, and to keep the genitals comfortable and slippery during sexual activities. It's common to find that you need to apply extra lubricant during sex, for both comfort and durability of the barrier.

Lubricant is easily washed off the genitals during regular bathing, though if you are prone to yeast infections, you may want to rinse it off sooner rather than later.

You can purchase lubricants at your local pharmacy (they're usually in the same area as condoms), obtain them at some sexual health clinics, or find them via Internet or mail-order suppliers.

Helpful Hints

▶ **Accept no substitutes.** Latex-safe lubricant is either water-based or silicone-based, and will indicate "for sexual/genital use" on the tube or bottle. While things like body lotions are acceptable for male masturbation, they are NOT acceptable for use with latex barriers during partnered sex. Body lotions, baby or cooking oils, massage oils or creams, and Vaseline should NEVER be used with condoms, gloves, or dams. Not only do many of these substances erode latex, and thus put it at risk of breaking or tearing, but most of them do not belong inside the internal genitalia, the vagina, or the anus, as they can cause infection.

▶ **Go sugar-free.** Many lubricants contain glycerin, which may create problems for those prone to yeast infections. Glycerin-free or low-glycerin lubes are available. Flavored lubricants should not be used vaginally or anally, as they contain more sugars, which can also create or exacerbate yeast infections.

▶ **There *is* such a thing as too much lube.** Way too much lube may help cause a condom to slip off. So, when using lube, no need to have a river of the stuff: just enough to be comfortable and moderately slippery.

Dental Dams

Dental dams are used for female-receptive oral sex (cunnilingus) or for anal oral sex (analingus).

How to use a dental dam:

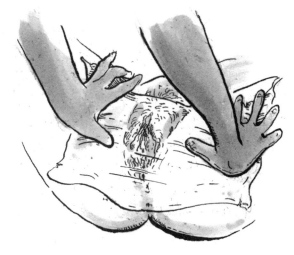

Most dams have a light talc coating, so first, rinse off the talc with water, as it can cause some irritation. Apply lubricant to the genitals where the dam will be placed. Then, open up the dam—it's like a little sheet of latex when opened—and spread it over the vulva or anus. You or your partner can then hold the dam in place with your hands during the activity.

Dental dams are often harder to find than condoms. While most online safer sex and sex toy suppliers sell them, many pharmacies that sell condoms and lubes do not. You can also obtain them at medical supply stores. If you cannot find a source for dental dams, you may also use cling film or plastic wrap as a dam. Do NOT use the type specifically designed for microwave use, as that sort has

small holes in it, so it will not provide adequate protection. You can use the plastic wrap the same way you'd use a dam. Additionally, cling film can be even more handy, because it comes in far larger sheets. For cunnilingus, you can actually wrap the cling-film dam around the wearer's thighs, so no one has to hold the barrier in place with their hands. There also are dam latex "hot pants" available for hands-free protection.

Helpful Hints

▶ **Use one side—once.** Always keep the same side of the dam or cling film against the body. You can't flip-flop dams and have them work effectively: only one side may be used. Dental dams cannot be reused, to be effective against the spread of disease or infection.

▶ **You can also make a dam out of a latex glove.**

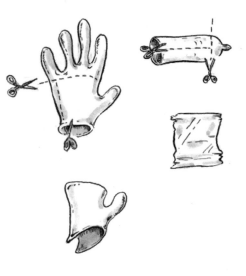

There are a few ways to do this: You can cut off the fingers and base and then cut lengthwise along the thumb and open it up (and you then have

s.e.x.

four finger cots as well). Or—and this is especially handy if you're performing manual sex and oral sex at the same time—you can put the glove on your hand, then cut a rectangular flap from the base to the fingers, and simply lift that up and cover the vulva while wearing the rest of the glove on your hand, or while fingers are inside the vagina, already gloved. You can also cut a glove's fingers off, then cut up lengthwise on the side without the thumb, and put your tongue inside the thumb to use the dam.

safer sex arts & crafts!

 WANT another way to use a dam for cunnilingus, hands-free? One of our volunteers at Scarleteen passed on these instructions to make a DIY dam harness:

■ Get a packet of garter snaps and any fabric that tickles your fancy (ribbons, silk cord, green monster fur–all available at most craft or fabric stores).

■ Take a dental dam (or piece of Saran wrap) of the sort/size you will be using. Attach a garter snap to each corner of the dental dam.

■ Position the dental dam over your crotch. Now, the fun bit: attach strips of fabric/ribbon to the other ends of the snaps and tie them around yourself so that they hold the dam in place. You can do this in almost any way you like. Two obvious arrangements are: (1) the bikini type, with just two strips of fabric going from front to back over each hip, or (2) the garter belt type, with a "belt" around the waist and four strips of fabric hanging down, each attaching to a strap. You can get as

artsy-craftsy as you like, or not: if you can't sew at all, you can use fabric glue, or just use ribbons, which you can tie.

■ Once you've got it all fixed together to your liking, you can use it, then simply unclip the snaps, toss away the dam, and you're done! You can snap in a new dam with the reusable belt anytime. You can also use existing underpants to make a dam harness by cutting out the crotch area, placing the dam where the crotch once was, and attaching the garter snaps that way.

▶ **Hold the chocolate.** Some dams come flavored, but as with flavored condoms or lubricants, these may bring on yeast infections. If you're prone to yeast infections, it's likely best to stick to unflavored dams.

Latex or Polyurethane (Nonlatex) Gloves

Gloves are used for: female (fingering, petting, or fisting) or male (handjobs) manual sex, or manual anal play. A glove can also be used as a dental dam.

How to use gloves:

Be sure to remove any serious jewelry from your hands before using gloves, and if you have long or sharp nails, it's a good idea to cut them first. Take the gloves out of the box or baggie they're in, and slide your hands into them, just like any other kind of gloves.

For manual sex, the gloves should be lubricated on the outside with latex-safe lubricant. When finished, toss the gloves in the garbage. A new pair of gloves should be used each time, when switching from one set of genitals to another, or from penis or vulva to anus.

your basic safer sex kit should contain:

- Unlubricated or lubricated condoms
- Latex-safe lubricant
- Latex gloves (or nonlatex for those with allergies)
- Dental dams (or, keep a nail scissors in your kit for cutting condoms or gloves to use as dams)

Possible Kit Additions:
- Finger cots
- Baby wipes (for quick cleanup of genitals, especially after using flavored lubes or condoms or silicone lubricants)
- Cranberry tablets (helpful to prevent UTI development)
- An over-the-counter analgesic, such as aspirin, acetaminophen, or ibuprofen (helpful for soreness due to vasocongestion)
- Aloe vera gel (handy for external genital irritation after sexual activities)

If you can't afford the basic supplies, you can't afford to be sexually active. Safer sex gear is going to be the least of your expenses. Basic sexual healthcare, which you NEED, at least once each year, costs money. Emergency contraception, in the case of a birth control failure, costs money. Treating an STI costs much more than protecting against one. If you're having heterosexual sex, an accidental pregnancy is going to cost you big bucks. So, if spending around twenty-five dollars every few months or so is more than you can handle, then—financially speaking—so is partnered sex.

To use a glove as a dental dam, see illustration above. You can also cut the fingers off gloves to make finger cots (see below), if you're only using one or two fingers for a sexual activity (such as light anal play, or clitoral stimulation during manual sex).

You can use a whole glove or just the fingers of it to cover shared sex toys, but latex gloves may NOT be used as a condom substitute.

Local pharmacies or megastores should carry latex and polyurethane gloves. They are also available at medical supply stores, or via mail order through catalog or Internet sources.

Helpful Hints
- ▶ **They're not just for dishwashing anymore!** Gloves are the bomb when it comes to vaginal manual sex, fisting, or anal play. It's not just a matter of providing STI protection; ragged fingernails or cuticles, and even small calluses, can make manual sex less pleasant (and cause abrasions or fissures), and gloves smooth all that out.
- ▶ **Accept substitutes.** Again, as with condoms and dams, if either you or your partner is latex-sensitive, nonlatex gloves are also available.

Finger Cots

Finger cots are used for: manual sex, when only a finger or fingers are being used, such as for anal play or clitoral stimulation. They can also be used to cover small sex toys (like remote vibrators).

How to use a finger cot: Easy-peasy. Just unroll the finger cot onto your finger or a sex

s.e.x.

toy, like a miniature condom. When you're finished with it, dispose of it. Finger cots may not be used as a substitute for condoms.

Finger cots are tougher to find than most other safer sex products, but can be obtained by mail order via condom suppliers, medical supply stores, and many sex shops. See page 211 for how to make finger cots out of latex gloves.

SAFER SEX, PART THREE: LIFESTYLE ISSUES

While anyone who is sexually active can contract STIs, the following lifestyle issues cause greater risks:

▶ **Multiple partners:** Of any sex, gender or orientation, simultaneously (such as in threesomes) or sequentially (having a string of partners one after the other). Think about it this way: someone who crosses a busy street a few times a day is more likely to get hit by a car than someone who crosses the same street once a month. Same goes with multiple partners: the more partners you have, the more possibilities there are for you to transmit or contract an STI. That's simple math.

▶ **Drug and alcohol abuse:** Due to shared needles, paraphernalia, or bottles (most folks know that shared needles create HIV and hepatitis risks, but did you ever think about oral herpes being passed around with that bottle?), but also due to increased risk-taking that often occurs while under the influence of drugs or alcohol. One reason that many people enjoy drugs or alcohol is the feelings of reduced inhibition they can produce, but that same effect can also lead to sex with unknown

partners, ditching safer sex practices and precautions, and engaging in other risky sexual activities that one might otherwise have avoided. In addition, it is common for date or acquaintance rape to occur when one or all parties are intoxicated. Being sober helps keep you safe, even from STIs.

▶ **Denial or secrecy:** People in denial about having sex tend to have sex less safely. For example, refusing to admit that you ARE sexually active (by staying "technically" a virgin); hiding from friends or family that you are sexually active in general; or being secretive about dating someone whose age, sexual orientation, race, behavior, and so on, may be seen as unacceptable can incline you to also be in denial about sexual responsibility and safety. The whole world doesn't need to know about everything that happens in your bedroom. However, if you can't be honest about it with yourself, your partner or partners, and those closest to you, your sexual health may be at a greater risk.

▶ **Poverty:** Because sexual healthcare and safer sex tools cost money, poverty and/or homelessness can increase STI risks when the basics to make sex safe are not affordable or available.

▶ **General poor health or poor self-image:** When you're unhealthy, malnourished, stressed out, worn out, or battling off existing infections or conditions, your body is at a greater risk. When you don't feel well physically, or don't hold yourself in high regard, you're more likely to make poor choices than when you're well and self-respecting.

▶ **It-can't-happen-to-me-itis:** Simply put: it CAN happen to you, and the more you convince yourself it can't, or take risks to test that theory, the more likely it is that it WILL happen. Statistically, if you're sexually active and haven't already contracted an STI, then one of your three or four closest sexually active friends has.

Gender, Orientation, and STIs

No one gender or orientation is immune to sexually transmitted infection and disease, and no one gender or orientation is responsible for the spread of STIs. However, there are some gender-specific differences and gender-specific concerns with STIs that are worth knowing about.

Men, of any orientation, are the greatest transmitters of sexual infections and diseases. There is a far greater chance of a woman contracting an STI from a man than the other way around. Because of the construction of the vulva and vagina, and because young women in particular have cervical cells that have not completely matured, young women are more susceptible to infection than men and older women, and thus are at the greatest risk of contracting STIs. Men can ejaculate into a woman's vagina, not vice versa; semen often carries STIs that female vaginal fluids do not or cannot transmit to men since they never really get inside the male genitals. Because of the construction of the male genitals, men are naturally less susceptible: except for its tip, the penis is covered in skin, which is more resilient and a less likely site for infection than a woman's vulva and vagina, which are primarily mucous membrane. Many STIs are not only asymptomatic in

men but also more difficult to screen for in men than in women, and fewer men than women seek out preventative sexual healthcare. Of course, if a man (or woman) does not inform a partner they currently have an STI, as many do not, risks also are increased.

Men and women who partner with men are at the greatest risk for most STIs. Men who partner with women are right behind those two groups. Women who partner with women are currently known to be at the least risk of STI transmission. However, due to biases and some data collection problems, we can't be too sure about some of this. For instance, it's likely that lesbians' risks are greater than are typically stated, because in much STI data, "lesbian" is defined as a woman who has NEVER had a male partner, which excludes a majority of lesbian women. Too, plenty of research and reporting is still biased in placing the greatest burden of STI transmission on gay men, even when that isn't factually so. Right now, the population with the highest global rates of HIV/AIDS is women who acquired the virus from male partners.

Women with male partners who do not engage in direct genital contact are at less risk for many STIs than women with female partners who do. Men who do not engage in receptive anal sex with other men are at far less risk of HIV infection than women who engage in vaginal intercourse with men.

EASY WAYS TO INCORPORATE SAFER SEX INTO YOUR SEX LIFE

Safe IS sexy. Knowing you're responsible, educated, and safe is empowering, and when you are sexually empowered, you're in the driver's seat of your sexuality. And

s.e.x.

being in charge of your sexual self is about as sexy as it gets.

Accentuate the positive. Condoms can help to maintain erection and fend off premature ejaculation. Female manual sex or anal play with a glove and lube usually feels a whole lot better and more comfortable. Vaginal intercourse using condoms and lubricant also usually feels better, since latex provides a smoother texture, and lubricant keeps everything from drying out and getting sore. And that's just the tip of the iceberg. Most people find that when they make an attitude adjustment about safer sex, they discover great things about it they never suspected.

Use safer sex as a tool to strengthen your relationships. Taking the initiative and sharing the responsibility for safer sex can really solidify the emotional bond between you and your partner. Take turns putting on the condom or holding the dam. Create a joint budget for safer sex supplies, and do the shopping and choosing together. Make a safer sex kit that is just for the two of you: create a cool case or container for it that's personalized, special, and fun. By all means, talk about it. Get tested for STIs every six months together. It doesn't have to be torture if you make a date of it. Go have a nice breakfast, go get tested, support one another while you wait for results, and when the results come in, do something together. Sex is about union and mutuality. Learning to communicate and cooperate when it comes to safer sex also helps us to communicate and cooperate in our relationship and in our general sexuality.

Make it fun. On the day you want to introduce condoms into your partnership, blow up a bunch of them like balloons. Or buy some glow-in-the-dark ones and don't tell your partner what they do until the lights go out. To introduce latex gloves and lube, you could borrow a stethoscope and play doctor. To start using a vaginal barrier, make an oh-so-stylish bikini out of the plastic wrap. If things get awkward as you're learning to use these things, let yourselves laugh about it—there IS something very funny about a glove that shoots across the room, or about a neon green condom, and sex is *supposed* to be fun.

"DON'T YOU TRUST ME?"

One of the biggest obstacles to sound safer sex practice is the issue of trust, and the assumptions some people make about trust and sex. Some people feel that being asked to use safer sex practices means that their partner doesn't trust them. Some people are of the mind that since they trust their partners, they don't have to be concerned about STIs.

Many STIs can be present, even for years, without a person knowing they're there. They may have no symptoms, or may not know that certain symptoms they're experiencing are due to an STI—especially if they don't get regular sexual healthcare and screenings. Some STIs, such as HPV and herpes, are still difficult to test for when they're asymptomatic, especially in men. Many people haven't ever had screenings. They might think that since an ex-partner was a "good" girl, there wasn't a risk, even with unprotected sex. An ex-partner of theirs may have lied about their sexual history, or said that

S.E.X.

they had tests done when they hadn't. Someone might not know that activities other than vaginal or anal intercourse carry disease or infection risks. And many people are so terribly afraid of having an STI, that they don't get screenings at all, even when they know they should; they just don't want to know, even though they may be endangering themselves and their partners with that avoidance and denial.

Trust is earned over time, not blindly given: if we just gave it to everyone, it wouldn't be very valuable. We trust somebody because they have shown us that we can, and the objects of our affection, attraction, or love shouldn't be exempted from the criteria we'd apply to anyone else, in terms of earning trust. Love should include trust, but it doesn't create it.

When we ask for safer sex practices, it's in the interest of protecting ourselves AND our partners as best we can, ensuring all our health and well-being, and having sex in an environment of safety and smarts. Anyone who is profoundly hurt or offended by that request either doesn't know the facts about STIs; is scared to deal with all that partnered sex entails; is embarrassed to admit that they don't know how to use safer sex tools, like condoms or dams; or may well NOT be trustworthy. Trying to make a partner feel guilty about asking for safer sex practices is unfortunately something that works all too well for a lot of people—people we really SHOULDN'T trust or be sleeping with. By making you feel bad about not trusting them, they're trying to make you forget that you have good reason not to.

Before you become sexually active with a partner, you should both already trust one another a good deal, and both partners should know that trust is present without

much doubt. When that's the case, and when both people are accurately informed about STDs and sexual health in general, trust really shouldn't be an issue or an obstacle, because taking care of one another is PART of trust.

 WE'RE all aware of the profound double standard that sends the message that it's more okay for men to be sexually experienced than women: sexually active men are studs or "players," whereas sexually active women are sluts or easy lays. That double standard makes some young women reluctant to keep safer sex supplies on hand, or ask partners to use them, for fear of seeming more sexually experienced than they are or want to appear. In *Slut! Growing Up Female with a Bad Reputation,* Leora Tanenbaum points out that the slut label is affixed more arbitrarily than most of us would think: not only to girls who are self-possessed sexually or are known to have been sexually active, but to girls who merely dress differently or don't fit into traditional roles, who have different social circles than others, or who have been victims of sexual assault. We can all agree that labels and double standards like this really suck. But not having what you need on hand to keep yourself safe and well isn't an effective counter to them or an effective way to avoid them. Put your health first: without it, you'll be in no shape to tackle your daily life, let alone pervasive social problems.

WHAT IF YOUR PARTNER WON'T PRACTICE SAFER SEX?

A partner who absolutely refuses to practice safer sex is refusing to be responsible and care for your health and well-being and their

S.e.x.

own. (Sadly, over the years at Scarleteen.com, many people have asked if THEY could contract something from a partner, yet they are unconcerned about whether a partner could contract an STI from THEM.) In short, a partner who will not practice sex safely and responsibly is a partner you need to say no to until they change their tune. Someone like that may likely be equally irresponsible, unsafe, and inconsiderate when it comes to other issues that affect you greatly: about having other partners or not, about caring for your feelings and emotional needs, about respecting your right to say no to certain sexual activities—the works.

Sometimes, partners may say no to safer sex because they just don't understand that unsafe sex is just that—unsafe—and that that lack of safety can't be fixed by just trust.

Someone who says no to safer sex the first time around may be someone worth talking to plainly about safer sex, about the risks involved with sexual activity. Now and then, a partner who says no can turn into a partner who says yes pretty quickly once they're furnished with accurate, honest, and compassionate information. But what if that person maintains their position of "no" to safety after you or someone else has furnished them with accurate information, and they know your rules for being safe? Time for you to say no, too: no to sex with them.

Sex that is safe on all levels involves sane limits and boundaries. We could give you all sorts of witty, smart answers to possible partner comments like "But it doesn't feel as good without a condom," or "I don't like condoms," or "You don't trust me," but the fact of the matter is that your best bet is to walk into any sexual situation with clearly communicated limits about safer sex, and not waver on them or get pulled into argu-

ments about practicing safer sex. More times than not, if you let a partner know, kindly and diplomatically, that you're just **not willing** to risk their health or yours for sex, and that if they want to have sex with you, they are going to need to do so safely, you'll find that people who are trustworthy, mature, and caring partners aren't going to balk at all.

Sure, that's not always as easy to do as it sounds. Someone you've got a major jones for sexually and/or romantically may make it hard to make or keep those limits. It can be a struggle even to keep your head intact when you've got a bad case of the super-duper in love woozies. Someone's arguments may sway you from doing what you know is best for yourself. If others in your peer circle are vocal about not practicing safer sex, or about thinking it's stupid, it can be hard to be the only one being safe and smart, and harder to be the first person to lay down the law to your partner. It's all too easy to give in, every now and then, if a partner whom you do trust, and who is normally safe and smart, suggests trying unsafe sex "just once to know how it feels." Trouble is, you can find out how chlamydia or herpes feels that way, too. (Hint: They don't feel good.) It can also be difficult to resist the emotional manipulation of someone who believes they're healthy and insists that you want to practice safer sex because you don't trust them. But remember, you can trust them all you want, but if they're walking around with genital herpes, unaware, trust isn't going to keep you safe.

Most people don't need to practice safer sex, or all portions of safer sex, with a given partner forever. Once you've been with a partner, monogamously (only with them), for at least six months; practiced safer sex during that time for all moderate-to-high-risk activities; and each had two full negative screens, your risks are pretty minimal. The two of you *can* then decide to try sex without latex barriers, if you like. What about any partner who's unwilling to take those really simple measures to keep you both as healthy as possible? That's not the right partner for anyone.

WHAT IF YOU DO GET AN STI?

Discovering you have an STI can be pretty intense, especially when you're young. It's hard enough to find out you're ill in any way, but with sexually transmitted diseases it can be even more difficult; you may feel ashamed, dirty, stupid, or naive. Because some STIs can have long-term effects, even change your life completely, or make you very sick, and because of how daunting it can seem to inform current and future partners about it, it can all be really scary. While it's okay to feel however you do, there really is no need to feel any of those ways. We're human: we get sick, and can get sick via any site on our bodies. Most illnesses can be treated and/or managed these days. We make mistakes, and sometimes mistakes carry consequences we have to deal with—and sometimes, things just happen. You may have contracted an STI even while being careful and practicing safer sex. Getting an STI doesn't mean you're a bad person, doesn't mean you're dirty, and it doesn't mean you have to live the rest of your life like a leper or a monk.

If and when you're diagnosed with an STI, the very first person to talk with is your doctor. Be sure to ask all the questions you have about:

▶ **Healing:** If a treatment is available, what are the directions? Are there any special cautions? Do partners also need to be treated at the same time? Do you need to abstain from protected sex while being treated? When should you start seeing improvements in symptoms with treatment? If you don't see improvements within a certain time, what should you do? Will you need more than one treatment? If so, when?

▶ **Dealing:** What are all the specifics about your particular STI? Are there long-term effects you need to be aware of and on the lookout for? Do you need to make any lifestyle changes in terms of your environment, diet and nutrition, exercise, or other elements? Will you need any extra healthcare in the future? Is there a counselor or support group in your area available to you? Are there high-quality resources for managing or finding out more about your specific disease or infection—books, brochures, or Web sites—that your doctor can refer you to?

▶ **Revealing:** Which partners do you need to inform besides your current partner: how many partners back? What should they be told? How might they have gotten or passed on the STI? Once treated, what extra precautions do you need to take with partners in the future? Do your parents need to be informed? If so, how do you want to do that with your doctor?

Our society has made STIs sound like the worst thing in the world to get, even though many STIs aren't any more dangerous than a common cold, so long as you have them treated quickly. The big STI panic is caused

s.e.x.

by a lot of different cultural ideas and situations: some STIs are or have been transmitted by infidelity; sex and the genitals are considered shameful or sinful in certain traditions or communities; and, more than anything, most people aren't very informed about STIs—they believe that most STIs are far worse than they actually are, or they believe that only "dirty" people, or people of low moral character, contract sexually transmitted diseases or infections.

Part of dealing with life with an STI involves dealing with those attitudes, which is unfortunate and sometimes difficult. The best approach to take is to furnish anyone putting that sort of thing on you with the real facts, with accurate, up-to-date information. And if that doesn't change their tune, then remind yourself that those messages and attitudes are coming from ignorance and have little or nothing to do with you personally at all.

Breaking the News

Telling current and/or recent partners, which needs be done when you discover you have contracted an STI, is rarely easy. If you care deeply about your partners, you may be upset with yourself for potentially getting them sick. If you've been in a relationship for a while and develop an STI, you may have to battle trust issues: Did your partner cheat? Did you? Was someone dishonest about their sexual history or about testing? If so, what now? If they deny it, can you fully believe them and get past your doubt?

With partners you've had for a while, the best bet is to be honest and complete in your information about the STI. Give yourselves plenty of time to talk, to process, to deal with emotional and physical consequences. You may have to deal with your partner's mistrust, anger, or upset for a while. Either or both of you may find that sex isn't all that appealing after a diagnosis, or that it's difficult to connect sexually for a little while. All of those things are normal. If you need help dealing with them, you can ask your doctor for resources or referrals.

If you acquired an STI from a partner you don't know very well, or haven't been involved with that long, telling them can be especially awkward. Sometimes, even tracking them down can be problematic, so just do what you can. If this was a very casual sex situation, you may feel angry at yourself, especially if the sex was unprotected, or if you chose to have sex when your judgment was impaired in any way. It's important to recognize that an STI is no more a divine punishment for having sex than a runny nose is a punishment from G-d-on-high for going outside in the winter. **STIs are just natural consequences of being in close, intimate contact with other people, like any other kind of human infection**. They happen to all kinds of people, in all sorts of situations: married, single, monogamous, polyamorous, young, old, rich, poor, straight, queer—the works. If you chose not to take preventative measures, then you made a mistake. Beating yourself up over it doesn't make you well again. It's nonproductive, and isn't likely to help you do what you need to, which is to stay well and simply make better choices for yourself next time. If you're angry at yourself, go ahead and entertain that for a bit, but be sure to take care of the practical things you need to, however awkward, and then put your energy into forgiving yourself, managing the consequences, and moving on, smarter and safer.

Continuing sexual partnership can be a hurdle when you have an STI. With something temporary and treatable, like chlamydia or BV, it's pretty easy in the long run, because it'll be gone completely before too long. Other infections and diseases that are not fully curable, and may or will stick around—such as herpes, HPV, or HIV—are more of a challenge, because you'll need to inform every new partner about it, before you become sexually active with them, and you may need to take extra precautions you aren't accustomed to. You may even find that some potential partners won't want to have sex with you, once they learn about the risk. That's their right, and logically you can probably understand it, but rejection, however sound or fair, still hurts. Fear of that rejection may keep you from wanting to be upfront, but it's a whole lot easier to deal with that rejection than it is to deal with a person who contracted an STI from you, when you KNEW you were putting them at risk for it, and didn't inform them. Living with rejection is easier than living with yourself for doing that.

Long-Term Dealing

Unfortunately, despite the prevalence of STIs, there aren't a lot of simple road maps for dealing with one. For the most part, it's very individual and involves some trial and error. But informed, honest communication will really serve you, and those involved with you, well. Taking care of yourself—physically and emotionally, presently and preventatively—is key. Seeking out and finding the emotional support you need, via friends, partners, family, or support groups for STI sufferers, is incredibly important, especially if you have an STI that may make you severely ill or threaten your life.

Remember that you aren't anything close to alone: again, over nineteen million people each year develop an STI.

Whether we like it or not, or accept it or not, STIs are common, normal, and prevalent, just like lots of other kinds of illness and injury. They aren't any better or worse for being sexually transmitted, and YOU aren't any better or worse a person for having an STI.

top ten bits of b.s. about stis

1. "Virgins" can't transmit or contract STIs.
2. Only vaginal intercourse is risky.
3. Most infections will clear up on their own.
4. Only people with more than one partner can get an STI.
5. AIDS is the most common STI.
6. Only semen can transmit STIs.
7. You can always tell when you or someone else has an STI by the symptoms.
8. Lesbians don't pass on or get STIs.
9. STIs are most prevalent in gay men or men with male partners.
10. If you love and trust your partner, it's safe to have unprotected sex.

SAFER SEX FOR YOUR HEART

When we get involved sexually, we are taking risks—physical *and* emotional—no matter what. There is no such thing as a no-risk sexual or love scenario, no matter your age or situation. Sexuality involves very deep intimacy and feelings, and when we explore those feelings, we take risks.

That isn't to say that all risks are bad to take. On some level, in order to discover

s.e.x.

things that ARE healthy for us, that are beneficial and bring us joy, we do have to take risks and chances. That's the case whether we're talking about a sexual relationship or trying out for the school basketball team, bungee-jumping or getting our first job. But taking risks that we know or suspect are foolhardy is risking too much for too little. Again, sex need not be harmful or hurtful. It can be a very positive and wonderful thing—and when it isn't, that may be because we are creating or continuing the situations and environments that make it negative for us and others. We all need to learn to avoid doing that, to be mindful of it, if we want our sexual lives and relationships to be healthy, happy, and of real quality.

And isn't that what we all want? So, go on and take a big risk—the risk of handling sexual relationships with care and patience, and with your whole health and well-being at heart, physical and emotional, personal and communal.

Taking care of your emotions, taking preventative steps to avoid heartbreak, and making sure that you and yours are safe from needless emotional harm is just as important as doing what you can to prevent infections and unwanted pregnancies. As you know, sexuality and sexual partnership aren't just physical. You might hear someone say they can have sex with "no feelings," but that's

pretty unlikely. You might also have heard that having sex is okay, but only in one kind of relationship, at a particular age, or in some other special scenario. Not true. You may have heard that only sex within marriage or a long-term monogamous relationship is safe emotionally, but that simply isn't so: people are no less likely to be hurt by sex within marriage than they are outside it. To care for yourself in ANY kind of sexual relationship with others—long-term or short-term, romantic partnerships or casual hookups—you need to be able to assess what is and isn't emotionally safe and healthy, for you and those you're involved with.

You can reduce emotional risks just as you can reduce physical ones. Learning to be on the lookout for emotionally dangerous, self-defeating, or destructive scenarios is important for absolutely everyone. It's that awareness that offers you the best protection from heartbreak and nasty emotional sexual side effects throughout your life, not the kind of relationship you're in.

When entered into with a solid basis of self-awareness, compassion, sound judgment, and accurate information, sex has no more capacity to cause emotional distress or hurt than anything else in life—and it has the capacity to be something empowering and beneficial, in any number of situations and relationship models.

10

hidden wounds:
preventing, identifying, and healing
from abuse and rape

HEALTHY, BENEFICIAL, AND consensual sex and sexual or romantic relationships are democratic: everyone involved always gets a vote. When either partner doesn't have an equal voice, or when one voice is dismissed, it is abuse. When one partner does not treat another with respect and care for their physical, emotional, and sexual well-being, it is abuse. We have the right to be and *should* be physically and emotionally safe in our relationships and our world. Abuse, reduced to its simplest explanation, is all about power and control: someone who's abusing someone else wants all the power and all the control—not a partnership of equals. An abuser seeks to rob another person of security, safety, joint ownership of their relationship, and full ownership of their own heart, mind, body and life.

- Around one out of every three high-school and college students has experienced sexual, physical, verbal, or emotional violence in dating relationships.
- Forty percent of girls aged fourteen to seventeen say they know someone their age who has been hit or beaten by a boyfriend.
- 8.5 percent of California ninth graders and 10.4 percent of eleventh graders with a boyfriend or girlfriend had been hit, slapped, or physically hurt by their partner within the past twelve months.
- Women ages sixteen to twenty-four experience the highest rates of intimate violence—nearly twenty per one thousand women.
- Ninety-five percent of all victims of domestic violence are women. Domestic violence is the single major cause of injury to women, more than muggings and car accidents combined.

Sometimes such behavior is taken seriously in our culture and our communities and recognized as abuse. At other times, abuse may be denied, dismissed, or shrugged off as unimportant or "just the way things are." All too often, the victim is blamed for rape or abuse, instead of the rapist or abuser. Many forms of abuse are based on socially accepted inequities between genders, ages, races, or social strata. Some kinds of abuse, or warning signs of abusive behavior—like irrational jealousy—are even thought of as romantic! In a world in which abuse is so prevalent and common, it's not surprising that sometimes a person who is abused is not even clear in their own mind about what has occurred.

- Every nine seconds, a woman is battered in the United States.
- A survey of adolescents and college students revealed that date rape accounted for 67 percent of sexual assaults.
- Six out of ten rapes of young women occur in their own home or a friend's or relative's home, not in a dark alley.
- In a study of 769 male students, grades seven to twelve in Wisconsin, 52 percent reported engaging in sexually aggressive behavior: 24 percent in the unwanted sexual touch of another teen, 15 percent in sexual coercion to initiate sexual activity, and 14 percent in assaultive behavior (use of physical force, threats of physical force, or using alcohol to gain sexual activity).
- Over 50 percent of high-school boys and 42 percent of high-school girls believe that there are times when it is "acceptable for a male to hold a female down and physically force her to engage in intercourse."
- One-half of all rape victims are raped between the ages of fourteen and seventeen.

- **Every two and a half minutes**, somewhere in America, someone is sexually assaulted.
- **One in six American women** is a victim of sexual assault, and one in thirty-three men. Ninety-nine percent of their rapists are men.
- A child's exposure to the father abusing the mother is the strongest risk factor of transmitting violent behavior from one generation to the next.

Statistics from: The Bureau of Justice Special Report, *Intimate Partner Violence,* 2005 National Crime Victimization Survey, *Adolescent Male Sexual Aggression: Incidents and Correlates,* Donell Marie Kerns, PhD; *Family Planning Perspectives,* "The Ninth Biennial California Student Survey"; "Teen Dating Violence," Anita Mitchell, *Protecting Sexually Active Youth* 4, no.1 (March 1996); *Report of the American Psychological Association Presidential Task Force on Violence and the Family;* Family Violence Prevention Fund, *First Comprehensive National Health Study of American Women,* the Commonwealth Fund; the L.A. Commission on Assaults Against Women; and RAINN.

· TYPES OF ABUSE ·

From a literal standpoint, to abuse is to harm or injure. From a broader viewpoint, what abuse is depends on what sort of abuse we're talking about. The most common categories of abuse are:

Emotional and/or verbal abuse: Behaviors that are used to emotionally control, dominate, manipulate, or intimidate a person. Emotional abuse can be threats, name-calling, belittling, criticizing, or using words or actions in an attempt to make another person feel stupid, small, crazy, ashamed, or worthless. Other aspects of emotional abuse can include: isolating a person by keeping them from friends or family; dismissing a person's limits and boundaries; intentionally withholding general approval or support; constantly laying false blame on a partner; attempting to control someone's appearance or their physical freedom through threats or belittling; profound possessiveness; or a pattern of harming someone then begging their forgiveness or shifting the blame for abuse onto them. Emotional abuse is often thought to be the most benign form of abuse; however, it has the capacity to harm just as deeply as any other type of abuse, and for many people who have suffered a range of different abuses, emotional abuse can carry the deepest scars, especially when it has occurred during childhood or adolescence.

Physical abuse: Physical abuse is intentional physical harm or injury. Hitting, slapping, punching, pushing, biting, kicking, choking, or burning someone purposefully are all physical abuses. Throwing things at another person, threatening physical harm, or physically restraining someone are also physical abuses. Not everyone who is physically abused will have obvious injuries or scars; you cannot always tell who is physically abused merely by looking, nor does a lack of scars, bruises, or broken bones mean that a person has not been physically abused.

Rape and sexual assault: Forcing someone to engage in any sexual activity or response they do not want, have not consented to, or are not in a position to be able to give consent to is rape or sexual assault. Force may be physical, but it may also be verbal or emotional, including coercion. When a rapist is known to the person who has been raped,

it is called acquaintance, partner/spouse, or date rape. It is rape if a person consents to a sexual activity at one point then later rescinds that consent—changes their mind and says no—and their partner continues with the sexual activity, despite their protests. It is rape ANY time one partner does not want to be engaging in sex and the other engages in it with them anyway.

Coercion: Coercion is also a form of sexual assault—for example, arguing for or initiating a sexual activity to the point that another person gives consent by being worn down. Sexual activity that is initiated under duress, or when someone is under the influence of drugs or alcohol, can also be rape and sexual assault. Sex that involves physical abuse; is sexual assault. Forcing a person to view pornography, to wear certain clothes or go without the clothes they wish to, to look at the genitals of someone else against their will, or to watch certain sex acts (like masturbation) against their will can also be classed as sexual assault, as can name-calling or other forms of emotional, verbal, or physical abuse during sexual activity.

Child abuse: Physical, sexual, verbal, or emotional abuse that occurs to a child. While teens and young adults are not children, not only may they be legally considered so in instances of abuse (if they are under the age of majority), but many teens and young adults are also survivors of child abuse. Those who were abused as children may be more likely to be abuse victims as adults, especially if they are not aware that their abuse as children was not normal or acceptable; when we grow up without healthy

s.e.x.

boundaries and behavior, it is far harder to learn them—or even know what they are—later in life.

Incest: A subset of child abuse, incest is sexual abuse within the family—rape and fondling, as well as voyeurism, sexual comments, forcing a child to masturbate, and exploitation such as child pornography or prostitution—by parents or guardians, grandparents, uncles or aunts, siblings, or extended family members. Incest is considered to be one of the most damaging forms of abuse because it often begins when the victims are very young, and because it happens at the hands of those the victim often trusts the most, and who are the most responsible for his or her care.

gender divides and abuse in same-sex relationships

 WHILE the overwhelming majority of all abusers are male, that does not mean abusers are ONLY male. In instances of emotional, physical, and sexual child abuse, some abusers are female, and even many male abusers were child abuse victims themselves. Domestic or partner abusers are also sometimes female.

Because of this gender divide, it's often assumed that abuse doesn't exist within GLBT relationships. Statistically, rates of domestic abuse in gay and lesbian partnerships are equal to those in opposite-sex relationships. That invisibility can make finding support even more difficult for GLBT victims and survivors of abuse than for their heterosexual counterparts. There are also challenges specific to GLBT people within abusive relationships: social isolation may be even greater; the

abuse may not be believed, or it may be assumed that it must be "mutual." People who are not yet out may have to come out in the process of reporting abuse and getting help. Because GLBT communities are often very small, reporting abuse usually means everyone in the community will know about the abuse and "take sides." For lesbians, as with heterosexual men, reporting abuse can be difficult because some women's organizations are reluctant to acknowledge that women can also be abusive. GLBT people often have to face homophobia in the process of reporting and seeking help with abuse, but lesbians may also have to face sexism, and for gay men and lesbians of color, racism as well. Transgendered people may have to deal with transphobia throughout.

If you're a victim or survivor of abuse that is less likely to be recognized or acknowledged (and that goes for within your family as well), do NOT let that stop you from seeking help and/or reporting the abuse. While it can certainly be extra-challenging to get help and support in these situations, it's always going to be better to deal with those challenges to get yourself safe and sound than to remain trapped in abuse. Check the Resources section of this book for organizations that help male or same-sex partnered victims of abuse, as well as women abused by men.

Sexual harassment: Sexual harassment can be sexual and emotional and/or verbal abuse. Sexual harassment in uninvited and unwanted sexual behavior, like being touched when you don't want to be, being the target of sexual name-calling or jokes, or continued sexual propositions or sexual attention after you've already said no. Sexual harassment is currently epidemic in some schools, and sometimes even comes from teachers or other school staff, not just fellow students. "Gay-bashing" is also a form of sexual harassment. For more on sexual harassment, see "Body of Evidence" in chapter 7.

Domestic, Partner, or Dating Abuse: Emotional, verbal, physical, and/or sexual abuse that occurs between sexual or romantic partners or spouses. The abuse may also include threats or injury to property, pets, children, or other family members, not just the spouse or partner. *Battering* is another term sometimes used to describe domestic abuse.

Hate crimes: Hate crimes are physical, verbal, emotional, or sexual abuse based on and motivated by intolerance or hatred of people of a given sexual orientation, race, gender, nationality, religion, age, or disability.

TAKING THE BLINDERS OFF : IDENTIFYING AND COPING WITH ABUSE

When intimate partnership or sexual activity is new to you, it all can feel a bit risky, even if you're ready. Learning to talk about sex and work out interpersonal issues with a partner can be hard, and take a long time to master. But some things can tip you off to potentially abusive patterns.

Are you in a relationship or partnership that you suspect may be emotionally unsafe or unhealthy for you or others? Give yourself a checkup.

Are you:

▶ Suffering from anxiety, stress, or depression, or having unusual physical symptoms, such as stomachaches, insomnia, changes in energy levels or appetite, a sudden drastic increase or decrease in sexual drive, or other physical symptoms that are not caused by an existing condition, illness, or outside situation?

▶ Putting other important relationships or goals of yours at risk because of your relationship?

▶ Taking risks that put you and yours in a position of sexual, physical, or emotional risk, or feeling that you must make many sacrifices to have or maintain the relationship?

▶ Feeling isolated from everyone BUT your partner, or having trouble thinking of others outside yourself and your partner(s)?

▶ Discovering that other important parts of your life are taking a backseat to your relationship or really suffering (your grades, your job, your family, etc.)?

▶ Feeling sad, frustrated, or upset with sexual relationships or encounters, far more than you find yourself feeling happy?

▶ Feeling you must keep sexual activity, tension, or emotional issues high and escalating to maintain the relationship, using sexual activity or other behavior to avoid or defuse relationship conflicts, "zoning out" during sexual activity, or feeling either predominantly passive or dominating during sex with your partner?

▶ Becoming unable to be autonomous and have a life and sense of self independent of your partner or a sexual relationship?

▶ Feeling bad about yourself in general, or specifically in regard to your sexual

S.e.x.

relationship or behavior?

▶ Doing things you really don't want to do but feel you have to, or pressing a partner to do so?

▶ Having trouble discussing, making, or enforcing limits and boundaries (sexual or otherwise), or respecting those of your partner?

▶ Making a lot of excuses for yourself or a partner?

If you're experiencing any of these things (and/or the sorts of things on page 120 in the danger signs checklist), find someone outside your partnership to talk to about the situation—someone who you feel can be objective, maybe a friend, maybe your religious leader or a teacher, maybe an aunt or uncle. Take some time alone, too, to really look at how you're feeling, and seek out trouble spots or conflicts. Finally, as long as it doesn't compromise your safety, talk to your partner, as well. Making a reality check with someone else and yourself, then talking to your partner, is pretty vital and a good management tool. Things like those listed here may be a signal that your sexual relationship or behavior isn't healthy and balanced, or may be doing you or a partner harm. Checking in with that possibility now and again is always a sound practice.

So much of the information we get about protecting ourselves, from the time we're very young, is about protecting ourselves from strangers, and yet, data appears every year that shows that, especially for women, abuse and assault are much more likely to happen with someone we know, mainly those closest to us. Maybe you've no doubt that what you're dealing with is abuse. Maybe you're not sure. For many people who have been or are being abused,

it can become very difficult to know, especially since many aspects of abuse are manipulative, unexpected, or even considered to be normal behavior; because our experiences or abusers may not resemble what we've been told about abuse or assault; or because we're just in denial.

It's typical to excuse or shrug off some of the initial abusive behaviors we might experience, or not to recognize them as abusive or potentially abusive.

To identify and step away from abuse:

▶ **Listen.** Sometimes, it can be difficult to accept that a parent is really concerned, not just overprotective or too rigid, or that a friend is worried about you, not jealous that you have a boyfriend or girlfriend, and they don't. Often, when the people who care about you voice concerns, it's for good reason. And if and when everyone around you is voicing the same or similar concerns, there's an incredibly good chance they're right. Listen to what the people you know care about you have to say. As always, trust your own instincts, and in cases of abuse, give your head more clout than your heart. Because all abuse includes emotional factors, it's typical for people's emotions to be confused and convoluted when they've been abused.

▶ **Tell.** Even if no one else notices what is going on, you can get help. Keep your eyes open for good opportunities. For example, a speaker who comes to your school to talk about teen relationship abuse is a great person to ask for help, and is also someone who will likely do their best to try and get you

s.e.x.

help, and get your school to be more aware and proactive. Tell someone you can trust: friends or your friend's parent, immediate or extended family, a teacher, coach, or school counselor, a neighbor. Someone you know may say something that makes it clear they have survived abuse or are strongly opposed to it: these are good people to tell and ask for help. You can also call a hotline or a community service for victims of abuse: your local phone book will have listings. There are Internet communities where you can post anonymously. You can also go directly to local community centers, shelters, police stations, or social service agencies. *Tell someone.*

▶ **Leave.** Once you get some trusted help, you can make a safe plan to take action. That may include making sure you have other people around to help keep you safe when you leave the relationship; making places where you may see your partner, like your school, safe for you; filing charges or requesting a restraining order against someone; and getting yourself the emotional support you need, via friends and family, counseling, or support groups. With any sort of abuse, it's easy to get stuck in a pattern of feeling at fault when your partner is abusive or angry, and taking to heart what they say. But every now and then there may be moments where your head says, "Bullshit," or "Wrong!" to an abusive partner. Use the strength those moments of awareness can give you and make those moments the ones to get out and get away.

You may have doubts throughout this process, miss your partner, or try to convince yourself that what happened wasn't really abuse, or that it was punishment you asked for in some way. There's often a lot of one-step-forward, two-steps-back stuff, in dealing with abuse. You may have a very confusing range of emotions, from anger to apathy, sorrow to incredible relief. Do your best to honor and explore all of those emotions. Ask friends, family, or your counselor for the support you need. You may feel that, since you got yourself into a situation of abuse or tolerated it, you've no right to ask them for help, but that isn't so: people who care for you will want to be there for you during a crisis, just as you'd be there for them. They may not always be as patient or available as you'd like them to be, so do seek out as many avenues of support as you can. Support groups specifically for abuse survivors can be especially helpful, since the people in them know exactly what you're going through. Healing from abuse is often a long process, and abuse leaves traces all over your psyche that you have to learn to navigate your way through. The help and support of those who have been there are often priceless.

Some people are reluctant to seek out therapy, counseling, or support groups for abuse (or assault), because they aren't ready to really face up to having been abused, don't want to "talk to strangers," to share what seems very private to them with someone else, or deal with the stigma still attached to therapy and counseling. You might also be concerned that a therapist or counselor is going to blame you for the abuse or tell you how to live your life, or even bash a partner for whom you still feel loyalty, despite the abuse. Almost always, those are misplaced concerns: a good, qualified abuse counselor will not do those

s.e.x.

things. Most of what they do is listen, ask questions, and help you to make your own choices and do your own healing, rather than trying to do it for you. You also don't have to work with just any counselor, support group, or therapist: shop around and wait to start therapy until you find someone who feels best for you.

An Exit Plan

Those in abusive partnerships are often advised to have vital items at hand as part of an exit plan, so that when they have an opportunity to leave, they are able to do so quickly and efficiently, without having to leave behind birth records, clothing, pets, or other essentials. Since most young adults in abusive relationships do not live with their abusers, your preparation for leaving may be less extensive. Just be sure, if you're not yet ready or able to leave, that when seeing your partner, you have these items with you, on your person, at all times: your basic identification (such as a driver's license or state ID), your house or car keys, your cell phone or address book, any medications you take, and your debit card, credit card, checkbook, and/or cash. That way, as soon as the opportunity or necessity of getting out presents itself, you'll be ready to go immediately.

You might also be reluctant to enter therapy or counseling because that may feel like a statement that there's something profoundly wrong with *you*. But therapy isn't about "fixing" people or about being "crazy." It's about having someone who is objective and fully present who will listen to you, who has experience with all the things you're dealing with, and who knows good tools for managing them. People who have been abused or assaulted often suffer from depression, post-traumatic stress disorder (PTSD), anxiety and/or panic attacks, self-injury, low–self-esteem, substance abuse, or a host of other disorders or issues that require help and support. The point of therapy isn't to fix you because you're broken, but to help you deal so that you can move on and have a life of real quality.

BREAKING THE CYCLE

It's true that someone who is abusive is a troubled person. So, an abuse victim may feel that by remaining with or going back to an abuser, they're helping that person or saving them from themselves. You may feel if you just love them enough, or stick around long enough, your abuser will miraculously get better and stop the abuse. Unfortunately, that's just not true. No abuser is helped by being enabled or allowed to continue abusing. Thinking that is akin to saying that someone who has a drug problem is best served by living in a crack den, or that someone with an eating disorder will get better if you let them starve themselves to death. No one can love the abuse away.

Study after study has shown very clearly that until the *cycle of abuse* is broken, a person who abuses will continue to do so. The cycle is most often stopped when a victim leaves their abuser, or when the abuser is imprisoned, or, more rarely, given long-term anger management classes or therapy. The harsh truth, though, is that most studies—explained in articles like Cheryl Hanna's

"The Paradox of Hope: The Crime and Punishment of Domestic Violence," in the *William and Mary Law Review*—have shown that the ONLY deterrent that seems to be effective to stop abusers is incarceration (being in prison, away from their victim) or a strong fear of it.

The abuser isn't the victim: the person being abused is, and that's whose needs always need to come first, because that is the person in the most acute danger and in the most need of help. It is NOT an abuse victim's responsibility to get help for their abuser: it's their responsibility to get help for themselves.

Does This Sound Like You?

▶ Do you feel the need to control people around you, especially those close to you?

▶ Does letting others take the wheel make you feel profoundly uncomfortable, angry, or insecure?

▶ Do you betray the trust of others, by sharing very private information or secrets, or by blackmailing in some way?

▶ Do you find it hard to be patient with, or empathetic to, the troubles of others?

▶ Do you have a hard time handling variance in opinion? When someone thinks something differently than you do, do you belittle, dismiss, or attack them?

▶ Are you prone to making fun of or teasing people?

▶ Do you often feel very jealous or possessive?

▶ Do you feel your partners must be cheating, lying, or betraying your trust? Do you accuse them?

---

did you know . . . ?

the cycle of abuse

Teens Experiencing Abusive Relationships, an organization founded by teen survivors and friends of survivors, explains the cycle of abuse, a pattern most abusive relationships follow, as a series of stages:

1. A **honeymoon stage**, which is a state when both partners are happy to be in a relationship, and at a point where the relationship is loving and enjoyable.
2. The **tension phase**, when the couple is getting into small arguments, and the abuser becomes frustrated with their partner.
3. The last stage is the **abuse stage**, where one specific incident leads to an explosion of anger.
4. The abuser quickly reverts to the honeymoon stage to make up for their behavior, and the whole cycle begins again.

So, "being really nice sometimes," doesn't mean abuse isn't happening. When "being nice" is what happens before and after abuse, it's just another part of the abuse.

s.e.x.

- Have you ever hit or pushed a partner? Have you grabbed their arm or held them tight while you were arguing? Are you prone to do, or want to do, things like that when you're angry or frustrated, rather than talking or walking away?
- Do you ever throw things, slam doors, or threaten your partner when you're angry? Do you feel unable to manage your anger in any way?
- Have you ever forced or coerced a partner into having sex with you, or made it difficult for them to say no? Do you ever do this now?
- Have you ever threatened to harm yourself, your partner, or those he or she cares for, if a partner leaves you or breaks up with you?

If any of that looks familiar to you, *you* may already be abusive or be on the road to becoming abusive.

Even if you were reared in an abusive environment yourself, and some abusive behaviors seem normal to you, or even if you've started to exhibit abusive behaviors, you are *not* obliged to become an abuser: you *can* head it off at the pass. Plenty of people like you have done so. If you're concerned about being abusive now or in the future, seek out counseling and support **now**. Learning different patterns of behavior isn't usually easy, but it is doable. You can ask your family doctor or a school guidance counselor to point you toward help and resources. Even if you've never exhibited abusive behaviors but are just concerned you might, perhaps because you grew up around them yourself, you can ask for help and seek out support. There's absolutely no reason to feel ashamed about those concerns: if everyone were that con-

cerned and aware, far fewer people would wind up abused.

the blame game

 YOU may have walked home alone against your better judgment. You may have been at a party and had too much to drink. You may have tolerated sexual teasing and taunting, or kept quiet about it. You may have gone along with someone and initially wanted to be with them, but changed your mind. You may have gotten involved with someone who had a history of abusive behavior. You may have stayed in an abusive relationship, even when you knew you should leave.

Even if any of these conditions were present, and even if you didn't make the best choices, the fault still lies with the abuser, not you.

Certainly, we all need to learn to protect ourselves and make choices that are in the best interest of keeping us safe. But even if we have not done so, or if we missed what, in hindsight, seem like obvious clues that we were in danger, it's not our fault. **Ever.**

If someone is trying to tell you it's your fault, or to tell someone you know who's been abused that it is their fault, or if the little voices inside your head are telling you it's your fault, understand that they are wrong. Just as the person who crashed their car into a tree is at fault, not the tree, the person at fault is the abuser, not the abused.

▪ PROTECTING YOURSELF FROM ▪ ABUSIVE PARTNERS AND RELATIONSHIPS

The hardest part of recognizing signals of an abusive relationship is that often, people mis-

S.E.X.

take the earliest signs of abuse for aspects of romantic love. Intense jealousy, possessiveness, and claims of ownership; defending your "honor" with bullying or verbal or physical intimidation; very traditional ideas about gender and the "place" of men and women; and extreme codependency or neediness are all strong indicators of a possibly abusive person, not someone in love in a healthy way.

Some other common early signs or symptoms can include: a history of violence or a criminal record, existing violence within someone's family, abuse of or dependence on drugs or alcohol, a fascination with weapons or with acts of violence, or extreme mood swings.

A big part of being able to protect yourself is being aware not just of someone else's behavior, but of your own. While people who are abused come from all walks of life, people who find themselves in abusive relationships often have some things in common: low self-worth and self-image; emotional, social, or economic dependency; social isolation; depression; and stress or anxiety disorders. Many abuse victims believe that abuse is something they deserve. They may blame themselves for the abuses they suffer; they may defend or excuse the person who is abusing them. So, in many ways, only entering relationships when you and your partner are both really able to handle them—when you already feel okay with yourself, when you feel 100 percent able to stand up for yourself and be independent, when you're not in a crisis, when you want to be with someone else rather than "have" someone else—is a big help when it comes to prevention. If you face issues like these, seeking out help through friends, family, or counseling rather than in romantic or sexual relationships is also helpful.

CAN'T HAPPEN TO YOU?

For some abused people who do not have a low self-image, who firmly believe that abuse is not okay, and know full well what it is, it may be incredibly difficult to accept that they're being abused, that they have "allowed" themselves to be abused. If that's your situation, the shame of being abused or staying with an abuser can run very deep. It's sometimes hard to really see the whole of abuse coming, so it's not uncommon to truly just wake up one day and realize you are in the thick of an abusive relationship without really knowing how you wound up there.

For others, accepting that their partner is anything other than a wonderful person who loves them is very hard. Some abused people feel that if they acknowledge or address abuse, they'll only be hurt even more, or they worry that their partner will be harmed. Plenty are convinced that, miraculously, their abusive partner will get better, possibly though their love.

Sadly, it's also not uncommon for friends or family to defend abusers or certain types of abuse, especially if they are survivors of abuse or abusers themselves, and they perceive abuse to be normal or acceptable. Denial of abuse is very common, from many different perspectives.

▪ PROTECTING YOURSELF FROM ▪ RAPE AND SEXUAL ASSAULT

STRANGER AND ACQUAINTANCE DANGER

When it comes to stranger danger, you know the drill: Don't walk in desolate or dark places alone or unaware. Be aware of and alert to your surroundings: try not to

s.e.x.

233

space out when you're waiting for the bus or train, walking home, or in potentially unsafe places. If your gut tells you you're at risk, you probably are. If you get a hinky feeling, change directions, enter a public place where you aren't alone for a while, or just leave whatever situation you're in without delay. Don't hitchhike or accept rides from strangers.

People who rape are opportunistic: they tend to choose their victims not by what they look like or how they're dressed, but by who is available and seems less resistant, whom they feel capable of overpowering and raping. Again, everything we know to date about rape confirms that, like all forms of abuse, it is about power and about control of another person, first and foremost.

Learning how to be quick, assertive, and vocal to fight back is the best protection you've got. You don't want to get into an argument or negotiate with a rapist, and you do NOT have to just cave in and take it if someone is coercing you into sex, or exerting verbal or emotional pressure, but not (yet) physical force. **Do all you can to just get away, and if you can't do that, then do whatever you can to defend yourself.**

If you even feel unsafe alone with someone, or they are clearly being pushy or aggressive about sex, get out without delay: if you're about to be assaulted, you don't have time to worry about your reputation or what someone might say to their friends. Firmly and loudly saying "No," screaming, or yelling can help. Kick, punch, scratch, bite, and use whatever objects your environment gives you, to put yourself in a position to get away from your attacker. In a situation where you're being attacked, your job is to survive and do everything you can to GET AWAY,

not to worry about the attacker's safety, or whether or not hitting is fair.

coercion: the slippery slope

A PARTNER might suggest a sexual activity that you feel an aversion to or anxiety about. Or it may be the other way around, with you wanting something that your partner is reluctant to try. Either way, if one partner pushes, pressures, argues, or manipulates the other into doing what they don't really want to, the reluctant partner has been coerced. They have not fully consented to that sex.

Consensual sexual activity **never** involves pushing or coercion, or one person doing something they don't very much want to. Consent is not "Well, maybe," "I guess so," or "Oh, all right, already!" Consent is a clear, enthusiastic **"YES!"**

If you want to do something your partner isn't sure about, you can certainly have a discussion about it, and if your partner is reluctant, point them to more information and let them know that they've got all the time in the world to think about it—and that "no" is still an acceptable answer. But when anyone is hesitant, taking "no" or "not now" at face value is the best policy. Entering into an activity either of you doesn't really want to do or is afraid of is a recipe for hurt feelings, broken trust, abusive patterns, and sexual and emotional trauma.

Self-defense classes rock, to teach you some practical basics of defense; to help you hone your reflexes so you are best able to act, even when you're feeling shocked or stunned (which is very common); and to up your confidence in your own ability to protect yourself. Often, communities and martial arts centers offer them for free or at a very low cost. Not only can many martial arts teach you self-defense skills that can

s.e.x.

save your life, they're often both a great workout and good self-esteem booster.

Most of all, trust your intuition. A little voice in the back of your head saying, "Hey, I don't feel safe" is a voice to pay attention to.

SLEEPING WITH THE ENEMY

The most prevalent risk of rape and assault isn't from strangers, but from people we know: friends and acquaintances, neighbors, family, boyfriends (and far more rarely, girlfriends), and the partners of other friends.

If you're in a casual situation where you're hanging out with a person who exhibits the sorts of potentially abusive behaviors described on page 231, excuse yourself casually if you can, then just get away or go home (on your own—don't let them drive you). Otherwise, ask a friend for help and/or call to have someone pick you up. On a date, someone who is uncomfortably affectionate, sexually pushy, or nosy, or who will not stop commenting on your body or sex appeal, is worthy of distrust. And when you know from the outset you're in a group of people you don't feel comfortable or safe with, trust your instincts: avoid those groups, and if you find yourself in them, get out.

When you go on dates with someone new, make sure a friend or parent knows that you're going, where you're going, and when to expect you to be home. If you discover that a person you're going to go out with has a history of sexual harassment or assault, cancel the date, no matter how cool or harmless that person may seem to you.

On dates or at parties, **do NOT get wasted out of your gourd**. Beyond putting a severe strain on your physical health, impairing your judgment with drugs or alcohol puts you at a higher risk of sexual assault.

Someone who is drunk or high cannot give full consent. Often alcohol and certain other recreational drugs incline people to act more violently or sexually than they would otherwise. So, whether you're a potential victim getting smashed, or are considering having sex with someone who is too drunk or high to know what they're agreeing to (or if you figure big parties are a good place to get laid), understand that under those circumstances, fully consensual sex is unlikely and rape happens all too often.

Date Rape Drugs
Even if you're just drinking soda, keep your glass with you at parties and on new dates, and pour your drinks for yourself. Some sexual predators put *date rape drugs* such as rohypnol ("roofies") or GHB into drinks to render a person unconscious or impaired, and then assault them. Go to large parties with friends, not alone; keep tabs on each other. If, for whatever reason, you feel you have been drugged or that any alcohol or drugs you have used have had a serious effect on you, call a cab or grab a ride and get yourself home or into medical care, immediately.

It's obviously easier to extract yourself from a potentially dangerous sexual situation with someone you have just met or barely know than it is with someone you are already close to: a good friend, boyfriend or girlfriend, or family member. It can also be easier to excuse or write off sexual abuse from people you are close to: maybe they just like

s.e.x.

"rough sex." Maybe they were confused, or just don't understand that what they're doing is wrong. Maybe you think you did something wrong to make them act that way. It's common to feel that rape from people close to you isn't "real" rape. There are plenty of ways you can try to rationalize sexual abuse from someone you care about: it is incredibly hard for anyone to swap the title of *boyfriend* for *rapist*.

It's typical for loyalties to feel divided when a friend, family member, boyfriend, or other person you know sexually assaults you. It's typical for victims of these kinds of attacks not to report them, seek out support, or even tell anyone else, because they don't want to hurt those they love, even though they have been hurt by them. Understand that no loyalty is owed to a rapist of any flavor. Some people feel so ashamed to have loved or stayed with a rapist that acknowledging the abuse and getting out seems scarier than continuing to be raped.

But the only sound way to deal with a partner who rapes you is to treat the situation as you would any other type of abuse: connect with those in your lives who seeing the abuse for what it is, and accept their support; tell someone; and leave the abuser and the relationship. The Rape, Abuse & Incest National Network (RAINN) reports that survivors of partner rape are more likely to be raped multiple times than stranger and acquaintance rape survivors, and that partner rape survivors are more likely to suffer severe and long-lasting physical and psychological injuries. Like any other kind of abuser, a partner, friend, or family member who rapes is not likely to stop, no matter how you behave or how much you love them.

WHAT TO DO IF YOU HAVE JUST BEEN RAPED

If you've been raped, you probably know that's what has happened. But if you were raped by someone known to you, or if the force involved was verbal or emotional, rather than physical, you may be uncertain. If you have the idea that you can't be raped or sexually assaulted, because you belong to a certain group or are a certain type of person—maybe because you're male, because you're careful, or because you feel you're unattractive—it may be harder to believe. As well, it's normal after a rape to be in shock, to want to deny it has happened, or to feel very confused about what exactly happened and how. But if you feel or know that what happened was something you did NOT enthusiastically want or agree to, that you withdrew agreement at any point, or that you expressly said no, you're dealing with rape.

The most important thing to do right after you are raped is to first get to a safe place, away from your attacker or the place of your assault. The very next best step is to contact someone who can help and/or support you immediately. If you are experiencing feelings of shock or emotional numbness, panic or fear, helplessness, or confusion—or are too injured to seek out help—you can also phone a rape hotline. For hotlines, see the Resources section.

If you can, get to or call a hospital or urgent care center, whichever you feel most comfortable with (and even if you are uninsured, you will be treated, so do not let worries about money be a deterrent). The hospital will handle calling the police for you, and if you want to have a friend or family member with you, you can ask them

s.e.x.

to make that call as well. If you're somewhere unfamiliar and without a phone, look or yell for help and ask someone, anyone, to call the police for you. Do not shower or change clothes, however much you'll probably want to: if you decide to press charges, you'll be removing very important evidence. Even if you do not know right away if you will want to press charges, it's important to have what you need to keep that option open.

In many cases, a rape counselor or rape crisis worker will also be available throughout the process of reporting. Some hospitals have what are called *SANEs—sexual assault nurse examiners*—who are trained expressly to deal with rape and assault. If a SANE or rape counselor is not present, you can ask for one, and ask to wait until one is available for the rest of your exam. That person is a powerful advocate and ally. They can help you deal with your initial emotions, talk you through the process, and give you important and accurate information about your options for reporting, pressing charges, getting counseling and joining support groups.

Pressing Charges

In the bigger picture, the more abusers and rapists who are reported and charged, the more awareness is created, and the more likely it becomes that our culture will take greater steps to address the incredibly widespread problem of abuse and assault. Reporting and pressing charges also often help a survivor obtain medical care and counseling; protective measures to prevent more abuse (a

---

what happens during a rape exam?

ONCE you are admitted into the emergency room or care center:

- Any overt general injuries (such as cuts or broken bones) will be tended to, and the doctor or nurse may ask you some basic questions, primarily to determine what healthcare you immediately need.
- You will receive an overall examination, including a genital exam and STI and HIV testing. The doctor or nurse will use a "rape kit," which is a collection of materials expressly designed for collecting evidence from a rape victim and her clothing. If you think you may have been drugged by your rapist or someone else, let your nurse or doctor know, so they can do the appropriate urine or blood tests. Photographs may be taken. An examination after a rape can feel very invasive, so express your needs, as best you can. If at any point you need anyone to stop the examination, all you need to do is say so.
- You should be offered preventative medications for some STIs, and emergency contraception if your rape presented a pregnancy risk and you are not on a hormonal method of birth control. If either is not offered to you, ask for it.
- When the police arrive, they should first determine if you're able to answer questions at this time, and may then ask you questions about your assault. . If YOU do not feel able to answer at that time, you may schedule the questioning for another time.

s.e.x.

---

restraining orders, for example), which are of particular concern when a rapist is known to the victim; and emotional closure.

But pressing charges isn't easy.

It often involves a lot of vulnerability, a certain loss of your privacy, and a few risks. For someone who reports and presses charges, it can be a very hard pill to swallow when an attacker or abuser is not charged. Having more people than your immediate circle be aware you've been raped or abused can be tough. Due to the laws in this country, rape trials are still not made easy on the victim, and they are often an arduous, emotionally trying process. Many people still hold the outdated and ignorant notion that, in some way, rape is the victim's fault. You may even hear this, if you go to trial, from the perpetrator's defense counsel. Rape trials take time, as well. Most rape prosecution cases in the United States take anywhere from a few months to over a year to complete, and take at least ten to twenty days to even begin the process.

Know that a person can also report or press charges after the fact, especially in the case of minors. If you were raped or abused some years ago and wish you'd reported it, chances are good that you can still do so. Because physical evidence is probably missing, those cases aren't as likely to result in convictions, but they can offer you some resolution and acknowledgment, help support someone else's case against the same person, as well as get a report on file to help protect others from the same person in the future.

In deciding whether or not to press charges, what's most important is YOU and your needs. It's up to you to decide to press charges or not, and it should ultimately be about what's truly in your best interest. It's a good idea to talk about this with someone supportive you can trust. You can also get good advice anonymously from a rape hotline or a local rape crisis center.

▪ HEALING AND DEALING ▪

One of the toughest things about surviving assault and abuse is finding resolution and closure. Reporting and pressing charges can help with that a good deal, in many cases. It's a very clear way of saying, firmly, that you have been harmed, a statement that is important to be able to make to yourself; shame often arises out of denial or feeling that one has to hide what happened. The victim of an assault or of abuse shouldn't be the one ashamed: they aren't the abuser. Above all else, rape is a crime, and prosecuting a criminal helps to keep that criminal from committing the same crime again, against you or against others.

Emotional support is crucial to healing. If you've been raped, counseling, or even talking about the assault, may seem like the last thing you'd want. However, it's often the most important thing you need.

While friends and partners can be very sympathetic about rape, someone who hasn't been through it, or isn't experienced with, or knowledgeable about, the issues involved in healing from rape is unlikely to be of great help to you. Braving it out on your own may also seem more appealing than talking about it with others. If it really feels that way to you at first, then it does: there is never a deadline on getting counseling or support for rape. Even if you don't want it right now, at any point you decide you need or want it, you can seek it out.

s.e.x.

if you know someone who has been raped:

- Help them to find safe space by asking what they need and doing your best to provide what you can.
- Believe and support them. The behavior of rape victims varies widely from person to person; being emotionally controlled or calm is just as common as weeping openly. If your friend has told you he or she was raped, believe them, and let them know that however they are feeling is okay.
- Listen without judgment: allow them to express any of their feelings, even the ones that make you uncomfortable, or that don't seem appropriate to you. If you know you have any biases or preconceived notions about rape, be self-aware and do not bring them to the table.
- Offer to be an advocate; in reporting, the legal process, or telling others, your friend may want and need an ally. Rather than giving advice, give your friend options and venues for help: hotline or support group numbers, offer to be with them for medical appointments, or talking to parents and other friends.
- Remember that this is about them, not you. It's normal to feel very upset or angry when someone we care about has been hurt, but we need to manage those feelings ourselves or with support and counseling elsewhere, not with our friend or partner who has been raped. It's also normal to feel that you know EXACTLY what they need to heal, but that's not helpful; instead, follow their lead and listen to what they are expressing that they need.
- Be patient, even over months or years. It takes time—sometimes a very long time—to process through and recover from sexual assault.

If you have a sexual or romantic partner who is a survivor of rape or other abuse, you'll also need to work out certain sexual and intimacy issues your partner may have. Your partner may have *triggers*—things that make them experience all the emotional effects of the abuse again—that you'll need to become aware of and work to avoid. There may be certain types of intimacy or sexual activities and dynamics that are off-limits for your partner, and/or it may take your partner a longer time to feel comfortable with certain types of intimacy. Forming trust may be more difficult for your partner. In many areas, you can find support groups or counseling for the partners of survivors, to help you best manage these issues, for your partner as well as yourself. For books about abuse for survivors and/or their partners, see the Resources section.

Be aware, however, that when you've been raped or abused and just don't deal with it, or put off dealing with it, your life can suffer pretty greatly. You may struggle with post-traumatic stress disorder (PTSD). You may struggle with triggers. It may be difficult to ever feel completely safe or fully trust others again. Your own sexuality, sexual partnerships, or other relationships may elicit feelings of shame or fear, rather than comfort or pleasure. Enjoying relationships of all types, and even living a normal daily life, can be really inhibited by denial or avoidance of a rape or failing to deal with it. When the rapist is someone known to you, especially closely, silence may even set you up for yet more sexual abuse from that same person.

s.e.x.

Learning what you need to feel safe—with others and even just in your own skin—what you're ready for at any given time, where you're at in your healing process, how to manage a whirlwind of different emotions, what are and are not healthy ways of dealing with sexual abuse and assault are all vital to your well-being. If your ways of coping are essentially just replacing one trauma or injury with another—for instance, via reckless or harmful sexual relationships, cutting, or other self-injury—you can find yourself in a never-ending cycle of agony.

To work through assault and come out whole and healthy, you've got to not only accept that it did happen, you've got to do the work—however unfair it seems—to heal.

STAND UP

The biggest single thing that perpetuates rape and all types of abuse is silence. All too often, not only does abuse go unreported, it goes unacknowledged altogether. Most people neither want to be victims nor want to be treated like victims.

So, don't be a victim. **Be a survivor.** Surviving, healing, and thriving takes long, hard work, strength, and bravery. It means standing up for yourself and telling someone when you've been abused or assaulted. It often means calling your abuser or attacker on what they did, through reporting and the legal system. It may mean working through abuse that happened some time ago, and that you'd rather not revisit. To heal, you've got to do the hard work. You have to look at all your feelings, even the ugly ones, and let yourself have them; you have to put the blame where it belongs; and you have to learn ways to cope with the effects of abuse, long- and short-term.

At the most basic level, surviving is refusing to allow an abuser to have continued power or control over you—to resist and reclaim your absolute and inarguable rights to physical and emotional safety, autonomy, and power within and for yourself. Survivors won't be silenced or shamed: they'll be strong and give themselves credit, care, and love—and require others to do same—for all they are and all they've done to survive and thrive. An abuser or attacker is a terrorist; a survivor of abuse or assault is a warrior.

to be or not to be . . . pregnant: contraception

CONTRACEPTION—BIRTH CONTROL—has existed for nearly as long as people have, but never in history have we had so many effective, safe, and accessible options as we do now.

Early attempts at birth control, such as resin barriers and vinegar spermicides, were precursors to modern methods, and people have almost always known that abstention was effective for prevention, although for much of history, most women didn't have that option. Until fairly recently, few women had the power or support to choose when they wanted to become pregnant (and sadly, this is still the case in some places and relationships). Even as recently as a hundred years ago, a bill was passed in the United States—the Comstock Law—that defined birth control information as *obscene*. Many people and couples were and still are pressured to reproduce, regardless of their

wishes. These scenarios, and the lack of safe, reliable, and accessible birth control, sometimes led (and again, sadly, still do) to infanticide or abandonment of unwanted children, domestic abuses, and unsafe or fatal abortions, as well as compounding the oppression of women. Today, some lobbies, communities, and cultures—often the same ones who bemoan teen pregnancy—still seek to block or reduce access to birth control, especially for young adults. Funding to provide and research birth control doesn't come close to meeting the needs of women, especially those living in poverty.

Unwanted pregnancy and childbearing can result in both private and public ills. From a global standpoint, we face real problems with lethal malnutrition and poor health in infants and children—even here in the richest nation in the world, which also happens to have the highest infant mortality and childhood poverty rates of any developed nation. Those problems are compounded by poverty, lack of education, unprepared or unwanted parenting, and the stigmas affixed to teen and single parents and their children. Unwanted pregnancy can seriously undermine your health and well-being, physical and emotional. Viewing partnered sex as a gamble tends to create crummy relationships, crummy feelings about oneself, and crummy parents. For much of history, women have been denied easy access to birth control as a means of controlling *them:* women's rights are deeply linked to freedom of reproductive choice. Whether it's done by a government, a culture, or a partner, keeping women from the power to choose whether or not to become pregnant keeps women from having sexual autonomy and truly giving consent to heterosexual sex.

 OBVIOUSLY, most of this chapter is directed toward women at risk of pregnancy, but if you're a guy having sex with women—or thinking about it— **read up!** This is about you, too. If you're a same-sex-partnered guy or gal who plans to stay that way? Lucky you: you don't need to worry about birth control! But you've probably got friends or siblings who do, and who could always use more folks around them in the know about birth control. So much sexuality information is passed peer-to-peer that the more accurate information anyone knows, the better. Do your pals a good turn and have a look!

Becoming pregnant—not just parenting— should be a *choice,* and one that has real bearing on the rights and well-being of all people, especially of women and children. When reliable birth control methods are used properly and consistently, and sex for both parties is fully consensual, few people will become pregnant before they are ready.

According to *Contraceptive Technology,* every year in the United States—which has the highest rate of teen pregnancy and births in the Western world—about **one in every nine women under nineteen who have been sexually active becomes pregnant**. That may seem like a lot, but it's been normal through all of history for women to begin childbearing in their teens and early twenties. At this point in history, teen pregnancy rates are some of the LOWEST they have ever been, with the United States seeing profound declines since 1950. But still, despite big developments in birth control methods and widely increased accessibility, the majority of young pregnancies *are* still unplanned or accidental.

Young adults—like older adults—get pregnant unintentionally or accidentally for several reasons. The biggest reason is simple: *birth control methods often weren't used at all.* With major health organizations like the CDC and the Guttmacher Institute releasing data that shows only about 30 percent of sexually active young adults using contraception regularly, and many young adults having intercourse for a year or more before seeking out contraception, it's pretty obvious how unplanned pregnancies occur. There are many reasons birth control may not be used: due to lack of information about birth control methods, how to obtain them, and when they are needed; lack of access to birth control; partner pressure not to use birth control; nonconsensual sex and rape; concerns about privacy and discovery; embarrassment or shame; denial (of being sexually active and at risk, for instance); and "it-can't-happen-to-me-itis."

Many young adults who do use methods of birth control use them sporadically or improperly; failure rates for many birth control methods are higher for young people than for older folks, and most methods' overall failure rates are far higher than they would be if methods were used properly and consistently. Teens who use condoms as birth control, for instance, too often use them improperly or after direct genital contact has already occurred. Younger women on the pill more often take pills late or skip pills than older women do. Some methods commonly used, such as withdrawal or spermicides, just aren't effective.

Young adults choosing to be sexually active with partners *are* responsible for their own choices, and most certainly SHOULD be responsible—and that means *both* partners—for birth control choices, including the choice not to be sexually active. But the fact of the matter is that a whole lot of the world doesn't help you do that very much, and the burden of birth control lies largely with women. As a result, choosing to be responsible about birth control involves way more effort and struggle than it should.

That doesn't change the fact that your reproductive choices are still just that: *yours.* Yours, not only to make in the first place, but to be accountable for and live with. And when you opt into being sexually active with opposite-sex partners, those choices start with using birth control. The ability to choose when and if you want a pregnancy is your **right**.

When it comes to being sexually active, everyone should be making sound choices about when it's right for them and when they're ready to manage all aspects of sexual activity, including, but not limited to, risking pregnancy. Sometimes, the best choice to make is NOT to engage in partnered sex. But sex is a normal, natural part of being human, and it's just as valid to choose to have sex and sexual partners. Unwanted or unplanned pregnancy is not a "punishment" for sexual activity: it's just a natural result.

pregnancy risks, plainly wrapped

 ANY direct, opposite-sex genital contact, or direct female genital contact with fresh semen, produces a risk of pregnancy. That means that unprotected intercourse that lasted twenty seconds carries a pregnancy risk, as does a penis rubbed on a vulva, or ejaculation upon the female genitals. Sperm don't have watches: they don't give a hoot how long you were going at it, or if you consider what you were doing sex or not. If there was direct, opposite-sex genital and/or seminal contact, you've got a risk of pregnancy. No one can accurately tell you which direct-contact scenarios are riskier than others, because variables are at play that most young adults can't account for—namely, your personal fertility level on a given day, determined by accurate daily charting—and other variables that no one can account for, such as chance and the somewhat random nature of pregnancy, which is influenced by general health, the viability of the particular male sperm, and the like.

s.e.x.

▪ NO BIRDS, NO BEES, NO BULL: ▪
How Conception Really Happens

A man produces millions of sperm cells every day, and they are microscopically small: it'd take a few hundred lined up in a row to be just one inch in length. When a man ejaculates, the semen normally has between 200 and 600 million sperm in it. Because sperm are so sensitive to the environment outside the testes, only about a couple of hundred of those sperm will be able to reach the female egg, and that is one reason the body produces so many. While it only takes one sperm to actually fertilize the egg, a couple of hundred "helper" sperm are also required to help usher that one in.

Sperm can not only come from ejaculate, but can be within pre-ejaculate, the fluid that comes from a man's penis before orgasm, when he is aroused. Generally, sperm are only present in pre-ejaculate when a man has recently ejaculated, but there's no practical way of knowing if it's in there or not at a given time.

In most healthy women, from a couple of weeks before menarche (first menstruation) begins and until menopause, one *ovum* (egg cell) is released each menstrual cycle from the ovaries into one of the fallopian tubes. Usually, only one tube at a time has a fertile ovum in it, though some women may release more than one ovum each cycle. If sperm pass through the vaginal canal and the cervix, some of them will go to one fallopian tube, and some to the other, seeking out that egg cell. Those sperm that find a live ovum surround it and try to penetrate the outer layer to fertilize it. If the ovum is healthy and fertile, and a sperm cell does penetrate and fertilize it, then the surface of the ovum changes so that no other sperm are allowed in. It's a bit like calling in to a radio station for a contest: once the fiftieth caller gets on the line, they just stop answering the phone.

What is formed in fertilization is a cell called a *zygote.* It contains forty-six chromosomes (the carriers of hereditary characteristics, like hair and eye color, body size, and genetic conditions), twenty-three from the egg, twenty-three from the sperm, so its new DNA structure is different from the structure of either the sperm or the ovum alone. Over the next few days, as the fertilized egg—called the *morula* at this stage of the game—progresses down the fallopian tube, it will divide several times, until it becomes a sixteen-celled structure called a *blastocyst.* If it implants in the wall of the uterus, around the tenth day, the endometrial tissue and developing *placenta*—a temporary organ formed with the outer cells of the blastocyst, which grows over time to nourish a growing embryo and fetus via the mother's bloodstream—begin producing new hormones (the same hormones pregnancy tests read for, one of which, hCG, is only present after conception).

It is at this point that you have a pregnancy. (To find out what happens after that, if a pregnancy is sustained, see chapter 12.)

PREGNANCY RISK Q AND A

Can a girl get pregnant if her partner ejaculates in his pants, in the bathtub, or across an interstate highway?

The MOST likely way to become pregnant is by direct vaginal contact with sperm. Sperm can live up to about twenty minutes

s.e.x.

what are your risks of pregnancy?

High to moderate: Unprotected vaginal heterosexual intercourse; intercourse with condom breakage or other birth control failure; ejaculation into the vulva; direct contact of male genitals with the female vulva without a barrier

Moderate to low: Unprotected anal intercourse (female receptive); vaginal intercourse with condom breakage or birth control failure just before menses; manual sex with direct ejaculate transfer (such as giving a handjob, then putting unwashed hands with semen on them directly in the vagina)

Low to none: Opposite-sex genital-to-genital contact or intercourse with a condom and/or other reliable birth control method; oral/genital fluid swapping (such as semen in the mouth, potentially swapped with deep kissing, then cunnilingus); "dry" sex

No risk of pregnancy: Kissing, cuddling, fondling, massage, or hand contact (such as shaking hands with a man who has recently touched his penis); oral sex; same-sex activity; masturbation (solo or mutual); activity with unshared sex toys; manual sex without fluid sharing

in an environment that is unfriendly to them, but they are basically pretty delicate creatures in the great outdoors. So, for instance, having unprotected anal sex where sperm can run right down into the vagina does create a pregnancy risk, but pregnancy isn't as likely as with unprotected vaginal intercourse. Same goes for scenarios like giving a male partner unprotected oral sex, having oral contact with semen, then kissing a partner, then having that partner engage in cunnilingus. Or sitting in a tub with a man who ejaculates in it, without actual genital contact: sperm really can't make it to the fallopian tubes through that many different bus routes. If there is a distinct barrier between a vagina and the penis, such as thick or impermeable clothing (like a few layers of denim or polyester), water, or an interstate highway, there is not a reasonable risk of pregnancy.

In addition, pregnancy cannot occur

from swallowing semen from oral sex, or from manual sex with no vulvar contact with fresh semen. The digestive system isn't directly connected to the reproductive system: sperm trying to get to the fallopian tubes through the stomach would be like you trying to get to class on time by walking through a brick wall.

What if the hymen isn't broken yet?

A woman can get pregnant at any time after her first menses (and in fact, first ovulation occurs two weeks before first menstruation, so pregnancy can technically occur before menstruation does). The state of someone's hymen is a nonissue. Even if a fully or partially intact hymen is present, nearly all hymens are perforate (have small holes in them), so that menstrual and vaginal fluid can flow through. Those holes will allow sperm through as well.

What if my partner says he/she is infertile?

It's rare for a teen or young adult to know their fertility status, because, barring certain medical conditions or diseases (such as PID, PCOS, eating disorders, Klinefelter's syndrome, or profound testicle injuries), most people who are not trying to become pregnant have not had tests to determine fertility. An adolescent claiming to be infertile, who also happens to be suggesting bypassing birth control, is probably either lying to you completely, ignorant about how fertility works, or confused about something their doctor told them. Unless you hear it from the doctor diagnosing infertility, assume your partner is fertile.

I've heard that the chance of becoming pregnant is the same as the chances of winning the lottery. True or false?

MOST accidental pregnancies occur in young adults within the first six months of having intercourse. Statistically, a heterosexually active teenager who does not use contraceptives has a **85 percent chance (0.85)** of becoming pregnant within one year. The chance of winning a state lottery jackpot is a mere 1 in just under 14 million, or .0000000716. Do the math.

▪ THE BIRTH CONTROL BREAKDOWN ▪

Different women have different birth control needs. For most, a method that is inexpensive and easy to use and obtain is most important. Some people are comfortable with hormonal methods, like the pill, while others don't want, or can't have, synthetic chemicals or hormones in their bodies. Some people need a constant birth control method, or want benefits some constant methods can offer, such as decreasing menstrual cramps or clearing acne; others just need something they can use occasionally.

Effectiveness and ease of use are generally the biggest factor in most people's birth control choices. Most barrier and hormonal methods are highly effective and easy to use: careless or erratic use is the single biggest factor in ineffectiveness or failure. Also, two methods—like condoms used with the pill, or a cervical cap with fertility charting—are usually better than one.

There are lots of options. If and when it's time to consider birth control, it's wise not to leap at one method just because it's what everyone else is using, or to assume that a method must be best because you've heard of it often or seen an aggressive advertising campaign for it.

Which birth control method is best for you is a very individual choice, and it may change a few times during your life (and involve some trial and error). Have a look at what's out there now, then talk to your gynecologist, doctor, or sexual health clinician to figure out what's most likely to be right for you. (Your doctor or nurse may even be able to tell you about new methods on the market that were not yet available at the time of this writing.) If your doctor or nurse is assigning you a method, rather than asking what you want and need, and exploring many options with you, then either advocate for yourself directly, or find a different doctor or clinician who will take

s.e.x.

more time and help you choose more effectively. What's best for them or what they think is best for a patient may not always be what the patient knows will work for them.

On the following pages, you'll find brief descriptions of all currently available methods, including approximate cost, where and how to get them, ease of use, common side effects, pros and cons, special concerns, and effectiveness. Effectiveness ratings come from a wide sample of groups, not from young people specifically. If we had data on effectiveness JUST based on teen and young adult use, many methods would be listed as less effective with typical use. For instance, according to Family Planning Perspectives, the failure rate of oral contraceptives (AKA, the pill) for adolescents may be as high as 15 percent because of inconsistent use, and for all contraceptive methods, young women experience a failure rate of about 47 percent in the first year of contraceptive use, whereas the overall failure rate for women over thirty is only 8 percent.

 WHILE it is always best to use the most effective birth control available to you, **using something is always better than using nothing.** While spermicides or withdrawal, for example, are not very effective used alone, they are much more effective than no birth control at all.

So, with any method you use, listen to your doctor or clinician's instructions carefully, and read the literature or inserts that come with your method: there are specifics to many methods that are not listed here, and birth control data, methods, and information tend to change or be updated pretty regularly. **Remember: For contraception to be effective, it must be used properly and consistently.**

cost ratings:

$: Cheapedy-cheap
(under $200 per year)

$$: Moderately priced
($200–$600 per year)

$$$: Big bucks (over $600 per year)

Bear in mind that costs may vary if your health insurance or national healthcare system covers or discounts the costs of any of the birth control methods. Cost estimates also are not merely for single-use: the estimates posted are for use over one year, assuming a user has sex around a hundred times in that year (the Kinsey Institute states that, in their studies, the average eighteen-year-old reports—which, like much self-reporting about sex, may be inflated—having sex 112 times per year). For instance, while a diaphragm costs more at the onset, in just a couple of months of use, it's cheaper than the pill.

The average rate of effectiveness is listed both for perfect use (when a method is used EXACTLY as directed) and for typical use (as most actually people use it), shown in how many women out of one hundred became pregnant using a given method in one year, with percentages. Effectiveness rates for typical use are based on the method a given person reports they have been using over a year, not for single episodes of use. So, for those who have reported using condoms as their birth control method, built into those rates are those condom users who sometimes don't use them. If you always

s.e.x.

use a given method, for all risks, and always use it properly, then *your* effectiveness for that method is the percentage shown for perfect, not typical, use.

ABSTINENCE

People who are not having ANY opposite-sex partnered sex do not need birth control: they are 100 percent protected from pregnancy. Refraining or abstaining from part-nered sex can be intentionally chosen expressly to avoid pregnancy.

We often hear that abstinence is the most effective method of birth control. However, that's not technically true. As noted in *Contraceptive Technology*, **about 26 percent of young adults "practicing abstinence" will become pregnant within one year**, which makes it about 74 percent effective in typical use—less effective than the typical use rates for almost any other method of contraception. If you're planning to use abstinence as your method of birth control, do yourself a favor and be realistic: If you're with a partner and are physically intimate at all—or are in any way half-hearted about abstinence—have a backup method of birth control around and available, just in case. You're no less abstinent if you have one on hand but still refrain from sex.

BARRIER METHODS

Barrier methods—condoms, diaphragms, cervical caps, Lea's Shields, and the contraceptive sponge—are those that work by preventing sperm from reaching or entering the vagina or cervix. Many people like barrier methods because they're easy to get and use, affordable, noninvasive, effective, and convenient. They don't interfere with fertility or the menstrual cycle, change your body chemistry or sexual response cycle in any way, or carry serious or long-term side effects. For people who can't remember to take pills on time every day, or who cannot or do not want to use hormonal methods, they're just the thing. Condoms also offer STI protection, which hormonal methods cannot. Some studies have suggested that other barrier methods, such as the diaphragm and cervical cap, may also provide *some* extra STI prevention, including protection from HIV, by protecting cervical cells from infection (though these should not be considered a sound method of safer sex).

Barrier methods may not work for those who feel uncomfortable with touching their genitals; who have a hard time communicating with partners; who don't want to "interrupt" sexual activity to insert a device, or ask partners if sex is on the menu for later, so as to insert the device in advance (though for people in those situations, part-nered sex isn't usually real smart, either). Barrier methods made of latex are not good choices for people who are latex-sensitive or allergic, but most of these devices do have latex alternatives.

Condoms (Male)

Effectiveness with perfect use: 2/100 or 98% effective

Effectiveness with typical use: 15/100 or 85% effective

Cost: $

What are they, and how do they work?

Condoms—thin latex or polyurethane sheaths—rolled onto the penis for any

s.e.x.

direct genital contact, work by preventing sperm from having any contact with the vulva, because semen is contained within the condom during both ejaculation and pre-ejaculation. For detailed instructions on how to use a condom, and more information on condoms, see page 207. Condoms fail if they are not used for all genital contact from start to finish, or if they break, tear, or slip off; they most often fail because they're not being used for all genital contact. If a condom fails, it will be fairly obvious, and emergency contraception (see page 259) can be used.

How and where do you get them?

A doctor visit isn't required to get condoms, nor must a person be of a certain age; in fact, condoms can be found all over the place: pharmacies, grocers, megastores, online vendors, student and community health centers, and clinics (where they can often be found at no cost). When buying condoms, be sure to avoid places where they may have sat on shelves or in hot or cold areas for a long time (such as in gas stations or vending machines), and store them properly yourself, away from heat or cold or places where they might get torn inside the wrapper.

Pros and Cons, Risks and Benefits

Some male condom users complain that condoms are not comfortable, or that they decrease sensitivity. However, that can usually be helped by shopping around: there are, right now, hundreds of different condoms available, and experimenting with different ring sizes, textures, or thicknesses can often solve this problem. Since condoms are worn by the male partner, he must be willing and able to use them, and it may take negotiation skills to make that happen. As well, for condoms to be most effective, they need to be used with an extra lubricant, so portability may be an issue.

The biggest benefit of condoms, male and female (see below), is that they are the **only** birth control method that also provides STI protection (and thus, for women, protection against cervical cancer). It's a very good idea to back up *every* other method of birth control with condom use, for that reason. Also, condoms are the ONLY inexpensive, fully reversible and easily accessible birth control for men: so for guys who want to be at the wheel of all aspects of their sexuality, condoms are a must.

Condoms (Female)

Effectiveness with
   perfect use: 5/100
   or 95% effective
Effectiveness with
   typical use: 21/100 or 79% effective
Usual cost: $$

What are they, and how do they work?

Female condoms are long polyurethane sheaths with rings, like the one at the end of a male condom, at both ends. A female condom is inserted into the vaginal canal, then the penis is inserted in the open end. As with male condoms, each condom is designed for one act of intercourse only, and it's removed after intercourse by twisting the outer ring and pulling the rest of the condom out of the vagina.

How and where do you get them?

The same places you'd get male condoms: pharmacies, grocers, online vendors, or health centers, though they may be harder to find

S.e.x.

than male condoms. As with male condoms, there is no legal age requirement regarding purchase, and a prescription is not needed.

Pros and Cons, Risks and Benefits

Some users find it hard to get the hang of using female condoms, or don't like the polyurethane material, which can feel or sound "scrunchy." Some women may also feel funny about the way the end of the condom "hangs" outside the vagina.

On the other hand, female condoms are nonlatex, so may be a good choice for those who are latex-sensitive or allergic. They are also a good choice for women whose male partners refuse to wear male condoms (though those *partners* may not be a good choice, period) or whose partners find male condoms reduce sensation for them. Too, unlike with male condoms, these don't require an erection for use. However, like male condoms, they also offer STI protection, which other methods do not. One more bonus of female condoms is that they can be inserted up to eight hours prior to intercourse, so for people who feel that male condoms kill the moment, female condoms can solve that problem.

Diaphragms/Cervical Caps

Diaphragm effectiveness with perfect use: 6/100 or 94% effective

Diaphragm effectiveness with typical use: 20/100 or 80% effective

Cervical cap effectiveness with perfect use: 9/100 or 90% effective

Cervical cap effectiveness with typical use: 16/100 or 84% effective

Usual cost: $, including exam and fitting

What are they, and how do they work?

A *diaphragm* is a latex, silicone, or rubber cup, about the size of your palm, that is inserted into the vagina before intercourse (even a couple of hours before, if you prefer) and used with spermicidal jelly. It is held in place behind the pubic bone, and covers the cervix to prevent sperm from entering; the spermicide kills any sperm that may wind up squiggling their way around the cup. Diaphragms are reusable, and can be used for a couple of years before they need to be replaced. The diaphragm offers protection during sexual activities for up to six hours, and needs to be left in place for at least six hours afterward up to twenty-four hours before it is removed because the sperm can remain viable, and if you took it out right away, rather than leaving it in to keep those sperm out of the cervix, it couldn't work. It can be used for multiple acts of intercourse, if extra spermicide is inserted into the vagina before each additional act.

A *cervical cap* is a reusable soft latex or rubber cup with a round rim, sized by a health professional to fit snugly around the cervix. It requires a fitting, is available by prescription only, and, like the diaphragm, is used with spermicide. Smaller than a diaphragm, it may be easier to use for some younger women. A cervical cap protects for forty-eight hours and can be used for multiple acts of intercourse within that time.

How and where do you get them?

Diaphragms and cervical caps require a fitting and prescription from a gynecologist or other sexual healthcare provider. If your sexual healthcare provider does not stock them in their office, you will simply take your prescription to any pharmacy to have it filled. The spermicidal jelly used for both methods can be obtained—without a prescription—from pharmacies, grocers, megastores, or online vendors.

Pros and Cons, Risks and Benefits

Wearing a diaphragm for more than twenty-four hours, or a cervical cap for more than forty-eight hours is not recommended because of the risk, though low, of toxic shock syndrome. Also, with prolonged use, the cap or diaphragm may cause an unpleasant vaginal odor or discharge in some women. For women prone to urinary tract, yeast, or bacterial infections, diaphragms or cervical caps may not be a good choice.

Some women also may not like using diaphragms or cervical caps because they find them difficult or awkward to put in, or because they don't like the accompanying spermicides. As with condoms, the biggest reason diaphragms and cervical caps fail is that they aren't applied properly, used all the time, or used for all genital contact, from start to finish—so if you feel like they're a drag to put in, then they're probably not a good choice.

But there are also a lot of pros. Both methods can be put in well before sexual activity, so they don't interrupt sexual activity. Diaphragms can also be for sex during menstruation (cervical caps cannot). Both can be used without replacement for a couple of years, making them one of the most inexpensive methods there is. Like other barrier methods, these do not pose the health risks that hormonal methods may pose, and may be used by women who cannot use those other methods due to health conditions. Both are comfortable once inserted, and neither partner is likely to feel them during intercourse or other sexual activities.

Lea's Shield

Effectiveness with perfect
   use: not yet available
Effectiveness with typical
   use: 15/100 or 85%
Usual cost: $

What is it, and how does it work?

Lea's Shield is a newer barrier form of contraception made of silicone: it looks a lot like an ellipse-shaped bowl, with a valve in the center, and a loop to help with removal. It is inserted into the vagina and held in place by the vaginal walls. Like diaphragms and cervical caps, it surrounds and covers the cervix to prevent sperm from entering, is used with spermicidal jelly, and can also be left in place, for up to forty-eight hours (and should be left in place for at least eight hours after intercourse).

How and where do you get it?

It may be obtained through a gynecologist or sexual healthcare provider, but does not require a fitting, so in some areas, it may also be obtained directly from a retailer.

Pros and Cons, Risks and Benefits

The pros, cons, risks, and benefits of the shield are similar to those of diaphragms and cervical caps: it's reusable, affordable, and convenient. It can be put in before sexual

s.e.x.

activity and left in place afterward; it also requires spermicide. Unlike the diaphragm or cervical cap, Lea's Shield also has a special drainage "valve" that allows for one-way flow from the cervix through the vagina, which may be helpful at preventing TSS and vaginal infections or irritations that are larger issues with diaphragms or cervical caps. Since it is made of silicone, latex-sensitive people can use the Lea's Shield, it resists odor better that latex barriers, and it can also be used during menstruation. Another obvious perk is that it does not require a fitting, as the other two methods do.

In trials of the shield, while a majority of women reported liking the shield, their male partners often reported being able to feel the device and disliking it.

Contraceptive Sponge

Effectiveness with perfect
   use: 20/100 or 80%
   effective
Effectiveness with typical
   use: 32/100 or 68% effective
Cost: $

What is it, and how does it work?

The vaginal contraceptive sponge is a device made of polyurethane that looks like a little white bagel. It contains spermicide that foams out from the sponge when it is used (you add water to it before inserting it, to produce the foam), and the device also forms a barrier to the cervix, so it works in two ways. It has a loop on one side for removal. Like a diaphragm, it should be left in place for at least six hours after intercourse, and removed no later than twenty-four hours after insertion, to prevent TSS and vaginal irritation from the spermicide.

When you're finished using it, you just pull it out and throw it away.

Where and how can you get it?

Where available (it has only recently been re-released in the United States), contraceptive sponges can be bought over the counter at pharmacies or megastores. No prescription or exam is required.

Spermicides

Spermicides come in many forms: foams, suppositories, tablets, film, creams, and jellies. Used alone, rather than with a barrier method, spermicides are not highly effective contraception, though certainly, they are better than using no contraception at all. They are only around 82 percent effective with perfect use, and around 70 percent effective with typical use. Family Planning Perspectives states that spermicides are one of the least effective methods of contraception. Spermicides may also increase STI risks in some users, because genital irritation due to spermicide can cause the genitals to become inflamed, and thus, more prone to infection—especially in younger women, who are always at increased risk of infection.

"Homegrown" agents sometimes thought to be spermicides, like lemon juice, vinegar, or castille soap, are even less effective, if they do anything at all.

Pros and Cons, Risks and Benefits

One sponge offers protection for up to twenty-four hours, even with multiple acts

s.e.x.

of intercourse. Sponges are also very inexpensive.

Because of the foaming that comes from the vagina with the sponge, it can be very messy and feel socially awkward for some users, and it is not a good choice for anyone sensitive to spermicides or prone to yeast infections. It may also carry risks of TSS if left in longer than advised.

HORMONAL METHODS

Hormonal methods all work by putting hormones into the bloodstream—via pills, patches, rings, injections, or subdermal (under the skin) implants—to alter the normal fertility cycle, making conception very unlikely. They may do any or all of the following: suppress ovulation (keeping eggs from being released each month), thicken the cervical mucus to make it difficult for sperm to reach the cervix and fertilize an egg, and/or prevent a thickening of uterine lining so that a fertilized egg cannot implant.

Hormonal methods are very effective, but only when used properly. Skipped or late pills or injections, or patches or rings used incorrectly or sporadically, can massively decrease the effectiveness of hormonal methods. Some medications, such as certain antibiotics and herbs, can also decrease the effectiveness of some hormonal contraceptives. Some hormonal methods are more reversible (easier to use without lasting effects, or to stop taking, allowing it to gradually leave your system) than others. One big downside of hormonal contraceptive use may be a false sense of security in terms of sexually transmitted infections. **Hormonal birth control methods provide no STI protection.** Combining a hormonal contraceptive with condom use is often the most effective birth control method there is for young adults, and also offers STI protection.

How to use your pill—and manage problems like late or missed pills—varies, so always be sure to ask your doctor about your brand, and read the inserts that come with your pill carefully.

for your health. . . .

 IF you're considering or starting any hormonal method, it is VITAL that you be honest with your doctor about anything that may create extra health risks for you in combination with a hormonal method. Are you a smoker, but keep that a secret from your doctor or gynecologist? When it comes to hormonal birth control, it can be a matter of life and death to fib about smoking. Women who smoke should NOT use most hormonal contraceptives.

Oral Contraceptives, AKA the Pill

Effectiveness with perfect use: less than 1/100 or 99+% effective

Effectiveness with typical use: 2.15/100–8/100 or 92–97%+ effective

Usual cost: $$, including cost of GYN exam

What is it, and how does it work?

The combined birth control pill—meaning that two different hormones, estrogen and progesterone, are both in the pill—is the most popular method of birth control in the United States. As long as a woman is taking her pills as directed and on time, every

s.e.x.

day of her cycle—generally in twenty-eight-day increments—the pill provides equally effective protection on every day of that cycle. When starting the pill, a backup method of birth control is advisable through the first cycle—one month—of use. A woman then takes one "active" pill—a pill with hormones in it—every day for twenty-one days, and then for the last week of the cycle, she takes one "inactive" pill—with only inert ingredients—during which time she will usually have a period (see below).

The pill works by suppressing ovulation, thickening cervical mucus, and/or impeding implantation.

Where and how do you get it?

The pill may not be obtained over the counter. It requires an exam and a prescription from your sexual healthcare provider, and you pick up pills at your pharmacy or health center each month, or in whatever number of cycles your pharmacist is willing to dispense them. Often, part or all of the cost of hormonal methods are included in health insurance plans or Medicaid, so costs may be lower that stated above.

Pros and Cons, Risks and Benefits:

Beyond a very high level of effectiveness, some benefits of hormonal contraceptives may include reducing PMS and menstrual cramps, lightening monthly flow, aid with acne, and reducing risks of many reproductive cancers, PID, and anemia. The pill can also help with menstrual irregularity, though it does not permanently "regulate" periods—in fact, since a woman taking the combination pill correctly isn't ovulating, the bleeding at the end of a cycle of pills isn't even truly a period, and is called, instead, "withdrawal bleed." Some women assume it does regulate

fertility cycles because, after being on the pill, their periods become more regular. But since it usually takes a few years of menstruating for cycles to become regular, what's more likely, especially if the pill was started in adolescence, is that periods have become more regular on their own, simply due to the passage of time while on the pill. It's normal, while on the pill, for monthly bleeding to be lighter than usual, and even to miss a period occasionally, or only spot.

The pill isn't right for all women. Some conditions that may make the pill a poor birth control choice, or prevent a doctor from prescribing it are: cigarette smoking, high blood pressure, liver disease, hepatitis infection, reproductive cancers; or a history of blood clots, unexplained vaginal bleeding, migraine headaches, or depression, Recent studies have also suggested that combined hormonal contraceptives, including the pill, may inhibit the normal growth of bone mass that occurs during puberty and is important for healthy adult development, so if you're under twenty, ask your doctor about bone mass.

All hormonal contraceptives carry similar possible side effects, to greater or lesser degrees, which often include loss of libido/decreased sexual desire, vaginal dryness, nausea, headaches, mood changes or depression, tender breasts, weight changes, missed periods or prolonged absence of menstruation, and/or spotting. Serious risks, which generally are rare in patients prescribed the pill wisely (taking into account factors that may increase risks) include liver and gallbladder disease, bone density changes (which may be more profound in younger women), blood clots, heart attack, and stroke. Risks and side effects are more likely with combined, rather than singular, hormonal methods.

Sometimes, the pill isn't the best choice for young adults, because remembering to take pills on time every day can be difficult—especially if the fact that the pill is being taken at all is being kept secret.

Other BCPs (Birth Control Pills): Seasonale

Seasonale is an oral contraceptive that is identical to the combination pill in contents and effectiveness. However, with Seasonale, active pills are taken for cycles of three months each, so that withdrawal bleed will only occur four times each year, rather than monthly. Other BCPs can also be prescribed for use consecutively, though Seasonale is currently the only one on the market expressly designed for consecutive use.

Progestin-Only Oral Contraceptives, or Minipills

Minipills are ever-so-slightly less effective than the combination pill because, rather than containing two hormones, they contain one: progestin. Minipills do not prevent ovulation as combined oral contraceptives do, but they still thicken the cervical mucus to make it unlikely for sperm to be able to travel to the uterus and fertilize an egg, and they also prevent the uterine lining from thickening, to make implantation unlikely should an egg be fertilized.

Minipills are a good option for women who want to use oral contraceptives, but can't take combination pills because of the risks estrogen presents in terms of blood clots, high blood pressure, headaches, or other issues. For smokers bound and determined to take oral contraceptives, minipills are safer than combination pills.

Menstrual Suppression

Seasonale suppresses—holds back—menstruation. Other BCPs can also be used to suppress menstruation, by skipping the placebo periods, and taking active pill packs back-to-back. Doing so may suppress bleeding for a cycle . . . or it may not. Sometimes bleeding still occurs, and sometimes a woman may experience spotting during the weeks afterward.

Medical organizations currently advise that a woman should not have fewer than four periods each year, and at this time, no data is available about the long-term effects of menstrual suppression, nor have specific studies been done on suppression in younger women. Given that (1) we don't have that data yet, (2) we do know of certain positive health benefits of menstruation, like helping to rid the vagina of bacteria, (3) hormonal methods pose extra risks to younger women in terms of bone mass (and those risks logically increase when more active pills each month are taken), it's advisable that you do this very infrequently, if at all, and always ask your doctor first.

The Ring

Effectiveness with perfect use: less than 1/100 or more than 99% effective

Effectiveness with typical use: 2/100 or 98% effective

Cost: $$, including cost of exam

S.e.x.

What is it, and how does it work?

The ring is a combination hormonal method that works the same way the pill does, and is used a lot like a tampon. It's small and flexible, and is inserted into the vagina once every four weeks: worn for three and removed for the fourth. A new ring is used at the beginning of the next cycle. The hormones are contained in the ring, which releases them into the bloodstream.

Where and how do you get it?

The ring is available by prescription, from your doctor, gynecologist, or sexual health clinic.

Pros and Cons, Risks and Benefits

The ring carries the same possible benefits, risks, and side effects as other combined hormonal contraceptives, and may be a good choice for women who want a low-maintenance hormonal contraceptive they do not have to remember to take daily.

Neither the woman "wearing" the ring nor her partner is likely to be able to feel it when it's been inserted correctly. Sometimes, the ring can slip out, but as long as it's reinserted right away, slipping won't make it less effective.

The Patch

Effectiveness with perfect use: less than 1/100 or more than 99% effective

Effectiveness with typical use: 8/100 or 92% effective

Cost: $$, including cost of exam

What is it, and how does it work?

The patch contains the same hormones as combined oral contraceptives, and works by delivering those hormones into the bloodstream through the skin, to suppress ovulation each cycle. The patch is a bit like a big Band-Aid, affixed to the skin in whatever area the user prefers (so long as it's an area that doesn't get very sweaty or is subject to a lot of friction, either of which could cause the patch to fall off), where it remains for one week before it is replaced with a new patch, in a new place on the body. As with birth control pills, most users will have one hormone-free week in the cycle, so for one week they don't wear a patch, but are protected from pregnancy during that week as they are when the patches are worn during the other three weeks.

Where and how do you get it?

The patch is available via prescription from your doctor, gynecologist, or sexual health clinic, and then with refills from your pharmacy.

Pros and Cons, Risks and Benefits

The patch is a good choice for women who want to use a hormonal contraceptive, but who have trouble remembering pills every day, and don't want to commit to a longer, less reversible form of hormonal contraception like Depo-Provera (see page 257). Patches are generally very resilient, and can be worn during bathing or showers.

However, if a patch user is late applying a new patch, she won't be effectively protected for that week. That is also the case if a patch falls off and stays off for a day.

Some people experience skin reactions to the patch. If a woman is trying to hide that she's using birth control, the patch may not be ideal. In addition, the patch has been shown to be slightly less effective for women who weigh more than 198 pounds.

Recently, it has also been suggested that the patch presents a risk of stroke higher than that of the birth control pill; fatality from any hormonal contraception method is extremely rare, but it is always something to consider when choosing a method.

Lunelle (Monthly Injection)

Effectiveness with perfect use: less than 1/100 or more than 99% effective

Effectiveness with typical use: less than 1/100 or more than 99% effective

Cost: $$, including cost of exam and office visits

What is it, and how does it work?

Lunelle is a combination hormonal contraceptive that is injected once each month. It contains estrogen and progestin, the same hormones found in combination pills. It's a good middle ground for those who want to use a hormonal method, but who have a hard time keeping to a regular schedule of pills or patches, and who do not want to commit to a longer-term hormonal method like Depo-Provera or an implant.

Where and how do you get it?

Your doctor, gynecologist, or sexual health clinician can prescribe Lunelle and inject it in their office. Some pharmacies can also handle giving the injections.

Pros and cons, risks and benefits

The big con is that a user cannot be late in getting her injections monthly, for Lunelle to be effective. So, if getting to the doctor or clinic once a month, without fail—and having the money to afford to— seems at all challenging, Lunelle won't be a good choice. Irregular vaginal bleeding is also a commonly reported problem with Lunelle, as are weight gain and water retention. Lunelle carries the same risks as other hormonal methods.

Pros include the fact that Lunelle is a very private method, in that no one will see your injections, as they might barrier methods or pills; it doesn't interrupt sex; and, as long as injections are received on time, it's foolproof from the user end.

Depo-Provera (Quarterly Injection)

Effectiveness with perfect use: less than 1/100 or more than 99% effective.

Effectiveness with typical use: less than 1/100 or more than 99% effective.

Cost: Around $$, including cost of exam and office visits

What is it, and how does it work?

Depo-Provera is an injection of the hormone progesterone only (no estrogen) that is given by a healthcare professional every three months, four times each year. It works in the same way birth control pills do.

Where and how do I get it?

Depo-Provera is available from your general doctor, gynecologist, or sexual health clinician.

Pros and Cons, Risks and Benefits

Depo has been shown in some studies to present higher risks of bone loss than other methods, so it is not advised for adolescent women, or young women who have not finished their growth. (For this reason, it's also advised that women of any age using Depo be sure to take a daily calcium supplement.)

For women who have finished growing, Depo is a good choice if they want a really low-maintenance method they don't have to worry about remembering about too often. Depo also works within just twenty-four hours of the injection. For women who can't take hormonal contraceptives with estrogen, such as Lunelle, Depo-Provera may be a good option. Like Lunelle, it also affords the user a high level of privacy in use, and is pretty goof-proof as long as injections are obtained on time every three months.

Depo is often best for users who already know that hormonal contraceptives work well for them, in general, without unwanted side effects, because once Depo has been injected, it's in the body for months, no matter what. If a woman has unpleasant side effects from Depo, such as constant spotting or bleeding, headaches, weight gain, or depression, she's stuck with them for some time, especially since it can take as many as eight months after the last injection for the body to clear itself of the Depo.

It's not unusual while on Depo-Provera to have extremely light bleeding or stop monthly flow altogether, which may be a benefit for some women, and a downside for others. Some women experience the opposite: persistent or constant bleeding or spotting, and around 70 percent of women report weight gain from Depo.

Implanon (Subdermal Implant, Once Every Three Years)

Effectiveness with perfect use: less than
     1/100 or more than 99% effective.
Effectiveness with typical use: less than
     1/100 or more than 99% effective.
Cost: Not yet available

What is it, and how does it work?

Implanon is a newly released, flexible plastic rod that is inserted by a healthcare professional under the skin of the arm. It works by releasing a hormone—etonogestrel—slowly, over time, into the body. Etonogestrel suppresses ovulation, thickening cervical mucus and altering the lining of the uterus to prevent pregnancy. Hormonal implants are the most effective method of hormonal contraception.

How and where do I get it?

Implants are only available via your doctor or gynecologist, who will insert the implant for you, and whom you will revisit after three years are up, for a new implant, if you wish to continue using the method. Your doctor or GYN is also the one would remove the implant at any time.

At the time of this writing, Implanon has not yet been studied in any women under the age of eighteen, so if you are a minor, it may not be an available or safe option for you.

Pros and Cons, Risks and Benefits

Unlike Depo, an implant can be removed immediately if a user just cannot deal with it, or no longer wants to. As with ceasing any hormonal method, it'll usually take your body at least a few cycles to get back to normal, but removal of the implant should cease many of the most intense side effects pretty quickly. It is very rare for patients to have any complications with insertion or removal.

As with Depo-Provera, women using an implant may have very unpredictable vaginal bleeding or spotting. And like any hormonal method, the implant has the usual possible side effects. The risk of ectopic pregnancy is also higher with Implanon than with other methods.

On the other hand, Implanon has the capability of making birth control a total no-brainer for up to three years. Like Depo, it does not contain estrogen, so is a hormonal option for women who cannot tolerate estrogens well, and it also works immediately, as long as it is inserted between days one and five of the menstrual cycle.

when on hormonal contraceptives. . . .

 IF AT any time, you are experiencing any of the following symptoms, it is very important that you call your doctor:

- Sharp chest pain, coughing blood, or shortness of breath
- Persistent pains in the legs or abdomen
- Severe headaches, dizziness, fainting, weakness, vision problems, numbness in the arms or legs, or vomiting
- Severe depression or mood changes
- Yellowing of the skin, lasting tiredness, loss of appetite
- Breast lumps or heavy vaginal bleeding

EMERGENCY CONTRACEPTION (EC)

While it's always best to use a reliable method of birth control, and preferably a backup, even reliable birth control sometimes fails. Sometimes things happen: Maybe we make dumb choices and use no birth control. Maybe we didn't have a say in the matter at all. Used to be that a hope and a prayer was all that was available in these situations. Now we have emergency contraception (and the hope and the prayer).

Emergency contraception can decrease the risk of pregnancy by 75–89 percent when used within 120 hours (five days) after a risk. It is inexpensive (usually between twenty-five and fifty dollars), carries very few side effects , and is easy to use.

There are two forms of EC currently available: emergency contraceptive pills (also known as the morning-after pill, the MAP, or Plan B) and the IUD.

The morning-after pill is the most common form of EC, and the easiest to use and obtain. It needs to be used within 120 hours after a risk, but the sooner it is taken, the more likely it is to be effective. ECPs are taken over two days: one pill the first day, another the second. The pills contain hormones—usually levonorgestrel—like standard birth control pills, but in a higher dose, and work the exact same way: by inhibiting or delaying ovulation, preventing fertilization of the egg, and/or inhibiting implantation of a fertilized egg. Its effectiveness and mode of operation have been verified by several studies, and reported in the *Population Council* and the *New York Times,* among other publications.

There are no known serious or long-term side effects from ECPs. Common side effects—which can last for several days, sometimes longer—are nausea or vomiting, headache, dizziness, breast tenderness, spotting, or fatigue. It's also common after taking ECPs for your period to begin a bit sooner or later than usual and be unpredictable for a couple of cycles. You may feel off-kilter or be a little out of sorts for a few weeks after using ECPs. Overall, most women taking ECPs do not need to stay at home in bed: you can go ahead with your normal daily life while taking them.

s.e.x.

is ec abortion?

ABORTION is the termination of a pregnancy. Emergency contraception helps prevent a pregnancy. EC is NOT abortion (nor are ECPs mifepristone, RU-486, or the medications used for medical abortion), because it can only work BEFORE pregnancy has occurred, just as birth control pills do, and it can only work if a pregnancy has not yet happened. It will not terminate a pregnancy if a woman is already pregnant. If that seems confusing, remember that pregnancy is not instant: it takes several days to occur, which is why EC can work sometimes even up to five days after a risk.

In many areas, ECPs can be obtained without a prescription: the United States now allows the sale of EC to women over the age of eighteen without a prescription. If you do not meet the age requirement, or live in an area where EC is not available over–the counter, you will need a prescription to obtain it. You can get that prescription by calling or seeing your regular doctor, gynecologist, general or sexual health clinician, or even by going into the emergency room or an urgent care center. It is common for an office visit to be required to get a prescription, and during that visit, your doctor or clinician will simply determine if you have had a pregnancy risk before prescribing (so be honest about what happened). If you are not current with your annual pelvic exams, they may suggest you have that exam at that time. If you ask, some clinics, doctors, or gynecologists may also be willing to give you a prescription for ECPs during your regular annual exam, to have on hand in advance, in case of emergency.

When you are given a prescription for ECPs, your doctor or clinician should give you clear directions for how to take them; if they do not, or you have additional questions, be sure to ask. You can also ask your pharmacist for additional information.

Some regular birth control pills can also be used as emergency contraception. To find out what pills to take in that instance, call the gynecologist, pharmacist, or sexual health clinician who prescribes your birth control pills for instructions, or see the Resources section of this book.

ECPs should not be used as regular contraception. There are no known dangers in doing so, but it's not as effective as many other methods of contraception, and would also be terribly expensive used regularly. ECPs also are not effective preventatively: you can't take them before sex for use as birth control.

Copper-T Intrauterine Device (IUD)

A copper IUD can also be used as emergency contraception, up to five days after a pregnancy risk, just like ECPs. As explained below, however, IUD use is not advised for younger women (especially those also at risk for STDs or STIs), and using ECPs is far simpler, less expensive, and less risky. However, using an IUD is more effective than ECPs, and if the IUD is right for you, it can also be left in place for as long as ten years to be used as ongoing birth control. For more information on IUDs, see page 262.

METHODS NOT GENERALLY RECOMMENDED FOR TEENS OR YOUNG ADULTS

Fertility Charting/Natural Family Planning (FAM)

Effectiveness with perfect use: 3/100 or
    97% effective
Effectiveness with typical use: 25/100 or
    75% effective
Cost: $

*Note: these effectiveness ratings are NOT specific to young
adult women, whose menstrual cycles have not become regular. These effectiveness ratings are for fully adult women.*

Natural family planning can be done by
several methods. The least effective is by just
counting the days in the cycle to estimate or
guess when ovulation might occur based
on average fertile times for all women
(sometimes called *the rhythm method*), or by
using online ovulation charts which only
count cycle days to estimate ovulation,
because there are no specific days during
which **every** woman is fertile or infertile.
Fertility varies among women: one woman
may be most fertile on the eleventh day of
her cycle, another on the sixteenth. Some
women even ovulate more than once per
cycle. During certain phases of the cycle—
namely, the final week of each cycle and
during menstruation—conception is generally *less* likely for most women. So, while
a majority of women are unlikely to be fertile just before and during menses, this
should never be assumed to be a given, and
there is a real risk of pregnancy any time a
woman has direct vaginal contact with
sperm, most commonly during heterosexual intercourse. There are times in a woman's
cycle (namely just around and during ovulation, when the mucus of the vagina is
most friendly toward sperm, and a fertile

ovum is available in the fallopian tube)
when she is *more* likely to become pregnant
than others, but she can technically get
pregnant because of live semen in the cervix
at nearly any time in her cycle, and as all of
our cycles differ, there is no one safe time for
everyone.

More effective is a combination of
observing and charting cervical mucus—
because its texture and consistency are different during different aspects of the
cycle—and taking basal temperature daily,
which fluctuates based on when a woman is
most fertile. There are also currently handheld calculators on the market that can be
used to chart and track fertility, and some
fertility Web sites do also use mucus and
basal temperatures to help a woman chart.

When used properly, FAM can be effective, and is a good choice for women whose
health, finances, or religion might prohibit
other methods—and/or for couples who
ARE prepared for a pregnancy. However, for
it to be effective as contraception, not only
does charting have to happen daily and consistently, but the results of the charting have
to be interpreted correctly, and unprotected
intercourse can ONLY occur on days
when, based on those results, a woman is
least likely to be fertile. Because FAM can
only give a woman information on when
ovulation probably occurred after her cycle
is finished, estimates are based on the previous cycle. For young women whose cycles
have not become regular yet, this isn't
workable.

FAM *can* be used very well as backup
birth control for younger women, if it is
used in this way: based on results, condoms
are used for times thought to be the least fertile, and then a woman *abstains from intercourse*

s.e.x.

completely during her most fertile times. And of course, young women can chart their fertility, even if they are not trying to use those results for birth control. Charting can allow a woman to become familiar enough with her cycles and their stages that when she's nervous about a possible pregnancy due to birth control failure, she may be able to recognize irregularities. Women using most hormonal methods cannot chart fertility, because if those methods are being used correctly, they are not ovulating.

IUDs

Effectiveness: less than
1/100 (perfect and
typical) or 99+% effective
Cost: Around $$

An IUD is a T-shaped device that contains either copper or the hormone progesterone. It is inserted into the uterus by a doctor or other healthcare professional. A string remains outside the cervix, which needs to be checked at least once each month to make sure the IUD is still in the proper place. Copper IUDs can remain in place for as long as ten years, progesterone IUDs for around one year. Strange as it seems for something that can work so well, doctors still aren't quite sure how the copper IUD works. It is generally thought that it prevents pregnancy because of an ionic reaction with uterine fluids, as well as by disrupting the movement of sperm. A hormonal IUD works by disrupting sperm and by thinning the uterine lining to impede implantation.

Typical side effects of the IUD include cramping during and a little after insertion, increased menstrual flow, and an increased risk of sexually transmitted infections. IUDs are generally not advised for women who have not previously been pregnant (whether they aborted the pregnancy or carried it to term), because it's often found that for those women, insertion is more painful, the device may not be as comfortable overall, and expulsion is more likely. Copper IUDS tend to cause longer and heavier bleeding and more cramping during periods.

Although IUDs are generally considered one of the most highly effective forms of birth control—both in perfect use and typical use, since once they're in, there are no pills to skip, or steps to forget—they're not for everyone. IUDs aren't advised for young women because the ideal user of an IUD needs to have a very low risk of STI transmission, because infections while an IUD is in place can result in severe health problems. Most sexually active teens have high risks of STIs due to both shorter relationships and a lack of safer sex practices, as well as incomplete cell development, which heightens STI risks, so teens generally aren't good candidates for IUDs.

The IUD may be a good choice for young women who:

▶ Have previously been pregnant
▶ Don't have those high risks
▶ Want a long-term method, but cannot take hormonal methods such as the pill or Depo-Provera
▶ AND are in a long-term relationship with decreased STI risks

Young women who do elect to use an IUD need to be VIGILANT about reducing their STI and infection risks.

Sterilization
(Female: Tubal Ligation)

Effectiveness: less than 1/100 or more
than 99% effective
Cost: $$$

Sterilization is highly effective, and it is per-
manent. The procedure works through a
safe surgery—often with a laparoscope, a
small telescope inserted through the navel—
that blocks the fallopian tubes by a cut or
seal so that they cannot reach the ovary and
be fertilized there. In some cases, tubal ster-
ilizations have been reversed, but that is not
often successful, and is incredibly expensive
to attempt, so the procedure should be con-
sidered permanent.

Because of this, it is generally only sug-
gested and/or offered to older adults who
have had plenty of time to be sure they do
not wish to ever have children. Some women
who have tubal ligation later regret it.

Sterilization (Male: Vasectomy)

Effectiveness: less than 1/100 or more
than 99% effective
Cost: $$$

Male sterilization is also highly effective,
although slightly less so than female sterilization, since some men who have had vasectomy performed do not realize it is not
immediately effective. It generally takes
around twenty ejaculations or so before the
body is rid of sperm, so a backup method
needs to be used for a little while after the
procedure until it is fully effective. In some
cases a vasectomy can be reversed, but not
always, and reversal is very costly.

Vasectomy is a safe surgical procedure
that blocks the vas deferens—the tubes
sperm pass through from the testicles to the
urethra during ejaculation—so that a man
still ejaculates, but his ejaculate no longer
contains sperm. Some men who have vasec-
tomies later regret their decision.

METHODS THAT SUCK (OR JUST REALLY SHOULDN'T BE CALLED BIRTH CONTROL)

Some methods just don't work at all, don't
work well enough to be relied upon, or are
just too risky to be worth it.

▶ **Withdrawal:** Also known as "pulling
out," withdrawal means that a man has
unprotected intercourse, but with-
draws (pulls out of the vagina) before
ejaculating. It is about 72 percent
effective, tops, and is one of the methods known to be far less effective for
teens and young adults.

Besides the possibility of sperm in
pre-ejaculate, most men—especially
younger men—can have a pretty hard
time anticipating when exactly ejaculation is beginning. They may withdraw after it's already begun, or get so
caught up in the feeling of orgasm
that they forget to do it altogether. As
is probably obvious, withdrawal also
offers no protection again STIs. It
stands to reason that during the baby
boom in the United States, the period
of the twentieth century when there
were more births than at any other
time—withdrawal was what a majority of people were using for birth control. Perhaps not coincidentally
(though other social factors were also

at play), the baby boom ended at about the same time as the advent of the birth control pill.

▶ **Chance:** Using no birth control at all puts women at an incredibly high risk of pregnancy. Within just one year of unprotected intercourse, the vast majority of young women will become pregnant, around 85 out of every 100, according to the World Health Organization. Having unprotected intercourse during your period isn't effective, either.

▶ **Douching or vaginal washing:** You can't rinse or wash sperm out of your body, because they are mighty fast, and water or soap can't make their way into the cervix.

▪ IT DOESN'T TAKE A VILLAGE . . . ▪ BUT SOMETIMES IT'S AWFULLY NICE TO HAVE ONE:
Birth Control Discussion with Partners and Parents

Anyone who needs birth control has at least one other person intimately involved in that need, so which method to use is often not a decision made solely by one person—and when responsibility for birth control is shared, it's always more effective. Ultimately, since the vast majority of birth control methods are female-directed, and because the person who could become pregnant carries the greatest risk of any reproductive choices, *the final choice on what to use should lie with the woman involved.* Single women who are not currently in relationships, and/or may have more casual sex partners, may make their birth control choices completely independent of anyone else.

If you're a minor, or a young adult living with your parents, financially dependent on them, or covered by their health insurance, some birth control options may also involve your folks. If you're a woman currently in an opposite-sex relationship, you and your partner may want to agree on a given method, especially if it requires his participation in using it correctly, and/or you may want to split the cost of birth control. If you're hooking up casually, birth control discussion should still be taking place. If you're male, you may want to help by paying for part of your partner's birth control method, helping her research which methods are best for both of you, and, in some situations, take responsibility for the burden of providing and insisting on birth control, if you don't want to become a father.

With every aspect of sex, discussion and communication are key to healthy, smart sexual choices and relationships—and birth control is certainly no exception.

DISCUSSION WITH PARTNERS

If you're female, the responsibility of birth control often largely lies with you. Since most methods of birth control go in your body, since you are the one who will need to deal with taking them, as well as any side effects, and you are the one who may become pregnant, it's **best** that you be the most responsible for doing what is best for you.

If you do currently have a sex partner, whether it's long-term or very casual, then you also have a partner to discuss birth control with.

With a casual partner:

▶ Discussion may be as simple as plainly stating what method you do use, and if it is condoms or involves backing up with condoms, making clear that you expect and require condom use with sex

▶ Discussion may also involve stating what choice you would make in regard to an accidental pregnancy, should your method or methods fail.

▶ If you're only using condoms and a casual partner refuses to, discussion will also involve drawing a line and opting out of sex with a risk of pregnancy with him. (Though it's safe to assume that a guy probably carries heavy STI risks if he refuses to use condoms, so you may want to opt out of sexual activity with him altogether.)

With longer-term or more committed partnerships:

▶ Discussions about birth control may be more involved. It's fair and sound to share birth control expenses or logistics, for instance. If you can't afford birth control all by yourself, or feel those expenses should be shared, this may be a requirement of your sexual partnership. Making it clear that one partner shouldn't always be responsible for reminders about birth control, or sexual policing when it comes to contraception, is also wise. And if you can't afford it and your partner can't afford to contribute, either, it may mean making plans to become sexually active at a later date, when you both can afford it.

▶ You may use more than one method over time, or tailor what you use more jointly, based on discussions about personal preferences, changing safer sex

habits, or greater desire or trust for shared responsibility.

If you're using nothing but condoms for birth control, with any sort of partner, a bit more negotiation and discussion is sometimes involved. You may have to step up in terms of insisting on it, reminding your partner when to put a condom on, or making sure you have plenty of them, and lubricant, on hand. If a partner complains about discomfort, you may have to experiment with different brands or types a bit until you find a condom that works. The same goes for a shared method such as abstinence or natural family planning, which requires your partner to abstain from sex completely or periodically, in order to be effective.

Sometimes, male partners may tell you that one given method of birth control is what they want to use most, even though it's really a method YOU will be using, taking, and largely responsible for. Let's say your boyfriend feels the pill is the best choice for both of you. You can research it and look into it, and weigh all the issues with it. You may come to an agreement on that. Or you may not. If you feel differently, you can certainly explain why (you don't want to take a pill every day, you don't like the side effects or health risks), but you shouldn't be engaging in huge arguments about it, because it's YOUR body it's all going in, not his. If he isn't comfortable with sex using any method but the one he has suggested—or doesn't want to use birth control at all—then he has the power to opt out of sex with you, and you with him. That's not a fun situation to be in, but being sexually active with a partner when you don't agree on a birth control method is a really bad idea. A sound golden rule is this: Whichever partner is more at risk for side effects and other consequences, or shouldering the most responsibility for birth control, gets the final say.

The same goes double for when you don't agree on using birth control at all. If a partner of any gender just plain refuses to use birth control, when either of you is not willing or prepared to deal with a pregnancy, then the only smart thing for you to do is flatly refuse to have sex with that person. Too, some young women who are hell-bent on becoming pregnant, or who just aren't comfortable discussing all these issues yet, are dishonest with their male partners about birth control—intentionally or by omission. Just as it wouldn't be at all okay for a male partner to force you into becoming pregnant (or for men as a ruling class to do so to women), it's equally not okay to manipulate a guy into becoming a parent when he doesn't want to in any way. Saying you're on the pill when you're not, or purposefully sabotaging birth control methods—by not taking your pills, for instance, or by popping holes in barrier methods—is both nonconsensual and seriously unfair. Even trying to convince a male partner to take risks he doesn't want to, or to go without birth control when he isn't ready or willing, just isn't okay. If you want to go without birth control, or talk about parenting, then talk about it responsibly and fairly, with respect and honesty, with the other person who'd wind up as a parent.

If the issue is just a simple lack of comfort with discussing birth control at all, either reevalute your readiness, and take a step back from sex until you *can* discuss it— or, if your reticence is due to feeling pressured or controlled by a partner, take a step back from *them*.

birth control issues to discuss with partners (the short list)

- **Effectiveness, ease of use, and availability:** Does what you both want work well? Can one or both of you easily access and use the method? Are both of you open to trying different methods?
- **Birth control backup:** Do you need it or want it? If so, what combined methods will you use?
- **Responsibility:** Whose is it? How will you work it together without unduly burdening one partner? How will you both pay for it?
- **Failure:** If birth control failed, what would both of you want to do? Are you in agreement on that? How might you handle it?

HEY, BOYFRIEND! MALE REPRODUCTIVE CHOICES

If you're a guy with a female partner, even though you're not the one who can become pregnant, you still get choices, and you should participate in birth control use and responsibility just as much as your female partner. Understand that many methods, such as hormonal birth control like the pill or Depo-Provera, which are used solely by women, carry risks and side effects (and they don't offer any STI protection). So, while it may seem to you that a given method is best and easiest for you, your partner may not feel the same way, since she's the one who needs to live with it, short- and long-term. For instance, she's the one who may have a diminished sex drive or less natural lubrication because of the pill, and the one who will need to remember to take it at the same time every day. If

s.e.x.

a given method seems like a good choice to you, by all means, bring it up for discussion, but know that the choice is primarily hers to make, and she's the best one to make it.

It might be difficult for you to understand the weight of birth control use for women, to comprehend how much a woman has to think about it, how much real estate it takes up in her head. However, it's not unlike safer sex practices, which you can know plenty about. Think about the flip-flopping that might sometimes go round in your head when you're making those choices—

*Do I **really** need to use a condom for oral sex?*

Can I get away with not using one for intercourse just this once?

Didn't I hear her ex cheated—what if she got a disease from him?

When do I ask her about it? How will she react?

Do I even have condoms with me tonight?

—the strong desire to avoid an STI, and even how sometimes, it just feels tiresome, or kills your buzz, to have to bring worries and practical issues to bed with you. Your girlfriend shoulders all that, like you, **and** all of those sorts of issues when it comes to pregnancy and birth control.

If you're in a long-term or committed sexual partnership with a woman, it's a great idea to suggest helping to shoulder aspects of birth control you can contribute to, like paying for it, helping with transportation to OB/GYN visits, or playing your part when it comes to using a given method.

It may also happen that you someday have a partner who isn't responsible about her part in birth control, or who wishes to become pregnant when you really don't wish to be involved in that. In those situations, the burden of birth control, via

condoms—or by vetoing sex if you don't agree with her about readiness for parenthood—may lie solely with you, and you have every right to insist that your OWN choices be respected. It's also completely okay for you to insist on backup via condom use, if you need or want it for your own security, even if your partner has told you she already uses an additional method. Of course, if you have any reason to believe you can't trust your partner to be honest about the method she's using, the best tack is not to sexually partner with her at all: trust is a pretty important and vital part of a healthy sexual partnership.

 SINCE you're unlikely to find a doctor who will advocate or allow vasectomy for young men, the only method you can use that is directed by you, or reliant upon you, is condom use. Beyond safer sex issues, condom use makes for an excellent birth control backup for any other method, so insisting on it and being in charge of that aspect of birth control can be an important role for you.

On the other hand, you may feel ready for parenthood when your female partner doesn't, or you may wish not to worry about birth control altogether. In other words, it may be you thinking about the birth control sabotage or behaving irresponsibly. Thing is . . . well, let's not tiptoe. That's not okay. If you're ready for sexual partnership, you need to also be ready to deal with birth control and to respect your partner's wishes when it comes to parenthood and birth control options. If you have a partner who wants to use condoms as birth control, and you just don't, then you

s.e.x.

need to just opt out of sex with her, rather than fighting or arguing about it.

You should be just as responsible for birth control as your partner is. No matter what kind of sexual relationship you're in, you still need to be bringing your half of birth control responsibility to the table, rather than assuming that your female partner is or must be solely responsible for taking care of it. That's not just an ethical issue, it's a practical one: if you don't, and a pregnancy does occur, your female partner can hold you legally responsible should she see a pregnancy through to term. So, even though it may feel like it's not your issue, and you do have limited choices in the matter, a good deal of responsibility does still lie with you, and to be a good partner, you need to step up and take charge of the aspects you can control.

DISCUSSIONS WITH PARENTS

If you're still a minor, are living at home, or are dependent on your parents financially (even just for healthcare), they may be people you've got to discuss all or some aspects of birth control with, too.

While some parents may not be especially jazzed that their teens are sexually active, most are going to be supportive of their teens having sex responsibly, which certainly includes using birth control for those with pregnancy risks. Some parents are even willing to help pay for those methods, or make sure you're able to obtain them.

Some parents will NOT be willing to pay for birth control methods and will insist that you're on your own with that. That's pretty fair: after all, if you're really ready for

partnered sex, some of that readiness is about the ability to be independently responsible for all aspects of sex, including paying for essentials yourself. Or, your parents may be willing to help, but with certain conditions attached, so you may have to do some negotiating with them, about with whom, where, when, or in what situations you're sexually active, about what methods you use, or about who will shoulder responsibility, financial and otherwise, should your birth control fail.

As in any other negotiations with parents about sex, it's smart not to be in a huge hurry or bring a lot of entitlement to the table. Be prepared to be cool and calm, and for loaded issues like birth control to take a few discussions, with plenty of time for both you and your folks to think things over and process, in between. Be prepared to make some compromises—understand that it's possible you may have to agree to disagree, or may be allowed to use a given method, but without their financial or emotional support.

what doesn't work, or really good ways to guarantee your folks won't support your birth control choices

- *"If you don't get it for me/pay for it, I'll get pregnant."* I really hope you're not saying this (especially after all that talk about personal responsibility in choosing to be sexually active). Blackmail of any sort is never very effective, especially when the one who'd pay for it most is the person threatening it. A better way of addressing that issue is to say *"I am choosing to be sexually active because I feel I'm ready, and I'm asking for your help* with birth control because I want to do this responsibly and not become pregnant."

- **"But you didn't use it, and see, you had me!"** Rubbing parents' faces in their own mistakes is a fine way to piss them off and make them really upset—not a good way to come to an agreement or get an endorsement. A better bet may be: *"I know that you had an accidental pregnancy, and I understand, but I don't want the same for myself, and I know I can avoid that by using reliable birth control."*

- **"Then I'll just get it myself and you'll never know."** The only thing this is good for is to pretty much guarantee your parents will henceforth not trust you, and your social and sexual life will suffer for it. This might be a better approach: *"I really want to be able to be honest with you about this: I hate being tempted to lie or hide things from you."*

- **"But <insert friend's name here>'s mother got it for HER."** Y'all know the drill on this one, and probably even know what your parent is likely to say about cliffs and friends jumping off them. Every parent gets to make their own parenting choices, based on what they feel is best for them, their family, and their individual child. If you really feel your friend's parent is making better choices, you might instead ask your parent if they would be willing to talk to that parent about why they made the choice they did First make clear—respectfully—that you understand they have their own opinions, but you would just like it if they could maybe take a listen to a different perspective and think about it.

There's a theme here you might have picked up on, whether you're discussing this issue with partners or parents, and that's honest, patient communication. It's certainly not always easy, especially with stuff as loaded as this is, but not only is being able to do that an important part of sexual readiness overall, it's also going to make your whole sexual life a lot easier and a whole lot better, now AND later. Birth control isn't the only issue where that comes in handy, but it's a biggie.

We tend to only think about reproductive choice in terms of what we do when a pregnancy has occurred, but birth control, choosing when and if we will become pregnant, is also reproductive choice—the most important one—and one that benefits from the support of everyone involved.

12

oh, baby!
conception, pregnancy,
and pregnancy options

IF A PREGNANCY has occurred, there are three basic choices to manage it: *parenthood, abortion, or adoption,* all of which are equally viable, legal, and valid choices, and any of which may be the best choice for a woman at a given time—and none of which is ever an easy choice to make.

Teen pregnancies account for about 25 percent of all accidental or unplanned pregnancies, and *the other 75 percent,* the great majority, *occur among legal adults of all ages.* So, no matter one's age, it's safe to say that if you're heterosexually active—even if you're not having intercourse, or not having intercourse yet, even if you're not the one who could become pregnant—it's wise to inform yourself about reproduction, pregnancy, and parenting, and to be familiar with all of the reproductive options, and their practical realities, in advance.

how long have you got to decide?

 FOR such a big choice, there isn't much time to make it, once a pregnancy has occurred:

■ A woman who chooses abortion has around **six weeks to three months** after pregnancy occurs before she is outside the window for safe, legal abortion. The later that choice is made, the fewer the options available, and the more traumatic or risky an abortion may become.

■ A woman who chooses pregnancy and parenting has around **two to four weeks after the first missed period** before needing to seek out prenatal care and start self-care for a healthy pregnancy for herself and her child. This is especially vital for very young women. The main reason there are higher physical risks, to mother and child both, with pregnancy in younger women is not physiological, but behavioral: lack of prenatal care, inadequate nutrition, lack of needed weight gain, and failure to make needed changes to some lifestyle factors (quitting drinking or recreational drug use, for example). Ideally, prenatal care should begin before pregnancy.

- A woman who chooses adoption can make that decision before or after the child is born. But to best secure a home for a child, make open adoption arrangements, and/or have prenatal care, childbirth costs, or living expenses during pregnancy paid for, it's best to start contacting adoption agencies and pursuing avenues to adoption **as soon as possible**. (However, the mother will still have the right to rescind her decision to give the child up for adoption up until the birth of her child.)

Obviously, if you have same-sex partners, you don't have to worry about accidental pregnancy. For gay and lesbian folks who do someday want children, for those with opposite-sex partners, and for any of us, this information is essential: after all, even if we can't become pregnant or never become pregnant, the vast majority of us will know someone else who does. Besides, we should all have a good idea of why our mothers can say *"I brought you INTO this world!"* with so much intensity.

(It should go without saying that if you're male and opposite-sex partnered, you need to read this.)

▪ HOW DO YOU TELL IF YOU'RE ▪ PREGNANT?

By taking a pregnancy test. There is no other way to know for sure early enough in the game to adequately consider the options.

Early symptoms, which aren't reliable to determine pregnancy, usually don't occur until at least a few weeks have passed, and most typically, after the first month. Some early symptoms can include: sore or tingly breasts, a missed period, general nausea, a feeling of tiredness, increased appetite, and/or having to urinate more often. However, since some of these symptoms can also be caused by stress, PMS, infections, or other illness, or can even take place psychosomatically (in your head), symptoms alone aren't sound to go by.

HPTs
Home pregnancy tests (HPTs) work by measuring for a hormone called hCG (human chorionic gonadotropin), which is secreted as soon as ten days after conception is complete. The most accurate results will be found at least two weeks after a risk, or at the first late or skipped period.

A home pregnancy test can be used either after a first missed period, or even as early as ten days from the suspected risk of pregnancy. A home test should be repeated one week later if it shows a negative result, and a period still hasn't arrived. The most reliable test is done by a doctor or clinician,

S.E.X.

so if a test shows a positive, a visit to a doctor or a clinic should be scheduled to verify the results. While home pregnancy tests are generally very reliable, positives should be verified professionally.

Some tests are more sensitive than others. You can tell which are more sensitive by looking at the box: those that say they are sensitive to a level of 20 mIU/ml (that'd be twenty milliinternational units of hCG per milliliter) are more sensitive or reliable than those that say they are sensitive at a level of 50 mIU/ml.

False positives are very rare. They may occur in instances where fertilization or conception have occurred, but will not continue to a full pregnancy; bear in mind that as many as half of all fertilizations will not complete to conception. They may also occur with women taking any drugs that contain hCG, such as fertility drugs. Hormonal birth control does NOT contain hCG. False negatives are more common, often because a test is taken too early, or read or taken incorrectly.

Blood tests can often detect hCG slightly earlier than home urine tests, so if the waiting is crazymaking, a blood test can be done as soon as six to eight days after a risk.

▪ REPRODUCTIVE OPTIONS: ▪
Parenting, Adoption, and Abortion

PARENTHOOD AND PREGNANCY

Pregnancy and Delivery Basics

For a healthy pregnancy, a woman will need regular prenatal care as well as good nutrition, plenty of rest and activity, reduced stresses, emotional support, and the practical and financial means to obtain all of those things. For a healthy pregnancy, childbirth, and child, teen or young adult mothers will need to be *more* dedicated to these issues than older women, not less.

If you or your partner is pregnant and thinking about bringing a pregnancy to term:

▶ Smoking, drinking, and recreational drug use need to be stopped, ASAP. A child's health may also be compromised if a woman was doing any of those things shortly before pregnancy or when she became pregnant, so a pregnant woman with a recent history of smoking, drinking, or doing drugs will need to be honest with her doctor and herself. Partners of pregnant women who do any of these things and plan to stick around should quit, either because of the way some of those habits can indirectly affect mother or child, or out of support and responsibility.

▶ If a pregnant woman has an eating disorder or chronically diets, that should be addressed with a doctor, because for a healthy child and pregnancy, gaining some weight is important, especially for younger women.

▶ It is also vital to practice safer sex if you're sexually active while pregnant, because STIs can create big health risks for a child during pregnancy and at birth, and young adult women are more susceptible to STIs.

Woman's Work

Labor and childbirth consist of three different stages: (1) labor (subdivided into early or latent labor, active labor, and a transitional

272

s.e.x.

Within the first few months of pregnancy—the first trimester—a woman may experience:

- Feeling more tired than usual
- General nausea or morning sickness
- Frequent urination, gas, constipation, and indigestion
- Physical and emotional symptoms similar to PMS

Often, after the first few months, emotional issues such as feeling irritable, unstable, or torn may pass, and into the second trimester, many women begin feeling better about being pregnant than they were in the first trimester, although hormonal changes and new frustrations—like not fitting into clothes, feelings about weight gain, fears and doubts, and other issues—may still cause moods to be erratic. Appetite will increase, and there may be food cravings as well as food aversions. Weight gain should also have begun by now, and *you will need to make a sincere effort to gain weight* during the rest of the pregnancy.

Once into the second trimester, many of the symptoms from the first few months will continue, and a woman may also experience:

- Greater fatigue or dizziness
- The pregnancy showing
- Swelling of the ankles and feet
- Changes in vaginal discharge, skin, and hair
- Enlarging breasts
- Headaches or sinus symptoms
- Backaches

Into the second trimester, fetal movement a woman can feel will also begin and increase through the months.

In the last few months of pregnancy, the third trimester, many of the symptoms from previous months will continue, and in addition, women will usually experience:

- Heavier vaginal discharges
- More intense back and body aches
- Some breast leaking
- Hemorrhoids
- Greater fetal movement
- Trouble sleeping
- Occasional contractions
- Shortness of breath
- Varicose veins
- Clumsiness
- Emotional issues, such as feeling tired of being pregnant, or worries about childbirth or parenting

phase), (2) childbirth or delivery, and (3) delivery of the placenta, or afterbirth. The whole process takes around fifteen to twenty-four hours, on average, for first-timers.

Early labor is the longest stage of labor and delivery, lasting many hours or even a couple of days, but is also the least intense. When short contractions—which feel like very intense menstrual cramps—start to occur within twenty to thirty minutes of one another over a period of a few hours, and the lapse between them gets progressively shorter, early labor has begun. Before that time, usually over a period of days, the cervix has been slowly thinning out (effacement) and dilating (opening), to about three centimeters.

When contractions are a few minutes apart and become stronger, **active labor** has begun, and it generally lasts a few hours. The transitional phase is usually the most difficult and tiring part of labor for most women: contractions are intense, longer and very close together. The cervix completes dilating during this phase, opening to around ten centimeters to be ready for delivery. Women in the transition phase may feel heavy pressure on the back, rectum, and bladder; body temperature tends to fluctuate erratically; and cramps, nausea, chills, shakes, and an overall feeling of exhaustion and/or serious moodiness or irritability are common and normal. Vomiting or bloody discharge may also occur.

When **delivery** begins, many women get a second wind, and are glad to be able to start pushing (if you bear down as you might when pushing out a bowel movement, you can get a vague idea of what pushing is like, sans baby). Is it painful? Pretty much always, to varying degrees. But pain during delivery is also often exacerbated by other factors—by being alone, if that isn't desired; by certain hospital environments or birthing approaches; by lack of preparation or knowledge of what's happening; by stress or anxiety, embarrassment, shame, or fear; and most of all, by the expectation of a lot of pain. So, it is often more painful for plenty of women than it should be, and the environment a woman is in, and her state of mind, count for an awful lot.

Midwifery

Before we had OB/GYNs, we had midwives; through most of human history, women have helped other women deliver their babies and sustain healthy pregnancies. Most of the practices Western doctors use today for childbirth are based on techniques women developed over the centuries through active learning. You can find references to midwives in the Old Testament. Midwives are still around today; you can see a midwife privately if you are pregnant, and some hospitals and healthcare systems even include midwifery among their available services, so ask your doctor or insurance provider about it. Too, if you're a young pregnant woman or teen who is struggling to afford or procure prenatal and delivery care—or dealing with discrimination in your prenatal care due to your age—midwives are often incredibly generous with their help and services for young women in need. For a few places to find a midwife, see the Resources section.

s.e.x.

With a vaginal birth, the doctor, midwife, or birthing coach or partner will aid with delivery and help the mother to keep pushing and stay as energized but relaxed as possible. While typical hospital deliveries have had women lying down, many are starting to catch on and adapt that posture to more natural positions that are helped by gravity, like partially sitting or squatting. When the baby begins to "crown," or its head first appears at the perineum, the birthing partner, midwife, or doctor will help ease the baby out of the vaginal canal as the mother continues pushing, until the entire infant is through the birth canal. The umbilical cord may be clamped, cut, or left in place until after the afterbirth has been delivered, and the infant will be given to the mother to hold, in most instances. Brand-new babies, even when cleaned off, rarely look like newborns in the movies: most retain a slightly wooly body hair called the *lanugo,* and they often look a little blue and pretty oddly shaped, including the head, which sometimes even looks conelike.

Vaginal delivery in full lasts an hour or two on average, but sometimes as little as fifteen minutes or as long as a few hours, especially if there are complications during birth.

The final stage of labor is the ***delivery of the placenta,*** or afterbirth—the tissue mass that provided nourishment for the infant during pregnancy. After delivery, the uterus will begin to contract again, and the mother will need to push just one or a few more times to expel the placenta. This generally takes five to ten minutes.

There aren't hard and fast rules on what a woman feels emotionally during labor and delivery. Most women are very glad when labor and delivery are over, not just because the exhausting process is complete and they can rest, but because for most, experiencing the whole process and giving birth to a child—and seeing their child—is seriously satisfying. But it's also normal for just-finished new moms to feel depressed or overwhelmed, or just plain tired.

C-Sections

A CESAREAN section—or c-section—is a surgical birth procedure in which an incision is made in a woman's abdomen and uterus to deliver a baby. A woman is given local anesthetic for a c-section, and the doctor removes the baby via the incisions.

Some women schedule c-sections, or plan on them in advance; other times they are done because of multiple births or vaginal birth complications. C-sections are also usually done with HIV-positive mothers, or mothers with genital herpes sores active during labor. Because it involves surgery, it carries more risks to a mother. Rates of cesareans are at a record high, and while there are good reasons for some women to have a c-section, many women's advocates, midwives, pregnancy and natural childbirth activists, and medical organizations such as the Kaiser Foundation have voiced concern about c-sections being done needlessly, or without enough—or accurate—information about options and risks to the mother.

If you're pregnant and planning to deliver, talk to your doctor or midwife in advance about your birthing options, and get the facts if you're thinking about a c-section delivery, so that you can make an informed choice.

It takes a few days to a few months after delivery for physical and emotional aftereffects to wear off. At first, mothers may experience physical effects like cramps, discharge

s.e.x.

(including *lochia*, postpartum bleeding that generally lasts for four to six weeks), exhaustion, and overall genital and breast soreness or discomfort A wide range of fluctuating emotions can occur, including postpartum depression (which can be a major long-term problem for as many as 25 percent of all mothers) and wild elation, and often swings between the two, as well as decreased libido. Within about six weeks, most women will return to feeling normal (albeit "normal" in the way that now includes life with a brand-new infant and a completely changed life).

Miscarriage: What It Is and Why It Happens

By medical definition, a miscarriage, or "spontaneous abortion," is a pregnancy that naturally (all by itself) ends before twenty weeks—the fifth month—of pregnancy. Experts believe that as many as 50 percent of all fertilizations or conceptions do NOT result in a viable pregnancy. Often, miscarriage occurs so early that women don't even know they've had one, or that they were even pregnant in the first place. Many of those incredibly early miscarriages aren't even technically considered miscarriages, but rather pregnancies that didn't complete.

It's estimated that of women who have become "fully" pregnant and know of their pregnancies, around 15–20 percent will miscarry. Most miscarriages are not preventable once pregnancy has taken place, and occur when the body is simply unable to sustain a healthy pregnancy. Miscarriage is the body's natural way to safeguard against an embryo or fetus that will be stillborn, deformed, or unhealthy, or a pregnancy that will put a mother's health at risk. Some factors that increase the possibility of miscarriage are:

▶ Lack of full sexual maturity or growth
▶ Poor nutrition
▶ Cigarette, drug, or alcohol use
▶ Hormonal imbalances
▶ Sexually transmitted infections or conditions
▶ Other reproductive or general medical conditions, like PCOS, uterine malformation, fibroids, lupus, congenital heart disease, severe kidney disease, diabetes, thyroid disease, or exposure to environmental hazards or radiation
▶ Stress or injury from sexual or domestic abuse

Symptoms

Early miscarriage is most common, and accounts for about 75 percent of all miscarriages. *Very* early miscarriage is rarely even noticed, nor does it have any visible symptoms, although some spotting or mild cramping may occur, and those are often mistaken for a period. You often can't have a very early miscarriage verified, so it's one of those situations where you simply may never know if you did or you didn't.

When miscarriage occurs after the first few weeks and is usually noticeable, symptoms often include mild to severe pelvic and abdominal cramps that may persist for more than a day, vaginal bleeding or spotting, sometimes including a passage of tissue from within the vagina, or a clear fluid drainage.

Early miscarriage rarely requires prompt medical attention or hospitalization. For most women, it is *physically* no more traumatic or intense than a period, if that. It's smart to see your doctor or gynecologist after a suspected miscarriage, however, to

s.e.x.

check up on your health and be sure you did fully miscarry. If, however, very heavy bleeding occurs or spotting lasts more than a week, if large clots are passed or a foul-smelling discharge is present, or if cramps are severe or a fever develops, seek medical attention.

No matter HOW a woman may have felt about a pregnancy, whether it was planned or unintentional, it is normal to experience feelings of grief, regret, guilt, and loss after miscarriage (and it's also normal not to feel upset). These feelings can be tricky when you're a young adult: friends, family, or partners may not have been happy you were pregnant in the first place, and may not be sympathetic. For women of all ages, grief and upset after miscarriage is usually worse than it might be, because of a lack of support or understanding from those around them, so seeking out support and emotional self-care is key.

---

teen pregnancy: not always an accident

A GOOD many teen pregnancies—about one in five—*are* intended or planned. According to Kristen Luker, in *Dubious Conceptions: The Politics of Teenage Pregnancy,* one reason that sex education hasn't reduced teen pregnancy rates as much as expected is that some young adults know full well what birth control is and how and when to use it, but *choose* not to, sometimes because they *want* to become pregnant.

In many cases, young women want to become pregnant for the same reasonable motivations older women have: they like and want children, want to be mothers, it feels right for them to do so, and/or they want to parent with the partner they're

with now. Sometimes, as with older women, the reasons aren't so great or responsible: to try to cement or force continuation of a relationship, to prove adulthood or sexual development, to try to fill emotional voids or quell loneliness, and/or to get attention they want but aren't receiving.

Maybe one of your goals in life is to be a mother, and there isn't a thing in the world that's wrong with that, as long as you understand that it isn't your only option, even if it seems that way. Even if you know that, and parenting is what you want, it'll keep. While few people will ever reasonably suggest that pregnancy and parenting are easy, both are easier when the woman involved is as prepared as she can be, physically, emotionally, financially, and practically. Since a BIG part of parenting is patience, if you just don't feel that you have the patience to wait to become pregnant and be a parent, chances are pretty good you also don't have the patience required to BE a parent.

There's no rule that teen mothers can't be good parents. Plenty of teen mothers ARE and have been good parents. But plenty of people who are or have been teen mothers will tell you that it would have been a whole lot easier for them to be better mothers, and happier people overall, if they'd waited, even just a few years.

Young Adult Parenting: Perils, Pitfalls, and Perks

Many people have the idea that they'll find a way to cope and can handle pregnancy and raising a child like a pro—sure that, for some reason, it'll be easier for them than it ever was for anyone before, even when they're totally unprepared. But more times than not, it ends up being more difficult than they imagine, especially for teens. That doesn't mean it's impossible to enjoy. Lots of young adults find parenting fulfilling, in spite of the challenges it brings. But wanting a child or loving a child isn't often enough preparation to ensure a healthy pregnancy—physically or emotionally—or readiness to parent well.

Teens and young adults CAN be good parents: as good as anyone else, of any age. There have always been many, many young adults who have been excellent parents, many who have *enjoyed* being parents and felt very good about the choice they made to be parents. If it's really what you want to do—and you're prepared to manage the realities of parenting—chances are good that you *can* do it and do it *well*.

So, if you're thinking about it, have a reality check, on the house.

You're 100 Percent Responsible for Your Child and Its Upbringing.

Sure, that means that the good stuff that happens, and all of your kid's accomplishments, are things you'll feel really proud to have had a hand in. But with responsibility comes accountability, something a lot of young people haven't yet had to deal with in any major way. In other words, if you are late to pick your kid up from day care, you're going to have to pay the late fees and deal with a bummed-out kid, and if you do it repeatedly, you may be asked to find another day-care center. The folks in charge aren't going to be real interested in whose fault it is, because it's your responsibility. If you have a partner who harms your child, you'll have to deal with both being and feeling responsible. If you make poor parenting choices, you and your kid have to live with them, as well as any long-term effects. You're also likely to be very emotionally invested in your child. So, when they're sick or unhappy, you're going to be scared and distracted. When you screw something up, you're likely to feel horrible about it. In many, many ways, your kids become your life. You're responsible and accountable for most of what your kid does, even through their teen years—legally, practically, and emotionally. Imagine the possibilities. All of them.

Those possibilities also include one parent NOT sticking around or actively parenting. That more often becomes a problem for women, but it can happen to men as well. And that leaves you not only dealing with child-rearing as a single parent, but also dealing with feelings of abandonment, betrayal, and heartbreak—at the same time you're trying to take care of your kid, or get through a pregnancy.

One reason choosing to be a parent is such a big deal is that you're not just making a choice for you, you're making choices for a person who can't make their own choices and who has to live with yours.

Parenting at a Young Age Can Be Really Lonely.

Young parents often feel incredibly isolated. You may (or may not) get plenty of attention, care, and company while you're pregnant, and in the first six months or so of your kid's life. But when all the showers and parties have passed, when the novelty of a cute baby has passed, a whole lot of young parents start to feel like they moved to Mars when they had kids. Many feel far more alone than they felt before they were parents.

Somebody to Love?

For a lot of women, one of the appeals of motherhood is the notion that someone—their child—will love them unconditionally.

But very often, especially once out of very early childhood, children DON'T behave as if they love their parents unconditionally. The unconditional love in a parent-child relationship is supposed to come from the parent, not the child.

Parenting Is Hard Work.

Just during your kid's first year of life, you can rest assured you'll have bags under your eyes the size of the Grand Canyon, you'll be pretty crabby, and your kid isn't going to say thank you for a couple of years. Postpartum depression—deep and sometimes debilitating depression after childbirth, which can sometimes last for months, during one of the most challenging stages of parenting—is common. Lactating and breastfeeding often hurts like the dickens. Babies often cry more than they gurgle cutely. Having to tend to someone's basic needs and functions literally 24/7—feeding, changing diapers, putting to sleep, entertaining—is exhausting, even with help, and always putting your own needs after theirs can make a parent feel like a walking bottle, rather than a person.

Kids Can Really Cramp Your Style.

You may be used to going out for a night with your friends, maybe needing to okay it with your folks, and come up with transportation and spending money. Now you'll need to find a reliable babysitter you feel safe with; try to afford extras when you often already can't pay for the basics; and reschedule things constantly because babies and kids tend to have schedules of their own that don't neatly coincide with yours. You may find that the things that are important to your friends aren't that important to you anymore—and that they're not very interested in what IS important to you, like your struggle to find good daycare, or the nights in a row you've spent with a colicky, screaming infant. Dating when you have a kid is difficult and often frustrating, and if you're co-parenting with a partner, you'll find that the two of you end up with very little alone time, and more challenges and conflicts in your relationship than you can shake a stick at. This is all the same stuff older people go through with parenting, but it's often harder when you are a young adult.

Juggling school, college, and/or work with a kid is also tricky, especially if you're single and young. It's hard to study when a baby is crying or a toddler decides to rip up your dissertation. Many schools do not make concessions for pregnant teens or mothers. Many employers aren't very understanding about letting you take time off because your kid is sick, or leave early to get to a day-care center before closing time. Even basic things you take for granted, like having the time to take a bath or shower, to take in a movie, to do your laundry, to talk on the phone with friends, or to sit down to eat a meal, will be compromised.

Kids Cost the Big Bucks.

Think the pregnancy test was expensive? Delivery alone—not counting prenatal care, or all the stuff you have to buy to prepare, like diapers and cribs—will probably cost around $10,000 for a normal, complication-free birth. In the first four years alone, raising a child often costs more than attending a four-year public college with NO financial assistance, grants, or scholarships whatsoever—something few people can afford. Children cost a LOT of money. Add their costs to the cost of taking care of yourself as well, and you can see why parents get so stressed out about money.

s.e.x.

You will need a reliable means to pay these costs. Your parents may be willing to help, but don't just assume they will, especially indefinitely. Not only isn't that fair—after all, they should get to decide when and if *they* want another baby—but they may or may not have the means to take care of the both of you. Your partner may be able to help, but remember that, whether you like it or not, he can up and leave at any time, and child support battles are the norm for single moms. Assuming federal or state aid will pay all the costs is also unrealistic. Many people aren't low-income enough, or don't meet other criteria to qualify for many programs—and even those who are eligible cannot come close to covering all of their costs with Welfare.

Kids Aren't a Cure-All.

If you have any major challenges in your life—an abusive partnership, depression, self-destructive behavior, an eating disorder, drug dependence, homelessness—they're likely to remain tough issues when you have a kid. Plenty of young parents find that dropping bad habits or patterns actually seems pretty easy when they first become pregnant, or at the beginning of their child's life. But it's typical for those issues to pop right back up in time. When they do, not only are they often even harder to manage and work through than before, but they directly impact someone besides you. How might your child be affected by growing up around an eating disorder, self-injury like cutting, or an abusive relationship? How are you going to manage putting your needs second when you're depressed? If your own parents or family had big challenges, take a look at how you think they impacted you. Even seemingly small issues, such as poor eating habits, or having a hard time making and enforcing

limits, can become pretty big problems when you're pregnant or parenting.

Kids also don't solve relationship problems. Not only do many young relationships not stand the test of time—but having a baby adds loads of extra stresses that make relationship longevity and harmony even more challenging. The vast majority of teen parents are and remain unmarried, and partners, even the father of your baby, can and do vacate the premises often enough.

Our Society Isn't Real Cool with Young Parents

If you're in your teens, parenting is going to be harder for you than it would be for someone just a few years older, and not just because of their better financial, health, or emotional status. A whole lot of people really look down on teen parents. Finding resources and assistance will be harder for you, and often you are going to have to fight for your right both to parent and to be treated like a parent. You'll be walking into parenthood with people assuming—even if you planned your pregnancy—that you're irresponsible. You're going to need to be able to strongly advocate for yourself and for your kid.

That may involve battling to get schools or workplaces to provide childcare or make allowances for your being a parent; it will probably mean working your buns off to obtain financial assistance, housing, school and work opportunities, healthcare, and emotional support. It may involve facing up to people who feel very confident that not only can you not be a good parent, but that you have no RIGHT to parent, and they may make it harder for you to do so. It may mean losing the support or presence of friends, family, or partners.

what they won't teach you in childbirth class
(from Aria, a Scarleteen volunteer and former teen momma)

1. Maternity clothes are tools of the Devil. A big stretchy panel on the front of your pants. Nightgowns with big slits in the front that do nothing for coverage. And some of the ugliest bras you've ever seen outside your grandma's dresser drawer. Get used to the "grandpa pants," because you'll be wearing them directly under your breasts until your baby comes. These, my friends, are what you should be shown when you're being taught abstinence in Health class.

2. When you're pushing during childbirth, sometimes your baby's head isn't the only thing that comes out. Imagine: downward pressure on your bowels as the baby moves south. Play with a Play-Doh Fun Factory, learn all about extrusion, and you'll understand what I'm talking about.

3. Newborn babies sometimes arrive complete with an impressive blanket of hair on their back and shoulders. Like those guys you sometimes see on the beach who you think are wearing sweaters.

4. Newborn baby heads are more moldable than clay. You may find yourself holding a little miniature Conehead. Or someone with a high ridge running down the center of their head. Don't worry; these go away within the first week or two. It's a great chance to try out all those adorable baby hats you've no doubt gathered in the last few months.

5. Modesty and Childbirth aren't very good friends. Toward the end, Childbirth gets so whiny and annoying that Modesty goes on vacation for a while.

6. You'll be amazed at how high your cervix seems when a doctor with big hands is checking it. Apparently, mine is located somewhere between my sinuses and my tonsils.

7. Remember all that lung capacity you lost in the last forty weeks? It comes back quickly and is one of the strangest sensations you'll encounter.

8. Remember all that bladder capacity you lost in the last forty weeks? It doesn't. And when you're lying in bed, sometimes you aren't aware that the tank is full. Be sure to remind yourself to get up at least once every three hours. You don't want to have to call the mop-and-bucket lady into the bathroom doorway. Believe me, I know.

9. You'll be told that it is not pain you'll feel during childbirth, it's pressure. This is true in the same way a tornado might be called an air current.

10. At all costs, avoid mirrors after you have your baby. That's a surprise best left for the safety and security of your own home.

11. You may not fall in love with your baby at first sight. This can take a while for some women, and is perfectly normal and acceptable. Your baby, however, will. Prepare to feel more needed than you have in your life.

12. Babies sleep more than you think. Don't always feel pressured to do the same. Not tired? Do something for yourself. Bathing will turn into an immeasurable joy.

13. Remember those periods you missed during your pregnancy? They're back. And they've brought friends. (For more on lochia, see page 276.)

if you're considering parenting . . .

- Talk to other parents at your school or workplace. Seek out young parents who currently have infants and toddlers (if you or friends don't know any, ask your school guidance counselor or job supervisor). Not only can you ask them about what it's like for them emotionally, you can also find out very practical things you need to know, like how the school, college, or job you're at handles young mothers. Do they provide day care? Is it safe and sound? What special programs and resources exist in your area for teen or young parents? What do you need to do to obtain those resources, and aid like funds and healthcare for young mothers and kids? How are your local hospitals with young mothers? What doctors, midwives, hospitals, or clinics would they suggest?
- Talk to your doctor, gynecologist, clinician, and/or nurse. About one-third of pregnant teens receive inadequate prenatal care; babies born to very young mothers are currently more likely to be low-birth-weight, to have childhood health problems, and to be hospitalized. And teen mothers sometimes have special health risks, so you'll need to be sure to spend extra time assessing your health. Healthcare pros can not only fill you in on health issues, but can also help hook you up with resources and support, and can also give you their unique perspective on what you'll be dealing with.
- Spend some time visualizing your life with a kid at every stage of the game: not just when they're babies, but when they're five, ten, or fifteen years old. Consider the goals you have for your life, and figure out how you might or might not be able to work toward

them while also parenting, with or without help or a co-parent.

Deciding to parent is a big deal for those of any age. People in touch with reality—whether they're seventeen or thirty-five—are often scared when they make that choice, because they have at least some inkling of how big a responsibility it is. So, it's normal to be scared (if you're not, at all, chances are you're not really seeing the big picture). It's also normal to feel grossly unprepared, even after the birth. Many parents of every age and social strata feel like hacks as parents, find that parenting is much more challenging than they thought it'd be, and worry about failing their kids. That's called caring.

That's a big list up there of challenges and pitfalls, which isn't to say that there aren't a lot of really great parts of being a parent. Kids are really cool, and they are often a whole lot of fun to be around. Parenting often makes *you* grow as a person, and you'll find that a child teaches you things no one else could. It's unique and special to be in a relationship with someone who is literally a part of you, and for whom you are the sun, moon and stars . . . for some of their life, anyway. Later on, they won't be so dependent and will be able to see your flaws (and likely let you know explicitly what they are), but even at that point, a strong relationship develops when you nurture it well, and one you will truly have for their whole life or yours.

If you've become a young parent, you may find that at the same time you're having to learn to take care of a baby, you're also having to learn to take care of yourself, and that's vital. *You* need care as well. It's important that you stay physically healthy and emotionally well; that the relationships you choose be beneficial, balanced, and healthy; that you get downtime by yourself or with your friends and partners. It's vital that you still follow your goals and dreams, and that besides becoming the parent you want to be, you also get to be the *person* you aspire to be.

The Adoption Option

Adoption in the present day is different than it used to be. For a long time, adoption meant that a birth mother was always required to give up all legal rights and responsibilities to her child, didn't ever know what happened to her child, and could nearly count on never finding out. For much of history until very recently, many birth mothers didn't even have a choice in participating in adoption at all. Things have become more flexible, and there are more options within adoption than there used to be.

The two basic types of adoption are:

▶ **"Closed" or confidential adoption:** A "closed" or confidential adoption means you relinquish all rights, and you do not meet the adoptive family. The family is generally given information about you, but it is largely very basic and health-oriented.
▶ **"Open" adoption:** Open adoptions vary in terms of how much or how little openness is involved. The least open allow a birth mother to choose the parents for her child, based on files of waiting families that she can look through. More open agreements may allow the birth mother to speak with potential parents or families via the phone or in meetings, to choose a family. The adoptive parents may be present during pregnancy and delivery, and agreements can even be open to the extent that a birth mother is allowed contact throughout a child's life, or may even be included within the adoptive family.

Adoptions can be arranged in many ways:

▶ Via licensed public or private adoption agencies
▶ Independently, with a lawyer or doctor making arrangements between you and the adoptive parent or family
▶ Privately, between yourself and a couple (although having a lawyer, even among friends, is highly advisable)

The birth mother's pregnancy and prenatal and postpartum costs are usually covered by the adoptive family and/or the agency, as well as her legal fees and basic living expenses during the course of her pregnancy. Expenses like fees for counseling or therapy may also be paid to the birth mother. In most areas, how much a birth mother can be paid is limited as to the actual amount, the time period, and what she can receive compensation for. So, in making decisions about how to manage a pregnancy, adoption is the one option where cost may not be a primary concern.

By law (in the United States), adoption records remain closed by default, and the adoptive family has full legal rights to the child. So, it's very important to really evaluate and discuss how much openness you want, and what you want that to mean, when considering adoption, if you need for

s.e.x.

it to be open. If you get to the point of making an agreement, you'll want to get all of that ON PAPER and get a lawyer involved who is experienced with adoption. Just be aware that even when it is on paper, if adoptive families change their minds in terms of how much access or contact a birth mother gets, the adoptive parents are favored by the law and adoption agencies. Open adoptions may still result in lack of access or contact with a child, sometimes permanently—something that occurs all too often, and that a birth mother will be unable to do anything about.

The Tough Stuff

Adoption is often very difficult for birth mothers. Many women become emotionally attached to their child during pregnancy, and some find giving the child up after birth to be very traumatic, short and long-term. That distress can be escalated when adoption is chosen not because it's what is really wanted, but because age, poverty, secrecy, or other issues make abortion or parenting seem impossible. This distress can be heightened further is a woman changes her mind early on (but not early enough to rescind the agreement), or has agreed to an adoption she was told or thought would be open, but that turns out not to be.

In terms of considering what's best for a child, most children who are placed in adoptive homes do well and have happy, healthy lives. There are many people in the world who want very much to be parents and can only do so through adoption. But a harsh truth is that in the United States alone, every year hundreds of thousands of children put up for adoption remain without permanent homes and enter the foster care system. That's more common with chil-

dren who were not placed for adoption as newborns or infants, for infants and children of color (African American, Hispanic, Native American, or biracial), and for special needs children.

To explore adoption, you can ask your doctor, guidance counselor, social services organization, or contact agencies on your own. It is also a good idea to talk to other birth mothers who gave their children up for adoption about their experiences. There are also national matching services, lists, and other resources available to seek out adoption services or private families.

ABORTION/TERMINATION

Abortion is a medical procedure performed to terminate a pregnancy. Legal abortion is performed within a clinic, hospital, or doctor's office, usually on an outpatient basis, and almost always within the first trimester of pregnancy. Legal abortion procedures are safe: statistically, health risks are much greater for carrying a pregnancy to term than for abortion. *No* long-term health problems have been found to be associated with legal medical or surgical abortion.

The only truly safe abortions are legal abortions. The majority of counties in the United States do not have a local provider, so you may have to travel past your own town or city to obtain one.

At this time, there are two main options for legal abortion: medical abortion or surgical abortion.

Medical Abortion

While not as widely available as surgical abortion, medical abortion—sometimes called RU486 or "the abortion pill"—is now available from many abortion providers. Medical abortion is effective up to around sixty days after the last menstrual period, or up until around ten weeks of pregnancy. It does not require surgery, but instead is a combination of drugs (usually mifepristone and misoprostol or methotrexate and misoprostol), given and supervised by a clinician, that causes a termination much like a miscarriage. The drugs do several things: stop embryonic cells from multiplying and dividing to continue a pregnancy, block hormones that would support a developing pregnancy, and cause uterine contractions that empty the contents of the uterus.

An injection of one drug is performed in the doctor's or clinician's office, while the other is inserted into the vagina a few days later, at home; OR the drugs are given orally, with one dose administered in the office, and the other a few days later at home. From a few days to a week after the first dose, the embryo and other products of conception pass out through the vagina. The experience will be very similar to early miscarriage: there will be some cramping and bleeding, from light spotting to heavier bleeding, and what is expelled may contain clots and/or the grayish-looking gestational sac created by the blastocyst. It does not contain the embryo; that is so small at the time medical abortion can be performed that it is unlikely to be visible. Cramps and bleeding are usually stronger than during a menstrual period. Side effects can include nausea, headaches, vomiting, or bowel problems, as well as continued spotting for a week or two. For a woman having a medical abortion, it is helpful and most safe if she arranges for someone else—her partner, a friend, family—to be on call for her, for emotional support, for material needs during the process, or for

transportation to an emergency room quickly, should her side effects be serious.

Medical abortions must to be coupled with follow-up visits to the provider to ensure that a full termination did occur and that the woman is in sound health afterward.

Medical abortions are not as effective as surgical abortions, and sometimes an additional surgical abortion will be necessary to successfully terminate a pregnancy.

abortion laws and minors

 ACCORDING to the National Abortion Federation, of teenage women who become pregnant, about 35 percent choose to have an abortion rather than bear a child. However, in many states, certain laws may restrict teen access to abortion, via policies that either require parents to be notified of a teen's intent to have an abortion (parental notification), or require a parent or guardian's written permission for an abortion to be performed for a teen (parental consent). Almost all of these policies have options for judicial bypass (for a teen to get a judge's permission for the abortion without parental involvement), and some states allow physicians to waive parental notification or consent. Too, court orders have prevented some states from enforcing these laws. If you are or know a minor woman seeking out abortion, you can find out what, if any, legal restrictions exist in your area either by calling your local abortion provider or sexual health clinic, or by referencing some of the abortion advocacy groups listed in the Resources section of this book.

Surgical Abortion

Surgical abortions—which are nearly always 100 percent effective—can be performed

s.e.x.

from the time a pregnancy is confirmed until the end of the first trimester. Sometimes, surgical abortion is performed after the first three months, but second-trimester abortions account for less than around 10 percent of all abortions. The type of surgical abortion performed—manual vacuum aspiration (MVA), dilation and curettage (D and C), or, more commonly now, dilation and evacuation (D and E)—depends on the length of the pregnancy and the specific situation. All are currently legal in the United States and Canada.

▶ **Manual or machine vacuum aspiration (MVA)** can be done within the first trimester, up to about thirteen weeks of pregnancy. This is the method most often used for abortions now, and manual aspiration can be used as soon as four weeks from the last menstrual period. During an aspiration, an injection first numbs the cervix with a local anesthetic. A woman can also elect to have a general anesthetic, which will put her under completely during the procedure.

The cervix is then dilated—with slim rods designed to slowly stretch the cervical opening—and a flexible tube is inserted through the cervix. That tube is either attached to an aspirating machine with a gentle vacuum, or, for very early abortions, to a handheld syringe. The contents of the uterus are removed through the tube with gentle suction. The entire procedure takes between five and ten minutes.

▶ **Dilation and evacuation (D and E)** can be done from about six weeks after the last menstrual period through the first trimester and sometimes into the second. Some abortion providers only use D and E for later-term abortions.

Local anesthetic is used, but painkillers or a general anesthetic can usually also be requested. The opening of the cervix is stretched with cervical dilators, just as with a vacuum aspiration procedure. Another sort of dilator may also be used, made of soft fibers that absorb moisture from the woman's body and expand overnight to enlarge the opening in the cervix. Sometimes a drug, misoprostol, may be used with the dilators to soften the cervix. Depending on what is used, how far along you are, and individual clinic policies and practices, you may be sent home overnight with a dilator or dilators in place, and with antibiotics to prevent infection. If so, you'll need to return the next day for the second part of the procedure.

After the cervical opening is dilated, a suction process will take place. With a suction curettage, or **dilation and curettage (D and C)**, there's a final step, which is to make sure the uterus has been completely emptied by using a curette—a small metal loop—to gently scrape the uterine walls. D and Cs are being used less often now for abortions, due to advancements in the suction tools and machines, as well as the use of ultrasound technology to ensure that the uterus has been emptied completely.

This process takes around ten minutes, not including the time it takes for dilation, or the night that may have passed.

Abortion Costs

Both medical and surgical first-trimester abortions cost about the same: currently around $450–$800 in the United States. Some insurance policies, or federal or medical aid, may cover some abortion costs, but generally only when an abortion is medically necessary rather than elective—that is, when a pregnancy puts the life of mother or child in danger. Some states and countries do provide funds for elective abortions for low-income women. There are also some grassroots sources for financial assistance for abortion for women who want an abortion but cannot come up with all the funds themselves. For information on abortion funds, see the Resources section.

What to Expect during an Abortion

How You Should Expect to Be Treated

▶ First and foremost, you should be treated with care and respect. Your privacy should be respected in every way. Generally, neither of these is a problem with abortion providers; providers and their staff take both of these issues very seriously.

▶ Throughout the process, you will be given counseling, and your counselor should respect whatever pace you need, even if you come in for an abortion and decide you do not want to go through with the procedure that day. It's important to be aware that you ALWAYS can opt out of the procedure, at any time before it begins, and staff at your clinic or doctor's office should make that clear. (And if you know from the onset that you want more involved counseling, because you are not sure about abortion yet, you can make an appointment for that all by itself: you don't have to schedule an abortion to receive abortion counseling.)

▶ You should be helped to feel as emotionally and physically safe as possible, and that usually includes heavy security for the clinic. The office or clinic where you have an abortion should be clean and sanitary. Your counselor, nurse, and/or doctor should explain your entire procedure to you, and be willing to answer any—and I do mean any—questions you have at any time before, during, or after the procedure. If you want someone with you, you are often allowed to bring them, although because of health, legal and safety issues, that person will only be permitted in the waiting room.

What an Abortion Feels Like

Medical abortion may cause heavy cramping at home that can be very uncomfortable, and bleeding will occur, but generally not a lot more than during a menstrual period. During surgical abortion, a woman is likely to also experience cramping, usually stronger than menstrual cramps, and may feel some strong "pricks" inside her pelvis, not unlike the sensation you feel in your mouth when a dentist gives you an anesthetic injection. Women who are more nervous, uncertain, scared, or conflicted are likely to experience much more pain or discomfort than those who are more relaxed and resolved.

s.e.x.

Common side effects that many women will experience following the abortion procedures include cramping, nausea, sweating, feeling faint, and, like women who have given full-term birth, depression. Less frequent side effects may include heavy or prolonged bleeding, blood clots, infection due to retained products of conception, dilators, or caused by an STD or bacteria being introduced to the uterus, which can cause fever, pain, abdominal tenderness, and possibly scar tissue. If postabortion side effects persist for more than a few days or are severe, call your abortion provider or your doctor immediately.

Unloading a Loaded Issue

Because abortion is still such a controversial issue among many people and politicians, it can be tough to choose it, or even think clearly and objectively about abortion as a choice. If you decide to get an abortion, you may even have to deal with protesters at your clinic, which can mean being called some pretty nasty names.

All sorts of women have abortions, across all racial, economic, age, marital, and other social lines. According to the Guttmacher Institute:

- ▶ About 80 percent of women who abort are over eighteen and unmarried.
- ▶ By the age of forty-five, about one in every three women will have an abortion.
- ▶ The majority of women who have abortions—about six in ten—are already mothers.
- ▶ The majority of women who have abortions do intend to bear and rear children in the future.

- ▶ The majority of women who have abortions subscribe to religious beliefs, and 70 percent or more of those women are members of Judeo-Christian religions, including Catholicism.

abortion trauma

MANY credible journals, such as the *Journal of the American Medical Association,* have stated that there is no data to support the idea or insistence that abortion is more emotionally traumatic for women than any other reproductive option. We have no logical reason to assume that any one choice is more or less traumatic for all women: in fact, studies support that the majority of women who freely choose abortion for themselves have positive, rather than negative, psychological responses, long-term.

There *are* some factors that are known to increase the possibility of emotional distress and trauma from abortion, listed in studies such as *Emotional Response to Abortion: A Critical Review of the Literature* and *The Psychosocial Factors of the Abortion Experience: A Critical Review* (see Bibliography). These include being of a very young age, lack of support from partners or community (including the world at large), pressure or coercion to abort, anxiety or distress before the procedure, moral or religious conflicts about abortion, preexisting mental illness or depression, a history of sexual abuse or assault, low self-esteem, and habitual avoidance of responsibility.

In other words, the sorts of factors that will make ANY reproductive choice more likely to be traumatic for a woman. In fact, the factors above are very similar to the at-risk indicators usually listed for women who give birth and are more likely to suffer from postpartum depression. So, remember, if you or someone you know is preg-

s.e.x.

nant and making a reproductive choice, it is vital that a woman's choice be just that: the option that she feels is best for her, first and foremost, and that she chooses on her own. And whatever her choice, emotional support throughout is crucial.

No matter what you believe, your feelings about abortion—especially when the possibility or event is actual and personal, rather than an abstract idea—may not be simple or line up predictably with your beliefs. Some women who generally are not comfortable with abortion as a whole may decide to have one in a given situation because they truly feel it is best for them. Some who are comfortable with abortion for others, or who have had abortions before, may, in a certain situation, feel it is not the right choice for them or their children. Plenty of women who do want children have an abortion at some point because they just don't feel capable or able to rear their children adequately at that time, due to relationship, financial, lifestyle, health, or emotional issues.

Few reproductive choices are easy, but right now, it's likely more difficult to choose abortion as an option because of all the personal and political biases against it. For that reason, it's important that if you DO choose abortion—just as is the case if you choose to parent or put a child up for adoption—you do so because you want to and feel it is the best choice you can make.

Where to Find Sound Help

If you're in the process of making a reproductive choice—whether it's parenting, adoption, or abortion—at some point you're going to need to go somewhere to get hooked up with the services you need. It's also often helpful to talk about options with someone who is objective, who isn't invested in the choice you make because they aren't an immediate part of your life and don't have an agenda of their own.

to tell or not to tell

 IT'S up to you whom you tell about a pregnancy, and when and if you tell them: you are not under any obligation, legal or otherwise, to tell family, friends, or partners about a pregnancy. Just be sure that, if you're waiting to tell a partner or parent, or not telling them at all, you're being fair about it. For instance, it's not fair to wait to tell parents you're pregnant until you show, if you expect them to help you with costs and parenting. Keeping an abortion from a partner to later hurt or manipulate them with it isn't okay. If you are carrying a child to term, a partner does have parental rights he's entitled to (unless you have reason to believe he will be harmful to you or your child), so a partner who is still around and staying around is one you're going to need to inform.

If you feel that telling a partner or parents about a pregnancy puts you in actual danger, then it is smart not to tell them yourself, but instead to seek out help, intervention, and support from appropriate resources such as local law enforcement or social services.

No matter what, be sure you tell *someone:* if not family or a partner, a friend, doctor, counselor, teacher, or someone else you trust to provide you support. No matter what choices you make, being pregnant is too tough to go it alone.

Research your clinic and counseling options to find the help best suited to you. Your best option is a center or clinic that

s.e.x.

provides a number of different services and that makes clear that ALL possible choices are acceptable, rather than pushing one choice. General sexual healthcare clinics—which provide a number of sexual health services, such as GYN exams, STI screenings, prenatal care, and abortion—are smart places to go. You can also talk to your gynecologist or general physician. School guidance counselors or student services centers may also offer reproductive option counseling. Any center or clinic you go to should be offering pretty extensive interviews and counseling before offering you services, and laying out what your choices are, to help you evaluate them. Any center or clinic you go to for counseling, once you've made your choice, should be wholly supportive of that choice. If your gut tells you something is amiss, trust it and find somewhere else to go.

Remember that you get to make this choice yourself, and come to your own conclusions about what's best. That's also the case even if you became pregnant intentionally with an eye toward parenting, then changed your mind: you are allowed to do that.

HOW TO TELL PARTNERS AND PARENTS ABOUT AN UNEXPECTED PREGNANCY

Let's say the pregnancy test just verified what you already suspected: you're pregnant. At some point, you may need to tell some people about this—your parents, your partner, or whoever it was that contributed the other half of the DNA, and possibly at least a friend or other trusted person so you can get some support and help.

▶ Take some time for yourself. Consider your options and get a good feel for what you think you'd like to do.

▶ Talk to a close friend or two. You'll need some support, preferably from people who are good listeners and aren't judgmental in terms of whatever your ultimate choice may be in regard to your pregnancy.

▶ Process it as thoroughly as you can in the limited time you have available. Call hotlines or visit pregnancy options counselors if you need to talk it out with someone who can be objective.

Telling Partners

There's no one right way to tell a partner pregnancy has happened, no special finesse, no golden phrase that'll make it all easier. How partners react is often pretty unpredictable. Someone you thought would handle it badly may take it like a pro and leap to your side, prepared to manage it all expertly. Someone you felt sure would be caring and involved may blow you off for a few days, or even completely. Even a partner you're very close to and have been with for a long while may be shocked.

Your partner may end up being a great ally for you in all this and tremendously supportive. But it's also common enough for pregnancy—or even a pregnancy scare—to be the beginning of the end of a relationship. It's entirely possible that your partner may greatly disappoint you, that disagreements about pregnancy may facilitate a breakup, or even that you'll find yourself adrift in this all by yourself. Your partner may try to blame you for the pregnancy, or be angry with you, even though you both were responsible. In abusive relationships, abuse usually increases with a pregnancy—and many abusive relationships that weren't physically abusive before become so. It's hard to look at, but according to the U.S. Department of Justice, the leading cause of death for pregnant women is homicide (murder), most commonly by an intimate partner. (So, if you're in an abusive relationship and think a pregnancy might make things better, please think twice.)

More typically, you'll see a range of behavior while your partner is processing all of this; they may need time to do that, just like you. While it's not easy to make allowances for crappy attitudes or bad reactions, especially when it's you who is pregnant, it often is necessary to give a person a little time to absorb and adjust.

When that adjustment happens, you can start talking about options, about what you want to do, and listening to their feelings. You can talk it out together as much as you need to, just bear in mind that it is ultimately YOUR choice. This is happening in YOUR body. So, how much a part of this they are is not just up to them, it's also up to you.

Trying to Understand Each Other

Men and women typically have disconnects about pregnancy: neither can really understand how the other feels. Men can't understand how it feels, physically or emotionally, to know you have something new growing in your body, or what it's like to have people you don't even know so invested in and opinionated about the choices you make about a pregnancy. Women might have difficulty understanding how men feel having so little control over the situation once pregnancy has occurred, what their experience is, since the pregnancy is not in their bodies. Communicating with each other as clearly as possible can be a big help. A pregnancy usually auto-matically ups the seriousness of any relationship: a partner who wanted a casual relationship may wake up to find that's no longer the case due to a pregnancy—a scenario that's far less tangible for many men until they've actually experienced it.

The reproductive choice you make may not be what your partner wants. That's a toughie, because it is *your* choice to make. Listen to each other. Understanding you don't need to defend your choice, just explain it as best you can, and listen to your partner's feelings. Know that you may have to agree to disagree, and that may be really hard. It may mean that you have to gather funds for an abortion on your own, or go through a pregnancy without the support or commitment of your partner.

Sometimes, it just takes longer for a partner to accept a choice and really deal with it. While you, as the pregnant person, don't really have that time in terms of what you have to do immediately, your partner does. So, you might need to make allowances for the fact that it doesn't feel, and isn't, as immediate for them as it is for you. If you're in a solid relationship and are having trouble dealing with a pregnancy, no matter the choice each of you wants to make, you might consider some counseling. Abortion and adoption agencies can usually provide counseling for both partners at a low cost, or for free, and if you're considering parenting, your OB/GYN or healthcare professional can probably suggest resources to get help, or even counsel both of you themselves.

Telling Parents

Telling parents is often trickier, especially if telling them you're pregnant also means telling them for the first time that you've been sexually active.

Your best bet is usually just to be as straightforward and honest as possible, and to prepare yourself for conflict or disappointment on the part of your parent. A parent is likely to be upset about a young pregnancy (even when it was planned). He or she may also be upset that you were sexually active at all.

Don't lie. If you didn't use birth control, or know you misused something or used something unreliable, say so. If the sex you had with your partner was consensual, don't say that it *wasn't*. And if it wasn't, don't say that it *was*.

Blaming a parent in any way for your unplanned pregnancy is also a bad idea. No matter what the situation, it's highly unlikely your parents forced you into bed with your partner. No one, ever, *has* to have any kind of consensual, partnered sex: it's optional, not compulsory, and if you didn't opt out when you should have, you are accountable, not your parents.

If you want help, **ask for it**, whether it's financial or emotional, whether it's about working things out with your partner or making the choice to continue or terminate your pregnancy. Understand that your parent can and may say no. While saying no to emotional support would be pretty lousy, saying no to financial help with pregnancy, abortion, or helping to care for your baby is fair and completely within their rights, especially if they're still financially supporting *you*. Expecting a parent to cover your pregnancy, parenting, or abortion costs, or expecting them to help with parenting your child, is expecting an awful lot. So, if you want help in those areas, you need to ask for it and discuss it, not assume you're entitled to it.

If the worst happens when you tell your parent or parents, there are ways to deal. If you get kicked out of your house, you can go to your partner or friend, another relative, or a neighbor. If all of those avenues are closed to you, you can go to your local police station, school, or community center to get hooked up with social services for temporary housing.

 ACCORDING to the National Campaign to Prevent Teen Pregnancy, around one out of every four teen mothers has a second child within just two years of her first. As obvious as it may seem to learn something from going without birth control, using an unreliable method, or using a reliable method incorrectly, plenty of people really don't.

So if you do **not** want to become pregnant again, make a sincere vow to ALWAYS use the most reliable method of birth control available to you, from this point onward, EVERY time you have any sort of sex with a risk of pregnancy. If you have a habit of winding up with partners who are lax about birth control, who refuse to use it or to cooperate with your birth control use—or you're a guy who is one of those partners—remember that someone who isn't ready to be responsible about sex in a way that supports the health and well-being of *both* partners isn't someone ready to have sex with a partner. If your partner is someone like that, it's really best to kick them to the curb.

FOR THE "DADS"

It's difficult to be involved in a reproductive choice that you had a part in bringing about, but that is not happening in *your* body. Ultimately, the reproductive choices your female partner makes are—and should be—HER

s.e.x.

choices. You may have input about certain reproductive options, and she may even work to make a choice you can both agree on—but she may also find that the best choice for her isn't the one you want. Again, while you had a hand in getting her there, pregnancy doesn't happen in your body, and the hard truth of the matter is that you can bow out at any time a whole lot easier than she can, socially and practically. Plenty of men do: in the United States, single mothers outnumber single fathers four to one, and the U.S. Department of Health and Human Services estimates that 68 percent of child support cases were in arrears in 2003.

There are also practical issues for male partners to bear in mind. You certainly can choose not to opt into parenting, but if she decides to bring a pregnancy to term, in most areas, you cannot opt out of financial support for the child that you helped create (another reason why, if you know you don't want to risk becoming a father, it's a good idea to make your own active reproductive choices by always using condoms, or opting out of intercourse). Even if a pregnant woman agrees to nonsupport from you financially, she can ALWAYS change her mind, at any time. Also, if you opt out of active parenting or child support at any time, and later change your mind, you may discover that being let back in is difficult, and sometimes, it's just not going to happen.

Ideally, before a pregnancy has occurred, you and your partner will have discussed what she and you think you'd like to do should one happen, so the both of you have some idea of what to expect from the other. Whether you have or you haven't, understand that trying to pressure a female partner into a certain reproductive choice just isn't okay. **It's her choice, not yours, however difficult that might be to accept.** You can certainly let her know what does feel best to you, and what you're capable of managing—money and/or support with adoption, abortion, or parenting, the ability and willingness to parent long-term or not. You can also let her know what you can't handle, or might need help dealing with: you're not nonexistent in this situation, after all. *You matter.*

Support services are available for the male half of any pregnancy, with whatever reproductive choice is made. If you're having a really hard time, seek them out (see the Resources section for some venues for support). In the case of a pregnancy being carried to term, you can ask your partner's doctor or prenatal clinic for a referral: there are often good support groups and free classes for dads-to-be. We hear a lot about "deadbeat dads," and young men who ditch their female partners when they become pregnant and carry a child to term. What we don't hear a whole lot about are the teen fathers who not only stick around, but also want to actively parent, of which there are also plenty. Some teen fathers find it difficult to be full participants: their girlfriend's parents may be wary or distrustful of them, and not let them parent actively; friends or family may knowingly or unknowingly encourage them in being inactive, or even ridicule them; or they may merely be given the role of paying for things and left out of caretaking. The expectation that guys will leave or blow off responsibilities may be so high that those who ARE trying to do their part may feel pretty defeated. If you do want to actively parent, you may have to be very proactive and clear about that, and work extra hard to get involved and stay involved,

s.e.x.

even when it's rough, or when people are asking you to prove things you really shouldn't have to. Seek out help and support where you need to, and don't be afraid to ask for it.

If you need support dealing with abortion or adoption, ask the abortion or adoption provider for help or resources for you, or phone your local sexual health clinic and ask for referrals.

Lastly, understand that women aren't the only ones who do or can make initial reproductive choices. *Every single time you have sex that carries a risk of pregnancy, you are making a choice.* Using reliable birth control properly is almost always a choice NOT to reproduce—and via condoms, you can make that choice for yourself, by yourself. Opting out of those risks altogether is also a choice you can control. If you know or feel that you just couldn't handle it if a pregnancy occurred, or that certain reproductive choices a woman might make with a pregnancy wouldn't be okay with you, then the right choice for you to make is to opt out of sex with pregnancy risks altogether. The reproductive choice that men have to make—which is just as vital as any that women make, and incredibly important—is to choose to create a pregnancy or not in the first place.

Be Pro-Choice!

Sexuality and partnered sex are about far more than reproduction, but for a majority of people, pregnancy—possible and actual—is a huge part of the sex they're having, even in efforts to prevent it.

The way human reproduction works can make it challenging to balance and equalize responsibility, power, effort, and awareness between men and women, when it comes to sex. There's a pretty profound difference, for instance, in going to bed with someone thinking, "Oh god, what if *I* get pregnant?" and going to bed thinking, "Oh god, what if I *get her* pregnant?" There's a profound imbalance when one partner is ultimately responsible for birth control, as well as for shouldering the biggest burdens should a pregnancy occur: making tough choices, quickly making big lifestyle and health changes, taking health risks, footing the bills, giving birth or having an abortion, informing everyone about a pregnancy, being the partner who is visibly pregnant to everyone, 24/7—and in case of rape, going through all of that while also fielding emotional and physical trauma. That is not to say that men who create a pregnancy—and certainly men who actively parent—have no burdens of their own, nor to say that having a child, or even being pregnant, is only a burden and never a boon.

Rather, *we ALL make choices about whether or not to reproduce,* even those of us with same-sex partners, even those of us with no partners at all. If we always mindfully make those choices, alone and together, and make an effort to share and own that responsibility as best we can, some of the inherent inequities in reproduction—physical, emotional, social, economic, and practical—can become far more balanced.

It's not as tricky as it sounds. As you've discovered, most birth control methods, when used correctly and consistently, are highly effective. There are plenty of sexual activities just as satisfying as heterosexual intercourse (and sometimes *more* satisfying). While some of those activities still carry STI risks, and safer sex will still need to be managed, one can easily choose to eradicate pregnancy risks altogether by engaging in them instead of activity with a risk of pregnancy—or, of course, by opting out of partnered sex or opposite-sex partnered sex altogether.

When that sort of ownership of responsibility is taken by all partners; when honest and open communication exists; when full, enthusiastic consent and choice of all partners is *always* a given; **and** when both partners make a conscious effort, always, to share all responsibilities in partnered sex, including owning and nurturing their own sexuality separate from a partner, it's actually incredibly easy to keep things balanced—and for the positive, preventative choices we actively—rather than passively—make to net positive, desired results.

s.e.x.

13

how to change the world
(without even getting out of bed)

DEAR YOU,

Well, here we are, at the end of this (very big, my apologies) book. Put your feet up. Have a cup of tea. Relax. Revel in the sunny afterglow of newly-acquired knowledge. I just want a few more minutes of your time before you shuffle off and ably explain to someone that the clitoris is so much bigger than they knew, pass on the fact that there's no fist in fisting, point out that there are more than two sexes, remark that, as easy as it feels, our bodies are sure doing a helluva lot of work to have just one little orgasm, or make a song out of the south-to-north trail of anal sexual anatomy to the tune of "Supercalifragilisticexpialidocious" (like so: "Pubococcygeus-rectum-anus-perineum").

In a better world, a more balanced, humanist place, your sexuality would be one of the least of your challenges. It would be something that grounded you in the body you live in, that sang the praises of your skin with you. It would be your solace, your source of extra energy, your way to amplify the joy of the good days and find an extra measure of comfort on the bad. It would bring you closer to yourself and to others in a unique, intimate way; it would be a powerful, individual tool of your self-expression. It would honor you and everyone else. It would always make you feel good, and you'd always feel 100 percent good about it.

I don't need to tell you that we don't live in that world: you know that already. Your sexuality—if you experience it honestly, earnestly, and wholly in this world—will probably be a challenge. If you're a young woman who wants to own it full-stop, you will be met with some resistance. If you are a young man who wants to reinvent your sexual role, you will probably have some areas of nonsupport. If you are in any way marginal in the eyes of the world at large—if you're female, of color, transgender, poor, pregnant, gay, lesbian, a young parent, bisexual, intersex, of size, disabled, not gender or heteronormative, etc.—then it's very likely that managing and owning aspects of your sexuality will often not come easy or receive latitude. Even for the most privileged person, who also has every other aspect of their life together, the way a lot of the world approaches sexuality can create challenges. That place where it can all be comfortable, easy, natural, and accepted is just not the world we live in. Yet.

Sometimes, when I'm having a bad day or a hard moment in the sexuality work I do, I stop what I am doing. I take a deep breath. I close my eyes. Then I picture every single person in the world healthy, happy, and whole in themselves and their sexuality: in body, heart, and mind. I picture a world without rape, sexual abuse, or domestic violence; in which safety, respect, and consent are simply givens. I picture a world where no one gets called a fag, a slut, a prude, or a pansy; where those jibes have no power. I picture a world without shame or guilt when it comes to shape, size, sexuality, or sexual or gender identity; where difference is embraced and celebrated, and where every voice is acknowledged. I picture a world without unwanted pregnancy, a world that isn't riddled with sexually transmitted disease, a world where we don't attack those different from us because who they are makes us question who we are. I picture a world where sexuality is necessarily nonexploitive, humane, and sacred . . . and a world

where no one has a coronary when some sixteen-year-old says they're ready for S.E.X. and feeling really good about it.

It might seem silly to you, but it always makes me feel a little better. If it weren't possible, if I knew it was nothing but a pipe dream, I don't think it'd do that. It's only because I know those things truly *are* possible—for me, for you, for everybody else—that I immediately feel more hopeful.

See, the world is made of people. (I know you know that part already, too.) And it's people who make it the way that it is, who choose to either start doing things a new, better way, or enable the same tired old crap.

I'm going to ask a favor of you.

I ask you to make that same picture in your head, and to consider being one of the many people who create that world: to recognize and claim the incredible power and potential that you have to not only make *your* world, but THE world, different—better—when it comes to sex and sexuality. Just as I'd suggest for your own sex life, I'm asking you to consider being active, not passive, thoughtful, not careless, compassionate, not cruel (to others OR yourself).

You can do this.

I ask this of you because I *know* you can do this. Some people before you have done an amazing job on this front. Others have mucked it up utterly. All of them had the power to do exactly what it is they did, just as you have the power to do whatever it is you're doing or will do.

Here's the beauty of the thing: this isn't that hard to do. You can do it just by claiming your sexuality for yourself, being its author, designer, and manager (and even when you stumble in managing it sometimes, as we all do); just by coming to it

S.e.x.

mindfully, with real care for yourself and others, you've won at least half the battle. Apply that same approach to how you regard and treat the sexuality of everyone else, and you've made a giant leap in helping us get to that better place. Hey—it's not every day that powerful activist work is so enjoyable. Seize that opportunity.

The American poet, essayist, humanist (and bisexual) Walt Whitman, in *Leaves of Grass,* said, "We convince by our presence."

This is what he meant.

At the start of this book, I asked something of you, too. I asked you to boldly **choose to create a healthy, happy, and fulfilling sexual life that is fantastic for you and for everyone else in it.**

You can not only do this, you can do it brilliantly. Be bold.

—Heather Corinna
November 15, 2006

s.e.x.

common sexually transmitted infections: stis from a to z

FOR information on how to safeguard your sexual health, protect yourself and partners against STIs, and deal with life with an STI, see Chapter 9, "Safe and Sound: Safer Sex for Your Body, Heart, and Mind."

▪ CHANCROID ▪

Chancroid is a fairly rare bacterial infection that produces genital sores. Reported cases of chancroid have declined steadily over the last decade or so, but it is believed to be often underdiagnosed and underreported. Chancroid is most common in men with multiple partners. It can make HIV transmission, and transmission of other STIs, more likely to occur.

How do you get it? Direct genital (penis, vulva, or anus) or oral contact with a chancroid sore.

How can you tell if you have it? Within a week or so after exposure, painful open sores on the genitals and/or swollen lymph nodes around the groin usually appear in men. In women, symptoms may be less obvious, producing more general complaints, such as painful urination or intercourse, rectal bleeding, or unusual vaginal discharge.

Chancroid is diagnosed by a healthcare professional either via a culture of a sore or through a blood test. Because chancroid sores are tricky to tell from other sores—herpes sores, for instance—getting a professional diagnosis is important.

How do you treat it? It is usually easily treated with antibiotics. Sometimes, scarring may result from the sores.

How do you avoid it? Safer sex practices offer protection against chancroid, as does keeping an eye out for any open sores on a partner's body or your own. If sores are visibly present, especially on areas that latex barriers can't cover, you should abstain from sexual contact until after treatment.

▪ CHLAMYDIA ▪

The most common sexually transmitted bacterial infection in the world, with as many as three million new cases every year in the United States alone, chlamydia is so common in young women that, according to the Centers for Disease Control, by age thirty, 50 percent of sexually active women have had chlamydia. Almost half of all chlamydia cases are in teens, and most people with chlamydia—as many as 50 percent of men and 75 percent of women—do not know they have it or have had it.

In women, chlamydia infects the cervix and can spread to the urethra, fallopian tubes, and ovaries. It can cause chronic bladder infections and pelvic inflammatory disease, ectopic pregnancy, and infertility. In men, it infects the urethra and can spread to the testicles, which can cause infertility. Chlamydia can also lead to Reiter's syndrome, especially in young men, which involves eye infections, urethritis, and arthritis. One in three men who develop Reiter's syndrome become permanently disabled.

How do you get it? Chlamydia is most often spread by unprotected vaginal or anal intercourse, oral sex, shared sex toys, contact during childbirth, and in rare cases, from hand to eye and other nonsexual contact.

How can you tell if you have it? Most people with chlamydia experience no symptoms. When symptoms are present, they may include pain or burning while urinating, unexplained vaginal bleeding or spotting, painful intercourse, abdominal pain or nausea, fever, or swelling or pain of the rectum, cervix, or testicles.

Chlamydia is diagnosed by a doctor with a urine or genital swab sample, and where cases of the throat are suspected, via a throat culture (swab).

How do you treat it? Chlamydia is usually easily treatable with antibiotics, and once treated is no longer present in the body and can't be passed to a partner unless you contract it again. However, it's very important that any partners over a two-month period be tested and treated. Reinfection (repeat infection) rates of chlamydia are very high, usually because male partners aren't treated, and/or during treatment, partners continue not to practice safer sex, so the infection just keeps getting passed back and forth.

How do you avoid it? Chlamydia is nearly always transmitted by sexual activity, so using latex barriers for vaginal, oral, and/or anal sex, or abstaining from sex, will almost always prevent chlamydia infection.

▪ CYTOMEGALOVIRUS (CMV) ▪

CMV is an extremely common herpes-type virus. CMV can create kidney problems, and is incredibly dangerous for people who have immune system problems or the AIDS virus. It infects more than half of all adults in the United States by forty years of age.

How do you get it? CMV is transmitted through body fluids through general nonsexual contact; vaginal, anal, or oral intercourse; blood transfusions or sharing IV drug equipment; bone marrow transplants; or from mother to infant during pregnancy, birth, or breastfeeding.

How can you tell if you have it? CMV often doesn't have obvious symptoms. When symptoms are present, they can resemble those of flu or mononucleosis (see page 307): swollen glands, loss of appetite, fatigue and general weakness, fever, night sweats, a persistent cough, or difficulty breathing. Pneumonia and an increased transmission rate of other STIs and diseases can also result from CMV infection.

CMV is usually diagnosed by a blood test, urine test, or chest X-ray.

How do you treat it? While symptoms can be managed with antiviral medications, no treatment is needed for CMV for those without any complications. Like many viruses, CMV can remain in the body for life. There is presently no cure.

How do you avoid it? Condoms provide protection against CMV during vaginal, anal, and oral intercourse, but it can also be spread by kissing or by non-sexual contact.

▪ GONORRHEA ▪

A bacterial infection, gonorrhea is very common: there are currently about forty million infected people in the United States, and about 75 percent of all reported cases occur in people under thirty. Rates of gonorrhea have been decreasing in the general population; however rates are rising among teens and young adults.

Gonorrhea appears in warm, moist places such as the cervix, uterus, fallopian tubes, rectum, urethra, mouth, throat, penis, or testicles.

How do you get it? Gonorrhea is usually transmitted by oral, vaginal, or anal contact, and can also be passed from an infected woman to her baby during childbirth. It can cause permanent infertility in both men and women. Women who have gonorrhea and do not treat it promptly may develop pelvic inflammatory disease (PID). Untreated gonorrhea in men can lead to infertility, prostatitis or epididymis, and/or narrowing of the urethra, which makes it difficult to urinate.

How can you tell if you have it? If a person has symptoms, they usually appear in the first week after exposure to gonorrhea, but many people do not experience symptoms, and sometimes symptoms appear a month or more after exposure.

s.e.x.

Men or women with a rectal gonorrheal infection may have unusual vaginal or rectal discharge, anal itching, genital soreness, unexplained genital bleeding, or pain when urinating. Gonorrhea of the throat—which is common, especially among people who engage in unprotected oral sex—is usually asymptomatic.

A doctor or nurse usually diagnoses gonorrhea with a swab test, for men or women.

How do you treat it? Gonorrhea is diagnosed from vaginal or penile discharge, and/or from cultures taken from the throat or rectum. It is treated with antibiotics. Treatment cures a gonorrheal infection, but a person can still contract it again, so it's important to treat *both* partners when one partner is diagnosed with it, so that if the infection is present in both, it doesn't keep being passed back and forth.

How do you avoid it? Gonorrhea is almost always sexually transmitted, so if you aren't sexually active, your chances of getting it are basically zero. If you are sexually active, you can prevent gonorrheal infection with basic safer sex practices and screenings: if two partners have had negative gonorrhea screens, and are monogamously partnered, they cannot contract gonorrhea.

▪ HEPATITIS ▪

Hepatitis A, B, and C are viruses that destroy the liver.

HBV (hepatitis B) is the form of hepatitis spread most commonly via sexual activity (although hepatitis A can also be transmitted by oral-anal contact, and hepatitis C may also be more commonly transmitted by sexual contact than previously thought). Internationally, one out of three people has been infected with the hepatitis B virus, and 400 million people are carriers of it. In the United States alone, one out of twenty people has been infected with hepatitis B, and there are over one million chronic carriers.

How do you get it? HBV is found in body fluids such as blood, semen, and vaginal fluid, so the most common ways HBV spreads are unprotected sex, sharing drug needles, and tattoos or piercings done with unsanitized tools. It can also be transmitted to an infant during childbirth or breastfeeding.

How can you tell if you have it? Soon after a person is infected, they might get flu-like symptoms such as fever, feeling very tired or easily winded, muscle and joint pain, appetite loss, and nausea or vomiting, but around half of all people infected with hepatitis B don't have any symptoms.

How do you treat it? There are treatments available to slow the development of hepatitis B, and the vast majority of people will fight HBV with natural antibodies and cure themselves over time, but a diagnosis is still very important, because some people never develop antibodies (and thus, will be carriers, always) and may develop liver problems or liver cancer later in their lifetime. Knowing HBV status is also vital when it comes to knowing if you can infect others.

How do you avoid it? The best way to prevent infection with hepatitis is to get the vaccine (available for both types A and B), so check in with your doctor to find out if you've had it (and chances are good that you have), and if not, ask for it. If you haven't been vaccinated against hepatitis, wear gloves any time you come in contact with body fluids (sexually or in work situations), don't share needles, make sure tattoos and piercings are done with fresh, new equipment, and practice safer sex.

▪ HERPES ▪

The herpes virus has been around since at least the ancient Greeks: *herpes* is the Greek word meaning "to creep or crawl."

There are two types of the herpes simplex virus (HSV): type 1 (HSV-1) and type 2 (HSV-2). Type 1 usually infects the mouth (cold sores are HSV-1), and type 2 usually infects the genitals.

Herpes is one of the most common sexually transmitted diseases. About one in five people in the United States over age twelve—more than 45 million people—is infected with HSV-2, the virus that causes genital herpes, although most are unaware they have it. Many do not have visible symptoms, and it is more common in women than men. It's acquired most commonly in adolescence, although symptoms may become more prevalent with age: young adults are at a very high risk of herpes. Since the 1970s, genital herpes infections have increased at least 30 percent, with the largest increase occurring among young adults.

At least 50 percent, and as many as 80 percent, of Americans have oral herpes (HSV-1) at some time, and most were infected in early childhood through non-sexual contact.

How do you get it? Both types can be transmitted sexually (through kissing and oral sex as well as through skin and genital contact), and HSV-1 is not limited to the mouth area: if a person with oral herpes performs oral sex, it is possible for the partner to get genital herpes. HSV-1 can also sometimes cause genital-area or anal-area lesions or sores.

Herpes viruses are spread by contact between an infected area of the body and an uninfected, susceptible area of an uninfected person's body. This means that herpes can be spread from ANY affected part of the body—penis, vulva, anus, mouth, eye, lips/face—with or without fluid sharing. If an active sore is on a hand or has contacted an object, it can also be transmitted that way; for instance, a person with cold sores could wipe their mouth with their fingers, then perform manual sex on an uninfected person and infect them that way.

Sexually, it is most often spread by unprotected vaginal, anal, or oral sex, manual sex, or kissing. Herpes is most contagious when someone has an active sore; however, it may also be spread when no sores are visible or perceived to be present. Safer sex practices and barriers offer protection, but barriers that do not cover the entire surface of the genitals, like condoms, cannot offer complete protection, even though they do reduce risks. It is possible to transmit the herpes virus even with protected sex.

How can you tell if you have it? *If you experience cold sores or fever blisters, you have*

S.E.X.

oral herpes, and can give it to a partner orally or genitally—something that is often not made clear to people with cold sores.

When symptoms are present with genital herpes, they're usually in the form of a rash or red blisters on the vulva, vagina, or cervix; on the penis, buttocks, or anus; or on the mouth and other areas of the body. It is generally sore or uncomfortable, and tends to recur (happen more than once). When someone first contracts herpes, they might also experience burning while urinating, swollen glands, fever, headache, loss of appetite, and tiredness. When these first symptoms do occur, it's usually within one month of initial transmission, but a rash or sores may not occur for years afterward, or may not be visible on the external genitals.

The primary symptom of oral herpes is cold sores, usually on or around the lips. However, as many as two out of three people with HSV-1, and almost half of all people with HSV-2, never show symptoms.

Either form of herpes can be diagnosed by a doctor, usually with a swab of an active sore or via a blood test.

How do you treat it? Herpes isn't curable, in that there isn't treatment to make the virus leave the body. Herpes symptoms and outbreaks—as well as the risk of transmitting it to a partner—can be reduced with oral medications, but the virus still remains in the body even when treated, and can be transmitted even when sores are not visible.

How do you avoid it? Most often transmission happens when there IS an active sore, or when a sore is just forming or healing. People with either form of herpes should NOT have oral or genital contact with others when sores are present or when they can feel the tingling sensation that often signals an approaching outbreak. Latex barriers help reduce the risk of herpes transmission, though not as well as they help prevent transmission of STIs spread by body fluids.

▪ HIV AND AIDS ▪

HIV (human immunodeficiency virus) is a type of virus called a *retrovirus* that changes a cell's DNA. The HIV retrovirus destroys the immune system and thus massively weakens the body's ability to fight disease and infection, even common infections like flus and colds. AIDS (acquired immunodeficiency syndrome) is an acquired syndrome, or group of symptoms, that is caused by infection with the HIV virus.

HIV causes AIDS, but AIDS is NOT an STI. AIDS is a condition that often develops as a result of HIV infection. HIV can be transmitted between partners; AIDS cannot.

HIV is not the most common STI, but it *is* the most lethal.

About forty thousand people in the United States become infected with HIV every year, and it is the fifth leading cause of death for the those under forty in the United States (Kaiser Family Foundation). Widely (and dangerously) misrepresented as a disease that only or primarily infects gay men, HIV currently infects women worldwide, especially women of color, at higher rates than men. Over forty million people worldwide have been infected with HIV, and over twenty-five million have died as a result, making it the deadliest epidemic in history.

At this time, no one has yet been cured of HIV or AIDS.

How do you get it? HIV is spread through body fluids (blood, saliva, semen, vaginal secretions, or breast milk) via unprotected anal and vaginal intercourse or oral sex (although transmission through oral sex is more rare), shared needles used for injecting IV drugs or body modification, accidental pricks with infected needles, blood transfusions, childbirth, or breastfeeding.

How can you tell if you have it? Initial infection may have symptoms that resemble mononucleosis or the flu within two to four weeks of exposure, but for most people, HIV infection does not show any symptoms for extended periods of time—and for some, it is asymptomatic for years. When symptoms are present, they may include sore throat, fever, mouth sores or ulcers, aching or stiff muscles or joints, headaches, diarrhea, swollen glands, rashes or eczema, yeast infections, tiredness, or rapid weight loss.

HIV is diagnosed with a saliva or blood test that looks for HIV antibodies. Because it can take up to three months or more for antibodies to appear, a negative test should always be repeated, and an annual or semiannual HIV screening is strongly advised for sexually active people.

How do you treat it? HIV cannot be cured, but it can be treated and managed through an aggressive combination of antiviral drugs, naturopathic remedies, nutrition, and consistent healthcare. Most HIV treatment acts to try to protect the immune system from further infection, and to fend off or slow the progression of HIV to AIDS.

How do you avoid it? HIV infection can be prevented by using condoms for vaginal intercourse, anal intercourse, or oral sex. Prevention methods also include decreasing your number of sexual partners; avoiding high-risk sexual practices like anal sex, oral-anal sex, or vaginal sex altogether; avoiding sex with those who use intravenous drugs, and not participating in IV drug use yourself; avoiding blood or urine contact with the mouth, anus, eyes, or open cuts or sores; and insisting your partners get annual or semiannual HIV screenings.

If, at any time, you know or suspect you may have been exposed to the HIV virus, talk to your doctor, as there currently are some medications, called antiretrovirals, that may reduce your risk of acquiring HIV after the fact.

▪ HUMAN PAPILLOMAVIRUS (HPV) ▪ AND GENITAL WARTS

HPV is likely the most common STI in the United States. The Guttmacher Institute reports that nearly three out of every four Americans between the ages of fifteen and forty-nine have been infected with HPV at some point in their lives, and some studies show that at *least* one-third of all sexually active young adults have genital HPV infections. Over five million new cases of HPV infections are reported every year in the

United States alone. There are more than seventy different known strains, or types, of HPV, some of which (around thirteen) are potentially cancerous and causes of cervical cancer, which kills over 200,000 women each year. HPV is often called genital warts, because when some strains are externally symptomatic, it appears as tiny cauliflower-like warts on the internal or external genitals. About two-thirds of people who have sexual contact with a partner with a wart-producing strain of HPV will develop warts, usually within three months of contact. Yet, only a teeny sliver of the U.S. population has genital warts; in most cases, HPV shows no external symptoms, although it is still present and highly contagious, and condoms do not offer complete protection against HPV.

It's still unclear if some HPV infections are temporary and may, in time, be cleared up by the body's immune system (although reactivation or reinfection would still be possible). Since there isn't yet a test or guaranteed way to know if a person has been able to shed the virus, it's safest to assume that someone who has had HPV can always infect others again.

How do you get it? Body fluids don't need to be shared for HPV to be spread. It is transmitted through genital contact, usually during vaginal or anal sex, and sometimes through oral or manual sex. Someone who is not sexually active is very unlikely to have HPV. Because latex barriers like condoms only cover part of the genitals, while using them absolutely does reduce the risk, they are not as helpful at preventing infections like HPV as they are with STIs transmitted by fluid sharing. So, it is possible to contract HPV from protected sex, but latex barriers make it far less likely.

How can you tell if you have it? Again, most HPV cases are asymptomatic: less than 1 percent of people with HPV have any visible symptoms. When symptoms are present, small, cauliflower-like warts may appear on the vulva, vagina, anus, or penis, inside the urethra, or in the throat, at any time from thirty days to years after infection. When warts are present, diagnosis by a healthcare provider is pretty simple, through a tissue sample, vinegar test, and/or visual exam of the wart or warts. When no visible symptoms exist, in women, a Pap smear may reveal precancerous conditions likely caused by HPV. A colposcope (a special magnifying instrument used to get a closer look at the vagina and cervix) may also be used to obtain a diagnosis. Currently, there is no clear HPV test for men. If a man's partner is infected, it is generally assumed that he is as well.

How do you treat it? The virus itself is not presently treatable or curable.

If warts are present, they can be removed by various methods, namely by being frozen off (cryotherapy) or burned off (electrocauterized), removed with a patient-applied solution, dissolved with acid solutions, or removed by laser surgery. Those methods are relatively painless, and are usually done in a gynecologist's or healthcare provider's office on an outpatient basis, not in a hospital, although people with more extensive warts may require surgery. Which method is used depends on the patient, the availability of methods, and the particular warts and strain in question. Even when warts are removed, the virus is still present in the body, and can be transmitted to partners.

How do you avoid it? To prevent HPV if you're sexually active, practice safer sex, including annual screenings and pap smears, even though latex barriers may not offer complete protection: it's a "can't hurt, can help" scenario. Avoiding genital contact with partners altogether is the best protection against HPV. Be sure, too, to stay up-to-date with yearly Pap smears, which can diagnose cervical cancer from HPV early enough for effective treatment.

There is now also a vaccine for HPV, which has so far been shown in trials to be nearly 100 percent effective at protecting patients against four of the most common HPV strains. To date, it is only available for women, and is recommended for women between the ages of nine and twenty-six, as early as possible—preferably by the age of eleven or twelve—before any exposure to the virus can occur. However, even for women above that age, or who have already been sexually active, the vaccine can still be used, although it may not be as effective. Be sure to ask your doctor about the HPV vaccine.

▪ MONONUCLEOSIS ▪

Mononucleosis, or "mono," is a general infection caused by the Epstein-Barr virus, spread in many of the same ways as a simple flu virus.

How do you get it? It's often called the "kissing disease," because it's spread

mainly by contact with saliva or mucus from someone with mono, and because mono is common in adolescents. But it can also be spread by sharing drinking glasses or silverware, or being coughed on by someone who has it.

How can you tell if you have it? Some lucky people with mono experience no symptoms. For most others, though, fever, a sore throat, swollen glands, headaches, reduced appetite, and exhaustion are common.

How do you treat it? Mono isn't treatable. As with a common cold, you just have to rest and wait it out—and that can take a week to over a month, unfortunately—but it's also not a serious threat to most people's health. Do see a doctor if you suspect mono, however, to make sure it isn't something else with similar symptoms that does need treatment, like strep throat.

How do you avoid it? Since mono is so often transmitted casually, and without sexual contact, the only thing you can really do to avoid it, besides living alone under a rock, is to be sure to avoid intimate contact with someone you know currently has or has been exposed to mono.

▪ NONGONOCOCCAL URETHRITIS ▪ (NGU)

NGU is a bacterial infection of the urethra in men (and more rarely, women), usually caused by another sexually transmitted infection, most often chlamydia. If left untreated, NGU can cause epididymitis in men, or

s.e.x.

PID in women, either of which can lead to infertility if left untreated. NGU affects around four to six million U.S. men each year, and is more common in younger men.

How do you get it? Usually through another STI transmitted via oral, vaginal, or anal sex.

How can you tell if you have it? Like many infections, NGU usually does not present obvious symptoms. If you have NGU genitally and do have symptoms, they may include genital discharges, pain or burning while urinating, itching, or genital soreness. Those with NGU of the throat may experience a sore throat.

A doctor can diagnose NGU through visible urethral inflammation (swelling) in men, a urethral swab or oral swab, and a Pap smear for women.

How do you treat it? NGU is treatable with a round of antibiotics. As with chlamydia, it's important that all partners be treated for NGU when one has been diagnosed with it.

How do you avoid it? To avoid NGU, either engage in safer sex practices for oral, vaginal, and/or anal sex, or abstain from partnered sex. Since NGU results from other infections, staying up-to-date with yearly STI screenings helps reduce the risk of developing NGU.

▪ PELVIC INFLAMMATORY DISEASE ▪ (PID)

Pelvic inflammatory disease is a serious bacterial infection of the female reproductive organs. Men cannot develop PID, and it is not contagious.

About one million cases of PID are reported in the United States annually, and 20 percent of PID cases are found in teens, who often are unable to get (or lax about) reproductive healthcare. When left untreated, PID can progressively infect other reproductive organs: the uterus, uterine lining, fallopian tubes, and/or ovaries. PID can result in chronic pain and ectopic pregnancy or permanent sterility. Of all infertile women, an estimated 15 percent are infertile because of PID.

How do you get it? PID usually starts in the vagina via an existing sexually transmitted infection. Gonorrhea and chlamydia are the usual cause of PID, especially when they are left untreated.

How can you tell if you have it? PID symptoms may include painful periods that may last longer than in previous cycles, spotting or cramping between periods, unusual vaginal discharge, pain or cramping during urination, blood in the urine, lower back or abdominal pain, fever, nausea or vomiting, and/or pain during vaginal intercourse.

PID is often difficult to diagnose, and it is widely thought that millions of cases each year go undiagnosed or overlooked. To diagnose PID, a pelvic exam is required that includes a Pap smear and a possible laparoscopy (a diagnostic procedure that can usually be done in an office visit), in order for your doctor or clinician to take a close look at your reproductive system. It is also imperative that you tell your doctor or clinician if you have been sexually active with a partner and what your sexual history has been, including any known or suspected sexually transmitted infections.

How do you treat it? PID is curable, but a person can become reinfected. It is often treated with a combination of antibiotics, bed rest, and a period of sexual celibacy. In more severe cases, surgery may be required, including the possible removal of some reproductive organs.

How do you avoid it? Safer sex practices, especially condoms during vaginal intercourse, offer a high level of protection from PID. Because untreated STIs are often at the root of PID, annual STI screenings greatly reduce the risk of PID.

▪ PUBIC LICE ▪

Pubic lice are sometimes known as "crabs." The condition is caused by very tiny parasitic mites that settle in the pubic hair and feed on human blood. About three million new cases of pubic lice are treated in the United States each year, but it is unknown how many people have it at any one time.

How do you get it? Pubic lice are usually spread through sexual contact (and latex barrier use doesn't help, since they live in the pubic hair, not on the genitals), but can also be transmitted through bed linens, towels, or clothes, because lice can live for twenty-four hours off a human body. It is unlikely that pubic lice can be spread by toilet seats, because the feet of lice are not designed to walk on or hold on to smooth surfaces.

How can you tell if you have it? The primary symptom of pubic lice is unmistakable: severe and constant itching in the pubic area, within about five days of infection. Some people also get blue spots where they were bitten. Scratching the itchy areas may spread the lice to other parts of the body that coarse body hair, such as the legs, armpits, mustache or beard, eyebrows, or eyelashes.

Public lice can be self-diagnosed, but not easily, as pubic lice can be confused with other sorts of mites. A doctor can best diagnose pubic lice with a skin sample and a microscope.

How do you treat it? Treating public lice is fairly simple: lotions and shampoos that will kill pubic lice are available from a doctor or pharmacy. A person with pubic lice will also need to clean anything that might have lice on it: dirty clothes, bed linens, towels, and the like need to be washed in very hot water. If something can't be washed, it needs to be put in a plastic bag for two weeks to kill the lice and keep them from hopping onto another body in the meantime. It's common to still be itchy for a bit after treatment. Calamine lotion or hydrocortisone creams can relieve itching.

Pubic lice do not cause anything more than discomfort and inconvenience, although people who scratch the bites may get bacterial infections.

How do you avoid it? Latex barriers with sexual partners don't make any difference to public lice. So, unfortunately, there's little you can do to avoid public lice, except avoiding close contact or linen sharing with someone you know has them.

S.e.x.

▪ SYPHILIS ▪

Syphilis, one of the oldest STIs out there, is a bacterial infection. There are currently fewer that forty thousand reported cases of syphilis in the United States, but there have been recent increases. People with untreated syphilis may develop neurosyphilis, a potentially serious disorder of the nervous system. Infants born to mothers with syphilis can be born with very severe mental and physical problems.

Interestingly enough, syphilis, with gonorrhea, was the target of one of the first abstinence and celibacy campaigns in the United States, during World War II. While nearly every other country furnished its soldiers with scads of condoms to protect them, the United States opted for a celibacy campaign. Guess whose country ended up with a syphilis epidemic peaking at over 100,000 cases?

How do you get it? Syphilis is spread through skin-to-skin contact, when someone touches a sore on a person who has syphilis. The sores are usually on the mouth, penis, vagina, or anus. Syphilis is usually transmitted during oral, vaginal, or anal sexual contact.

How can you tell if you have it? Syphilis has been called "the great imitator" because many of its signs look like other diseases. It is also difficult to know if someone has syphilis because a person might not have any symptoms at all. There are considered to be four stages of syphilis:

1. **Primary:** The first symptom of syphilis is an ulcer that forms in the area where the person was exposed, one to six weeks after exposure. Many people don't notice these if they are painless or hidden inside the mouth, anus, or vagina. These ulcers usually disappear in a few weeks on their own, but the person still has the infection and can pass the disease to other people during this stage.

2. **Secondary:** A skin rash of large, coin-sized sores is the symptom of secondary syphilis. There are infectious bacteria in the sores, so anyone who touches them can be infected. Mild fever, headache, sore throat, and hair loss are also secondary symptoms. These symptoms usually go away in a few months, but recur for up to two years, and again the person is still carrying the bacteria and can infect others.

3. **Latent:** During this stage, there are often no symptoms at all, but the infection is still present, although during this time the infected person will likely not infect others.

4. **Tertiary/Late:** People who are infected for a long time may start to have many severe problems. The bacteria can damage the heart, eyes, liver, brain, bones, and joints. People can become mentally ill, go blind, develop heart disease, or die.

Syphilis is serious business.

It is screened for with microscopic examination of fluid from sores, blood tests, and/or examination of spinal fluid. It's important that the partners of anyone diagnosed with syphilis also be treated, and that anyone treated be retested after treatment to be sure it worked.

s.e.x.

How do you treat it? Dangerous as it is, it's very easily cured and treated: just a single dose of penicillin can usually cure a person who has had the infection for less than a year. So, annual STI screenings are important: if you're tested once a year, you can rest assured that there's no way you'll be walking around with syphilis for longer than that, even if you've taken sexual risks.

How do you avoid it? Syphilis is generally only transmitted through unprotected sex, so you can prevent syphilis with standard and constant safer sex practices, or by abstaining from sexual contact with others.

▪ TRICHOMONIASIS ▪

Trichomoniasis ("trich"), infection with the *Trichomonas* parasite, is one of the most common STIs, mainly affecting women sixteen to thirty-five years of age. In the United States, it is estimated that five million people become infected with trichomoniasis each year.

How do you get it? *Trichomonas* lives in warm and damp environments like the vagina, urethra, or bladder. It is usually sexually transmitted via direct genital contact, but occasionally is spread by sharing damp towels, washcloths, or bathing suits.

How can you tell if you have it? Only about half the women with trich have any symptoms. When symptoms do develop, usually within one to several months, they may include: a yellow-green, foul smelling vaginal discharge; vaginal itching or redness; pain during intercourse or urination; and/or a frequent urge to urinate. Even fewer men with trich have symptoms than women; pain during urination and ejaculation, discharge from the urethra, and/or a frequent urge to urinate are some symptoms that may be present in infected men.

Doctors diagnose trich by examining genital discharge under a microscope, and/or with a genital exam.

How do you treat it? Antibiotics for infected people and their sexual partners usually cure the infection, but a second round of antibiotics is sometimes needed. It is also helpful to wear cotton underwear and avoid wearing pantyhose during treatment.

How do you avoid it? It is spread via direct genital fluid contact, so if you aren't sexually active, you aren't likely to acquire trichomoniasis. If you are sexually active, latex barriers during genital sexual activities offer excellent protection against trich.

s.e.x.

bibliography
and recommended resources

▪ PARENT INTRODUCTION, ▪
CHAPTERS 1–4

Chapters covering general sexuality; sex and culture; anatomy; body image and self-esteem; general health; masturbation, arousal, and orgasm; fantasy and pornography

BOOKS AND PRINT SOURCES AND RESOURCES

Angier, Natalie. *Woman: An Intimate Geography.* New York: Anchor, 2000.

Bartle, Nathalie, and Susan Lieberman. *Venus in Blue Jeans: Why Mothers and Daughters Need to Talk About Sex.* Boston: Dell, 1999.

Blank, Joani. *Femalia.* San Francisco: Down There Press, 1993.

Bornstein, Kate. *Hello Cruel World: 101 Alternatives to Suicide for Teens, Freaks, and Other Outlaws.* New York: Seven Stories Press, 2006.

Boston Women's Health Book Collective. *Our Bodies, Ourselves for the New Century: A Book by and for Women.* New York: Touchstone, 1998.

Brashich, Audrey D. *All Made Up: A Girl's Guide to Seeing Through Celebrity Hype and Celebrating Real Beauty.* New York: Walker Books for Young Readers, 2006.

Brumberg, Joan Jacobs. *The Body Project: An Intimate History of American Girls.* New York: Vintage Books, 1998.

Cohen, Joseph. *The Penis Book.* New York: Broadway Books, 2004.

Cornog, Martha. *The Big Book of Masturbation: From Angst to Zeal.* San Francisco: Down There Press: 2003.

Costin, Carolyn. *The Eating Disorder Sourcebook: A Comprehensive Guide to the Causes, Treatments, and Prevention of Eating Disorders.* New York: McGraw-Hill, 1999.

Delacoste, Frederique, and Priscilla Alexander. *Sex Work: Writings by Women in the Sex Industry.* San Francisco: Cleis Press, 1998.

Dodson, Betty. *Sex for One: The Joy of Selfloving.* New York: Three Rivers Press, 1996.

Drill, Esther, et al. *Deal With It! A Whole New Approach to Your Body, Brain and Life as a gURL.* New York: Pocket Books, 1999.

Ensler, Eve. *The Good Body.* New York: Villard Books, 2004.

Espeland, Pamela. *Life Lists for Teens: Tips, Steps, Hints, and How-Tos for Growing Up, Getting Along, Learning, and Having Fun.* Minneapolis, MN: Free Spirit Publishing, 2003.

Gottlieb, Lori. *Stick Figure.* New York: Berkley Trade, 2001.

Grant, Linda. *Sexing the Millennium.* New York: Grove Press, 1995.

Hite, Shere. *The Hite Report on the Family: Growing Up Under Patriarchy.* New York: Grove Press, 1996.

Hornbacher, Marya. *Wasted: A Memoir of Anorexia and Bulimia.* New York: Harper Perennial, 1999.

Houppert, Karen. *The Curse: Confronting the Last Unmentionable Taboo: Menstruation.* New York: Farrar, Straus and Giroux, 2000.

Jamison, Paul H. "Penis Size Increase between Flaccid and Erect States: An Analysis of the Kinsey Data." *Journal of Sex Research* 24, nos. 1–4 (January 1988).

Jukes, Mavis. *The Guy Book: An Owner's Manual.* New York: Crown Publishers, 2002.

Kempadoo, Kamala, and Jo Doezema. *Global Sex Workers: Rights, Resistance, and Redefinition.* New York: Routledge, 1998.

Kipnis, Laura. *Bound and Gagged: Pornography and the Politics of Fantasy in America.* Durham: Duke University Press, 1999.

Kirberger, Kimberly. *No Body's Perfect: Stories by Teens about Body Image, Self-Acceptance, and the Search for Identity.* New York: Scholastic Paperbacks, 2003.

Komisaruk, Barry R., Carlos Beyer-Flores, and Beverly Whipple. *The Science of Orgasm.* Baltimore, MD: The Johns Hopkins University Press, 2006.

Lopez, Ralph I. *The Teen Health Book: A Parent's Guide to Adolescent Health and Well-Being.* New York: W.W. Norton & Company, 2003.

Luciano, Lynn. *Looking Good: Male Body Image in Modern America.* New York: Hill & Wang, 2001.

Malamuth, Neil, and James Check. "The Effects of Aggressive Pornography on Beliefs in Rape Myths: Individual Differences." *Journal of Research in Personality* 19 (1985).

McKoy, Kathy. *The Teenage Body Book.* Rutherford, NJ: Perigee Trade, 1999.

Moore, Thomas. *The Soul of Sex.* New York: Harper Perennial, 1999.

Muscio, Inga. *Cunt: A Declaration of Independence.* Seattle, WA: Seal Press, 1998.

Nagle, Jill. *Whores and Other Feminists.* New York: Routledge, 1997.

Netter, Frank H. *Atlas of Human Anatomy.* Philadelphia: Saunders, 2002.

Paley, Maggie. *The Book of the Penis.* New York: Grove Press, 2000.

Parker, William H., and Rachel L. Parker. *A Gynecologist's Second Opinion.* New York: Plume Books, 2003.

Planned Parenthood Federation of America, Inc. *The Planned Parenthood Women's Health Encyclopedia.* New York: Crown Trade Paperbacks, 1996.

Reinisch, June M., and Ruth Beasley. *The Kinsey Institute New Report on Sex.* New York: St. Martin's Griffin, 1991.

Salmansohn, Karen. *The Clitourist.* New York: Universe Publishing, 2001.

Weschler, Toni. *Cycle Savvy: The Smart Teen's Guide to the Mysteries of Her Body.* New York: Collins, 2006.

Wykes, Maggie and Barrie Gunter. *The Media and Body Image: If Looks Could Kill.* London: Sage Publications, Ltd., 2005.

Zaviacic, Miland and Beverly Whipple. "Update on the Female Prostate and the Phenomenon of Female Ejaculation." *The Journal of Sex Research* 30, no. 2 (May 1993).

ONLINE SOURCES AND RESOURCES

About-Face
Combating negative and distorted images of women and girls in the media
http://www.about-face.org

American Academy of Pediatrics Circumcision Policy Statement. *Pediatrics* 103, no. 3 (March 1999): 686–93.
http://aappolicy.aappublications.org/cgi/content/full/pediatrics;103/3/686

ANRED: Anorexia Nervosa and Related Eating Disorders, Inc.
Information about anorexia nervosa, bulimia nervosa, binge eating disorder, and other less well-known food and weight disorders
http://www.anred.com

BBC News, "Breast Implant Suicide Link," March 7, 2003.
http://news.bbc.co.uk/1/hi/health/2826933.stm

BodyPositive.com
Boosting body image at any weight
http://www.bodypositive.com

BodyQuest
Interactive explorations of human anatomy
http://library.thinkquest.org/10348/

The Centre for Menstrual Cycle and Ovulation Research
Research center with a mandate to distribute information directly to women about changes through the life cycle, from adolescence to menopause
http://www.cemcor.ubc.ca/

Diana Russell
Academic expert on pornography and violence against women and girls
http://www.dianarussell.com/

GladRags
Source for alternative menstrual products
http://www.gladrags.com/

The Intersex Society of North America
Working to end shame, secrecy, and unwanted genital surgeries for intersexed people
http://isna.org

KidsHealth
General pediatric and adolescent health information
http://www.kidshealth.org/parent/

Lunapads
Source for alternative menstrual products, including Lunapanties
http://www.lunapads.com

Males with Eating Disorders
ANRED's FAQ on eating disorders in men and boys
http://www.anred.com/males.html

Many Moons
Source for alternative menstrual products and menstrual pad patterns
http://pacificcoast.net/~manymoons/

Medline Plus: Circumcision
http://www.nlm.nih.gov/medlineplus/circumcision.html

The Museum of Menstruation & Women's Health
The history of menstruation and women's health
http://www.mum.org/

National Eating Disorders Association
Largest not-for-profit organization in the United States working to prevent eating disorders and provide treatment referrals
http://www.nationaleatingdisorders.org

The National Women's Health Information Center, U.S. Department of Health and Human Services
http://www.4woman.gov

The National Women's Health Information Center, U.S. Department of Health and Human Services: Frequently Asked Questions about Douching
http://www.4woman.gov/faq/douching.htm

Self-Injury
Self-injury resource run by a young self-injurer
http://www.self-injury.net

She Loves Sports
Information and support for women's athletics
http://www.shelovessports.com/

The Something Fishy Web Site on Eating Disorders
Comprehensive ED clearinghouse and support forum
www.something-fishy.org

U.S. Food and Drug Administration: Breast Implants Home Page
http://www.fda.gov/cdrh/breastimplants/

Chapters covering gender; sexual orientation and identity; relationships

BOOKS AND PRINT SOURCES AND RESOURCES

Bass, Ellen, *Free Your Mind,* New York: Harper Paperbacks; 1996

Bell, Chris, and Kate Brauer-Bell. *The Long-Distance Relationship Survival Guide: Secrets and Strategies from Successful Couples Who Have Gone the Distance.* Berkeley, CA: Ten Speed Press: 2006.

Bell, Ruth. *Changing Bodies, Changing Lives: A Book for Teens on Sex and Relationships.* 3rd ed. New York: Three Rivers Press, 1998.

Ben-Ze'ev, Aaron. *Love Online: Emotions on the Internet.* Cambridge, UK: Cambridge University Press, 2004.

Bronson, Howard, and Mike Riley. *How to Heal a Broken Heart in 30 Days: A Day-by-Day Guide to Saying Good-bye and Getting On with Your Life.* New York: Broadway Books, 2002.

Brownsey, Mo. *Is It a Date or Just Coffee?: The Gay Girl's Guide to Dating, Sex, and Romance.* Los Angeles: Alyson Books: 2002.

Canada, Geoffrey. *Reaching Up for Manhood: Transforming the Lives of Boys in America.* Boston: Beacon Press, 1998.

Cote, James E., and Anton L. Allahar. *Generation on Hold: Coming of Age in the Late Twentieth Century.* New York and London: New York University Press, 1996.

Daldry, Jeremy. *The Teenage Guy's Survival Guide: The Real Deal on Girls, Growing Up, and Other Guy Stuff.* Boston: Little, Brown Young Readers, 1999.

De Rougemont, Denis. *Love in the Western World.* Princeton, NJ: Princeton University Press, 1983.

Easton, Dossie, and Catherine A. Liszt. *The Ethical Slut: A Guide to Infinite Sexual Possibitilites.* Oakland, CA: Greenery Press, 1998.

Elkind, David. *All Grown Up and No Place to Go: Teenagers in Crisis.* Cambridge, MA: Perseus Books Group, 1997.

Fausto-Sterling, Anne. *Myths of Gender: Biological Theories About Women and Men.* New York: Basic Books, 1992.

———. *Sexing the Body: Gender Politics and the Construction of Sexuality.* New York: Basic Books, 2000.

Ford, Michael Thomas. *The World Out There: Becoming Part of the Lesbian and Gay Community.* New York: New Press, 1996.

Foucault, Michel. *The History of Sexuality: An Introduction.* New York: Vintage Books, 1990.

Fox, Annie, and Elizabeth Verdick. *The Teen Survival Guide to Dating and Relating: Real-World Advice on Guys, Girls, Growing Up, and Getting Along.* Minneapolis, MN: Free Spirit Publishing, 2005.

Gilligan, Carol, and Lyn Mikel Brown. *Meeting at the Crossroads.* New York: Ballantine Books, 1993.

Gray, Mary L. *In Your Face: Stories from the Lives of Queer Youth.* Haworth Gay and Lesbian Studies. New York: Haworth Press, 1999.

Hanh, Thich Nhat. *True Love: A Practice for Awakening the Heart.* Boston: Shambhala, 2004.

Hatchell, Deborah. *What Smart Teenagers Know . . . About Dating, Relationships, and Sex.* Santa Barbara, CA: Piper Books, 2003.

Hooks, Bell. *All About Love: New Visions.* New York: Harper Paperbacks, 2001.

Huegel, Kelly. *GLBTQ: The Survival Guide for Queer and Questioning Teens.* Minneapolis, MN: FreeSpirit Publishing, 2003.

Hutchins, Loraine, and Lani Kaahumanu. *Bi Any Other Name: Bisexual People Speak Out.* Los Angeles: Alyson Books, 1991.

Jacobson, Bonnie, and Sandra J. Gordon,. *The Shy Single: A Bold Guide to Dating for the Less-Than-Bold Dater.* Emmaus, PA: Rodale Books, 2004.

Jennings, Kevin, and Pat Shapiro. *Always My Child: A Parent's Guide to Understanding Your Gay, Lesbian, Bisexual, Transgendered or Questioning Son or Daughter.* New York: Fireside, 2002.

Jones, Jennifer T., and John D. Cunningham. "Attachment Styles and Other Predictors of Relationship Satisfaction in Dating Couples." *Personal Relationships* 3, no. 4 (December 1996).

Kaufman, Moises. *The Laramie Project.* New York: Vintage Books, 2001.

s.e.x.

Levy, Ariel. *Female Chauvinist Pigs: Women and the Rise of Raunch Culture.* New York: Free Press, 2005.

Mapes, Diane. *How to Date in a Post-Dating World.* Seattle, WA: Sasquatch Books, 2006.

Ochs, Robyn. *Bisexual Resource Guide,* Boston, MA: Bisexual Resources Center, 2001.

Orenstein, Peggy. *Schoolgirls: Young Women, Self Esteem, and the Confidence Gap.* New York: Anchor Books, 1995.

Patterson, Charlotte J., and Anthony R. D'Augelli. *Lesbian, Gay, and Bisexual Identities and Youth.* New York and London: Oxford University Press, 2003.

Pollack, William. *Real Boys: Rescuing Our Sons from the Myths of Boyhood.* New York: Owl Books, 1999.

Queen, Carol, and Lawrence Schimel . *Pomosexuals: Challenging Assumptions About Gender and Sexuality.* San Francisco: Cleis Press, 1997.

Shandler, Sara. *Ophelia Speaks: Adolescent Girls Write About Their Search for Self.* New York: Harper Paperbacks, 1999.

Solot, Dorian, and Marshall Miller. *Unmarried to Each Other: The Essential Guide to Living Together As an Unmarried Couple.* New York: Marlowe & Company, 2002.

Stallings, Ariel Meadow, *Offbeat Bride,* Emeryville, CA: Seal Press, 2007

Sullivan, Jim. *Boyfriend 101: A Gay Guy's Guide to Dating, Romance, and Finding True Love.* New York: Villard Books, 2003.

Tanenbaum, Leora. *Slut! Growing Up Female with a Bad Reputation.* New York: HarperCollins Publishers, 2000.

ONLINE SOURCES AND RESOURCES

About.com
About: Teen Advice
Friendships and fitting in
http://teenadvice.about.com/cs/friendships/

All Girl Army
Young feminist blogging and community
http://www.allgirlarmy.org

The American Civil Liberties Union (ACLU)
Includes reproductive rights, GLBT rights,
HIV/AIDS, and youth rights divisions
http://www.aclu.org

American Psychological Association
Resolutions Related To Lesbian, Gay and Bisexual Issues:
http://www.apa.org/pi/reslgbc.html

Answers to Your Questions About Sexual Orientation and Homosexuality:
http://www.apa.org/topics/orientation.html

Appropriate Therapeutic Responses to Sexual Orientation:
http://www.apa.org/pi/lgbc/policy/appropriate.html

Discovery Health's Teen Relationships Index
http://health.discovery.com/centers/teen/relationships/relationships.html

Families Like Mine
Abigail Garner's site to decrease isolation for people whose parents are lesbian, gay, bisexual, or transgender, and to bring voice to the experiences of these families
http://www.familieslikemine.com/

Fetto, John, "First Comes Love" (Teen Dating Statistics), *Advertising Age:* American Demographics, June 1, 2003
http://www.adage.com/americandemographics

GayTeenResources (GTR)
A site "dedicated to the simple principle that LGBT youth should have a place they could go to online without worrying about being hit on, being outed to family or friends, and where they can find help and links to resources that could offer additional assistance."
http://www.gayteenresources.org

The Gender Public Advocacy Coalition (GenderPAC)
Works to ensure that classrooms, communities, and workplaces are safe for everyone to learn, grow, and succeed—whether or not they meet expectations for masculinity and femininity
http://www.gpac.org/

GLAAD

The Gay and Lesbian Alliance Against
Defamation
http://www.glaad.org/

GLBT Historical Society

Collects, preserves, and interprets the history of
GLBT people and the communities that support
them
http://www.glbthistory.org/

HRC: The Human Rights Campaign

America's largest civil rights organization working
to achieve gay, lesbian, bisexual, and transgender
equality
http://www.hrc.org/

Lambda Legal Defense and Education Fund

National organization committed to achieving full
recognition of the civil rights of lesbians, gay men,
bisexuals, transgender people, and those with HIV
through impact litigation, education, and public
policy work
http://www.lambdalegal.org/

The National Organization for Women (NOW)

The largest organization of feminist activists in the
United States
http://www.now.org

OutProud

Resources for queer and questioning youth
http://www.outproud.org

Parents, Friends and Families of Lesbians and Gays

Provides opportunity for dialogue about sexual
orientation and gender identity, and acts to create a
society that is healthy and respectful of human
diversity
http://www.pflag.org

Technodyke.com

Dynamic lesbian community Web site
http://www.technodyke.com

Teen Relationships Website

For teens, by teens: relationship information and
support
http://www.teenrelationships.org/

Teen Voices

Web site for Teen Voices, the magazine for teens, by
teens
http://www.teenvoices.com

Tolerance.org

Tests for hidden biases
http://www.tolerance.org/hidden_bias/index
.html

Transsexual.org

Transsexuality information and support
http://transsexual.org

The YMCA (Young Men's Christian Association)
http://www.ymca.net/

The YWCA (Young Women's Christian
Association)
http://www.ywca.org/

▪ CHAPTERS 7–9, 11–12 ▪

Chapters covering sexual readiness; choices
and sexual activities; sexual health and safer
sex; contraception, reproductive options,
and pregnancy

BOOKS AND PRINT SOURCES AND RESOURCES

Basso, Michael J. *The Underground Guide to*
Teenage Sexuality. 2nd ed. Minneapolis, MN:
Fairview Press, 2003.

Beckmann, Charles R. B. *Obstetrics and Gynecol-*
ogy. Philadelphia: Lippincott Williams &
Wilkins, 2002.

Blank, Hanne. *Big, Big Love: A Sourcebook on Sex*
for People of Size and Those Who Love Them.
Oakland, CA: Greenery Press, 2000.

———. *Virgin: The Untouched History.* New York:
Bloomsbury USA, 2007.

Bolles, Edmund Blair. *The Penguin Adoption*
Handbook. New York: Penguin Books, 1993.

Boston Women's Health Collective. *Our Bodies,*
Ourselves: Updated and Expanded for the 90's.
Gloucester, MA: Peter Smith Publisher, 2005.

s.e.x.

Bright, Susie. *Full Exposure: Opening Up to Sexual Creativity and Erotic Expression*. New York: HarperCollins, Harper San Francisco, 2000.

————. *The Sexual State of the Union*. New York: Touchstone, 1998.

Carmody, Moira. *Ethical Erotics: Reconceptualizing Anti-Rape Education. Sexualities* 8, no. 4 (2005).

Coles, Robert. *The Youngest Parents: Teenage Pregnancy As It Shapes Lives*. New York: W. W. Norton & Company, 2000.

Comfort, Alex. *The Joy of Sex*. New York: Crown Publishers, 2002.

Davis, Deborah. *You Look Too Young to Be a Mom: Teen Mothers Speak Out on Love, Learning, and Success*. New York: Perigee, 2004.

DePuy, Candace, and Dana Dovitch. *The Healing Choice: Your Guide to Emotional Recovery After an Abortion*. Minneapolis, MN: Fireside, 1997.

Dodson, Betty. *Orgasms for Two: The Joy of Partnersex*. New York: Harmony Books, 2002.

Eisler, Riane. *Sacred Pleasure: Sex, Myth, and the Politics of the Body—New Paths to Power and Love*. New York: HarperCollins, Harper San Francisco, 1996.

Hite, Shere. *The Hite Report: A National Study of Female Sexuality*. New York: Seven Stories Press, 2003.

————. *The Hite Report on Male Sexuality*. New York: Ballantine Books, 1987.

Jacobs, Thomas A., and Jay E. Johnson. *What Are My Rights?: 95 Questions and Answers About Teens and the Law*. Minneapolis, MN: Free Spirit Publishing, 1997.

Joannides, Paul. *The Guide to Getting It On!* Waldport, OR: Goofy Foot Press, 2004.

Kerner, Ian. *He Comes Next: The Thinking Woman's Guide to Pleasuring a Man*. New York: Regan Books, 2006.

————. *She Comes First: The Thinking Man's Guide to Pleasuring a Woman*. New York: Regan Books, 2004.

Lancaster, Roger N., and Micaela DiLeonardo. *The Gender/Sexuality Reader*. New York: Routledge, 1997.

Langdridge, Darren, and Trevor Butt. "The Erotic Construction of Power Exchange." *Journal of Constructivist Psychology* 18, no. 1 (2005).

Lindsay, Jeanne Warren. *Teen Dads*. Buena Park, CA: Morning Glory Press, 2000.

Lindsay, Jeanne Warren, and Jean Brunelli. *Your Pregnancy and Newborn Journey: A Guide for Pregnant Teens*. Teen Pregnancy and Parenting series. Buena Park, CA: Morning Glory Press, 2004.

Lorde, Audre. *The Uses of the Erotic: The Erotic As Power*. Tucson, AZ: Kore Press, 2000.

Luker, Kristin. *Abortion and the Politics of Motherhood*. California Series on Social Choice and Political Economy. Berkeley, CA: University of California Press, 1985.

————. *Dubious Conceptions: The Politics of Teenage Pregnancy*. Cambridge, MA: Harvard University Press, 1997.

Marr, Lisa. *Sexually Transmitted Diseases: A Physician Tells You What You Need to Know*. Baltimore, MD: Johns Hopkins Press, 1998.

Matcher, Robert A., et al. *Contraceptive Technology*. New York: Ardent Media, Inc., 2004.

Morin, Jack. *Anal Pleasure and Health: A Guide for Men and Women*. San Francisco: Down There Press, 1998.

————. *The Erotic Mind*. New York: Harper Paperbacks, 1996.

Murkoff, Heidi, et al. *What to Expect When You're Expecting*. 3rd ed. New York: Workman Publishing Company, 2002.

Newman, Felice. *The Whole Lesbian Sex Book: A Passionate Guide for All of Us*. San Francisco: Cleis Press, 2004.

Oumano, Elena. *Natural Sex*. New York: Plume Books, 1999.

Ponton, Lynn. *The Sex Lives of Teenagers: Revealing the Secret World of Adolescent Boys and Girls*. New York: Plume Books, 2001.

Ryden, Janice, and Paul D. Blumenthal. *Practical Gynecology: A Guide for the Primary Care Physician*. Philadelphia, PA: The American College of Physicians/American Society of Internal Medicine, 2002.

Shorto, Russell "Contra-Contraception." *New York Times,* May 7, 2006.

Shusterman, Lisa Roseman. "The Psychosocial Factors of the Abortion Experience: A Critical Review." *Psychology of Women Quarterly* 1, no. 1 (September 1976).

Silverberg, Cory, Miriam Kaufman, and Fran Odette. *The Ultimate Guide to Sex and Disability: For All of Us Who Live with Disabilities,*

Chronic Pain and Illness. San Francisco: Cleis Press, 2003.

Silverstein, Charles. *The Joy of Gay Sex*. 3rd ed. New York: HarperCollins, 2004.

Soll, Joseph M., and Karen Wilson Buterbaugh. *Adoption Healing . . . A Path to Recovery for Mothers Who Lost Children to Adoption*. Baltimore, MD: Gateway Press, Inc., 2003.

Southern, Stephen. "The Tie That Binds: Sadomasochism in Female Addicted Trauma Survivors." *Sexual Addiction and Compulsivity: The Journal of Treatment and Prevention* 9, no. 4 (2002).

Stotland, Nina L. *Abortion: Facts and Feelings: A Handbook for Women and the People Who Care About Them*. Arlington, VA: American Psychiatric Publishing, 1998.

Sundahl, Deborah. *Female Ejaculation and the G-Spot*. Alameda, CA: Hunter House Publishers, 2003.

Tone, Andrea. *Devices and Desires: A History of Contraceptives in America*. New York: Hill and Wang, 2001.

Turrell, S. C., et al. "Emotional response to abortion: a critical review of the literature." *Women & Therapy* 9, no. 4 (1990).

Venning, Rachel, and Claire Cavannah. *Sex Toys 101: A Playfully Uninhibited Guide*. New York: Fireside, 2003.

Weschler, Toni. *Taking Charge of Your Fertility*. New York: Collins, 2006.

Williams-Wheeler, Dorrie. *The Unplanned Pregnancy Book for Teens and College Students*. Virginia Beach, VA: Sparkledoll Productions, 2004.

Winks, Cathy, and Semans, Anne. *The Good Vibrations Guide to Sex: The Most Complete Sex Manual Ever Written*. San Francisco: Cleis Press, 2002.

Wiseman, Jay. *SM 101: A Realistic Introduction*. Oakland, CA: Greenery Press, 1998.

Wolf, Naomi. *Misconceptions: Truth, Lies, and the Unexpected on the Journey to Motherhood*. New York: Doubleday, 2001.

Zilbergeld, Bernie. *The New Male Sexuality*. New York: Bantam Books, 1999.

ONLINE SOURCES AND RESOURCES

The Abortion Access Project
Seeks to ensure access to abortion for all women by increasing abortion services, training new abortion providers, and raising awareness about the critical importance of abortion access to women's lives
http://www.abortionaccess.org

Abortion Clinics OnLine (ACOL)
Extensive directory of abortion providers and clinics in the U.S.
http://www.gynpages.com

Ann Rose's Ultimate Birth Control Links
Extensive information on birth control methods
http://www.ultimatebirthcontrol.com

Babeland
Sexuality information, safer sex supplies, books, and toys
http://www.babeland.com

The Body
A comprehensive multimedia AIDS and HIV resource
http://www.thebody.com/basics.html

Boonstra, Heather, "Teen Pregnancy: Trends and Lessons Learned."
The Guttmacher Report on Public Policy 5, no. 1 (February 2002)
http://www.guttmacher.org/pubs/tgr/05/1/gr050107.html

Breastfeeding.com
Information, support, and attitude
http://www.breastfeeding.com/

Centers for Disease Control and Prevention
http://www.cdc.gov/

The Center for Reproductive Rights
Legal advocacy organization to protect reproductive rights
http://www.reproductiverights.org

Condomania
Condoms and safer sex supplies
http://www.condomania.com

s.e.x.

Contraceptive Choices
Emory University's OB/GYN department page with extensive information on birth control, pregnancy, and abortion
http://www.gynob.emory.edu/familyplanning

Dailard, Cynthia, "Legislating Against Arousal: The Growing Divide between Federal Policy and Teenage Sexual Behavior."
Guttmacher Policy Review 9, no. 3 (Summer 2006)
http://www.guttmacher.org/pubs/gpr/09/3/gpr090312.html

Family Planning Perspectives
A journal of result results concerning all aspects of family planning
http://www.jstor.org/journals/00147354.html

The Feminist Women's Health Center
Comprehensive and accessible information on birth control methods, abortion and pregnancy, sexual health, and other topics regarding women's health
http://www.fwhc.org/

Gay and Lesbian Medical Association (GLMA)
Resources to help GLBTs find nondiscriminatory healthcare
http://www.glma.org/

Girl-Mom
Active, supportive community for teen parents
http://www.girlmom.com/

Good Vibrations
Sexuality information, safer sex supplies, books, and toys
http://www.goodvibes.com
Guttmacher Institute, *Facts on American Teens' Sexual and Reproductive Health*
http://www.guttmacher.org/pubs/fb_ATSRH.html: 09/2006

HipMama
Political commentary, community, and ribald tales from the front lines of motherhood
http://www.hipmama.com

The Journal of the American Medical Association
http://jama.ama-assn.org/

The Kinsey Institute
Data from Alfred Kinsey's studies
http://www.indiana.edu/~kinsey/research/ak-data.html

Momdadimpregnant.com

NARAL: Pro-Choice America
The nation's leading advocate for privacy and a woman's right to choose
http://www.prochoiceamerica.org/about-us/

The National Campaign to Prevent Teen Pregnancy
Working to drastically reduce the rate of unwanted teen pregnancy
http://www.teenpregnancy.org/

National Network of Abortion Funds (NNAF)
Providing financial aid for abortion services to women in need
http://www.nnaf.org/

Not-2-late.com: The Emergency Contraception Website
Constantly updated, comprehensive information on emergency contraception, including a location finder for EC
http://ec.princeton.edu/

OB/GYN.net
"The universe of women's health"
http://www.obgyn.net/

Ott, Mary, et al. "Greater Expectations: Adolescents' Positive Motivations for Sex."
Perspectives on Sexual and Reproductive Health 38, no. 2 (June 2006)
http://www.guttmacher.org/pubs/journals/3808406.html

Our Bodies, Ourselves
The blog of the Boston Women's Health Collective
http://www.ourbodiesourblog.org/

Planned Parenthood
Current, comprehensive information on sexual health, sexuality, and contraception; includes a locator to find Planned Parenthood clinics
http://www.plannedparenthood.org/index.htm

Population Council 11, no. 2 (May 2005)
"Emergency Contraception's Mode of Action Clarified"
http://www.popcouncil.org/publications/popbriefs/pb11(2)_3.html

Childbirth.org*Extensive information on all aspects of pregnancy and childbirth*
http://www.childbirth.org/

San Francisco Sex Information
Information and referral switchboard providing anonymous, accurate, nonjudgmental information about sex via phone or e-mail
http://www.sfsi.org/

The Sexual Health Network
Dedicated to providing easy access to sexuality information, education, support, and other resources
http://www.sexualhealth.com

▪ CHAPTER 10 ▪

Chapter covering abuse and rape

BOOKS AND PRINT SOURCES AND RESOURCES

Bass, Ellen, and Laura Davis. *The Courage to Heal: A Guide for Women Survivors of Child Sexual Abuse,* 3rd ed. New York: Collins,1994.

Bean, Barbara and Shari Bennett. *The Me Nobody Knows: A Guide for Teen Survivors.* San Francisco: Jossey-Bass, 1997.

Brownmiller, Susan. *Against Our Will: Men, Women, and Rape.* New York: Ballantine Books, 1993.

Cook, Philip W. *Abused Men: The Hidden Side of Domestic Violence.* Westport, CT: Praeger Trade, 1997.

Davis, Laura. *The Courage to Heal Workbook: A Guide for Women and Men Survivors of Child Sexual Abuse.* 1st ed. New York: Collins, 1990.

DeBecker, Gavin. *The Gift of Fear.* New York: Dell Books, 1998.

Feuereisen, Patti and Caroline Pincus. *Invisible Girls: The Truth About Sexual Abuse—A Book for Teen Girls, Young Women, and Everyone Who*

Cares About Them. Emeryville, CA: Seal Press, 2005.

Haines, Staci. *The Survivor's Guide to Sex: How to Have an Empowered Sex Life After Child Sexual Abuse.* San Francisco: Cleis Press, 1999.

Hanna, Cheryl. "The Paradox of Hope: The Crime and Punishment of Domestic Violence." *William and Mary Law Review* 39 (1998).

Katz, Jackson. *The Macho Paradox: Why Some Men Hurt Women and How All Men Can Help.* Naperville, IL: Sourcebooks, Inc., 2006.

Levy, Barrie. *In Love and in Danger: A Teen's Guide to Breaking Free of Abusive Relationships.* Emeryville, CA: Seal Press, 1998.

Morgan, Robin. *The Demon Lover: The Roots of Terrorism.* New York: Washington Square Press, 2001.

Murray, Jill. *But I Love Him: Protecting Your Teen Daughter from Controlling, Abusive Dating Relationships.* New York: Regan Books, 2001.

Ristock, Janice. *No More Secrets: Violence in Lesbian Relationships.* New York: Routledge, 2002.

Simmons, Rachel. *Odd Girl Out: The Hidden Culture of Aggression in Girls.* Orlando, FL: Harvest Books, 2003.

Snortland, Ellen B. *Beauty Bites Beast: Awakening the Warrior within Women and Girls.* Pasadena, CA: Trilogy Books, 1998.

Warshaw, Robin. *I Never Called It Rape: The Ms. Report on Recognizing, Fighting, and Surviving Date and Acquaintance Rape.* New York: Harper Paperbacks, 1994.

ONLINE SOURCES AND RESOURCES

Break the Cycle
"Empowers youth to build lives and communities free from dating and domestic violence"
http://www.breakthecycle.org

Date & Acquaintance Rape (University of Buffalo)
http://ub-counseling.buffalo.edu/violenceoverview.shtml

Home Alive
Women's advocacy group for self-defense and awareness
http://www.homealive.org

National Youth Violence Prevention Center
Working to prevent violence committed by and against young people
http://www.safeyouth.org/scripts/index.asp

Rape, Abuse and Incest National Network (RAINN)
Abuse and rape information clearinghouse, support network, and information hotline
http://www.rainn.org

Teens Experiencing Abusive Relationships (TEAR)
Relationship abuse organization and site founded by a teen survivor
http://www.teensagainstabuse.org/index.php?q=mission

See It and Stop It
The Teen Action Campaign's site to address and combat relationship violence
http://www.seeitandstopit.org/pages/

▪ SUGGESTED BOOKS FOR PARENTS ▪ AND PARENTS-TO-BE

Gore, Ariel, *The Hip Mama Survival Guide.* New York: Hyperion Books, 1998.
———. *Whatever, Mom: Hip Mama's Guide to Raising a Teenager.* Emeryville, CA: Seal Press, 2004.
Kindlon, Dan, and Michael Thompson. *Raising Cain: Protecting the Emotional Life of Boys.* New York: Ballantine Books, 2000.
Leach, Penelope. *Children First.* New York: Vintage Books, 1995.
Levine, Judith. *Harmful to Minors: The Perils of Protecting Children from Sex.* Minneapolis, MN: University of Minneapolis Press, 2002.
Medhus, Elisa. *Raising Children Who Think for Themselves.* Hillsboro, OR: Beyond Words Publishing, 2001.
Pipher, Mary. *Reviving Ophelia: Saving the Selves of Adolescent Girls.* New York: Riverhead Books, 2005.
Roffman, Deborah M. *Sex and Sensibility: The Thinking Parent's Guide to Talking Sense About Sex.* Cambridge, MA: Perseus Publishing, 2001.

Weil, Zoe. *Above All, Be Kind: Raising a Humane Child in Challenging Times.* Gabriola Island, BC: New Society Publishers, 2003.

▪ SEXUALITY BOOKS FOR ▪ YOUNGER READERS

Blank, Joani. *A Kid's First Book About Sex.* San Francisco: Down There Press, 1993.
Blank, Joani, and Marcia Quackenbush. *Playbook for Kids About Sex.* San Francisco: Down There Press, 1981.
Gravelle, Karen. *What's Going on Down There?: Answers to Questions Boys Find Hard to Ask.* New York: Walter & Company, 1998.
Harris, Robie H. *It's Perfectly Normal: Changing Bodies, Growing Up, Sex, and Sexual Health.* Cambridge, MA: Candlewick Press, 2004.
Loulan, JoAnn and Bonnie Worthen. *Period.: A Girl's Guide to Menstruation.* Minnetonka, MN: Book Peddlers, 2001.
Madaras, Lynda. *The "What's Happening to My Body?" Book for Girls: A Growing Up Guide for Parents and Daughters.* New York: Newmarket Press, 2000.
———. *The "What's Happening to My Body?" Book for Boys: A Growing Up Guide for Parents and Sons.* New York: Newmarket Press, 2000.
Mayle, Peter. *"What's Happening to Me?" A Guide to Puberty.* New York: Lyle Stuart, 2000.
———. *Where Did I Come From?* New York: Lyle Stuart, 2000.

▪ TOP-TEN YOUNG ADULT AND ▪ GENERAL SEXUALITY AND SEXUAL HEALTH INFORMATION WEB SITES

Advocates for Youth
http://www.advocatesforyouth.org

Guttmacher Institute
http://www.guttmacher.org

Go Ask Alice
http://www.goaskalice.columbia.edu

s.e.x.

American Social Health Association: I Wanna Know
   http://www.iwannaknow.org

Scarleteen
   http://www.scarleteen.com

Sex, Etc.
   http://www.sxetc.org

SIECUS: The Sexuality Information and Education Council of the United States
   http://www.siecus.org

Teenwire
   http://www.teenwire.com

Planned Parenthood
   http://www.plannedparenthood.org

The Kaiser Foundation
   http://www.kff.org

▪ TOLL-FREE CRISIS HOTLINES ▪

Alcohol & Drug Abuse Crisis Line: 1–800–234–0420

Centers for Disease Control National STI Hotline: 1–800–227–8922

Eating Disorders Awareness and Prevention: 1–800–931–2237

Emergency Contraception Information: 1–888-NOT-2-LATE

Gay, Lesbian, Bisexual, and Transgender Youth Support Line: 1–800–850–8078

Gay & Transgender Hate Crime Hotline: 1–800–616-HATE

National Abortion Federation Hotline: 1–800–772–9100

National Domestic Violence Hotline: 1–800–799-SAFE

National Suicide Prevention Hotline: 1–800–273-TALK

National Youth Crisis Hotline: 1–800–442-HOPE

Planned Parenthood, Inc.: 1–800–230-PLAN

Pregnancy Helpline: 1–800–848–5683

Rape, Abuse, Incest National Network (RAINN): 1–800–656-HOPE

Self-Injury Hotline: 1–800-DONT CUT

Teen Helpline: 1–800–400–0900

Teenline: 1–800–522-TEEN

S.e.x.

index

s.e.x.

s.e.x.

s.e.x.

s.e.x.